Dementia in Nursing Homes

Sandra Schüssler • Christa Lohrmann
Editors

Dementia in Nursing Homes

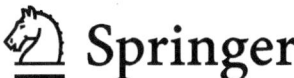 Springer

Editors
Sandra Schüssler
Medical University of Graz Institute
of Nursing Science
Graz
Austria

Christa Lohrmann
Medical University of Graz Institute
of Nursing Science
Graz
Austria

ISBN 978-3-319-49830-0   ISBN 978-3-319-49832-4   (eBook)
DOI 10.1007/978-3-319-49832-4

Library of Congress Control Number: 2017940194

© Springer International Publishing AG 2017
This work is subject to copyright. All rights are reserved by the Publisher, whether the whole or part of the material is concerned, specifically the rights of translation, reprinting, reuse of illustrations, recitation, broadcasting, reproduction on microfilms or in any other physical way, and transmission or information storage and retrieval, electronic adaptation, computer software, or by similar or dissimilar methodology now known or hereafter developed.
The use of general descriptive names, registered names, trademarks, service marks, etc. in this publication does not imply, even in the absence of a specific statement, that such names are exempt from the relevant protective laws and regulations and therefore free for general use.
The publisher, the authors and the editors are safe to assume that the advice and information in this book are believed to be true and accurate at the date of publication. Neither the publisher nor the authors or the editors give a warranty, express or implied, with respect to the material contained herein or for any errors or omissions that may have been made. The publisher remains neutral with regard to jurisdictional claims in published maps and institutional affiliations.

Printed on acid-free paper

This Springer imprint is published by Springer Nature
The registered company is Springer International Publishing AG
The registered company address is: Gewerbestrasse 11, 6330 Cham, Switzerland

Contents

1   **Introduction**   1
       Sandra Schüssler and Christa Lohrmann

2   **Meaningful Activities**   5
       Jennifer Wenborn

3   **Patient-/Person-Centered Care**   21
       Kathryn A. Weigel

4   **Psychosocial Interventions**   29
       Evelyn Finnema, Cora van der Kooij, Rose-Marie Dröes,
       and Linda Wolter

5   **Challenging Behavior in Nursing Home Residents
     with Dementia**   55
       Martin Smalbrugge, Sandra A. Zwijsen, Raymond C.T.M. Koopmans,
       and Debby L. Gerritsen

6   **Inclusion and Support of Family Members in Nursing Homes**   67
       Hilde Verbeek

7   **Pain in Dementia**   77
       Sandra M.G. Zwakhalen

8   **Staff Training and Education**   89
       Eira I. Klich-Heartt

9   **Communication in Dementia**   105
       Paul Watts and Stephen J. O'Connor

10 **Polypharmacy in Nursing Home Residents with Dementia**   123
       Rob J. van Marum

11 **Quality of Life of People with Dementia in Nursing Homes**   139
       Martin N. Dichter and Gabriele Meyer

12 **End-of-Life Care and Advance Care Planning in Dementia**   159
       Stephen J. O'Connor

13 **Depression in Nursing Home Residents with Dementia** 179
    Debby L. Gerritsen, Roeslan Leontjevas, Sandra A. Zwijsen,
    Raymond T.C.M. Koopmans, and Martin Smalbrugge

14 **Delirium** 191
    John P. Gilmore and Kathryn A. Weigel

15 **Dementia Care in Nursing Homes Requires a Multidisciplinary
    Approach** 203
    Jos Schols and Tinie Kardol

16 **The Prevention and Reduction of Physical Restraint Use
    in Long-Term Care** 219
    Jan Hamers

17 **Care Dependency** 229
    Ate Dijkstra

Introduction

Sandra Schüssler and Christa Lohrmann

Abstract

This chapter provides background information about dementia. In addition, the methodology and the results of both the systematic literature search in international databases and the ensuing online survey with international experts in dementia, upon which the topics of this book were selected, are presented.

Worldwide, dementia is a great strain on health-care systems, because it is increasing at a rapid rate. Globally, there are now more than 46 million people with dementia, and this number will increase to more than 100 million by 2050 (Prince et al. 2015). The worldwide costs of dementia are also increasing. In 2015, approximately 818 billion US dollars were spent on the treatment and care of dementia patients, and this will rise to one trillion US dollars in 2018 (Prince et al. 2015). These costs are higher than for other chronic diseases, like heart disease, stroke, or cancer (Prince et al. 2013). Currently we have no treatment to cure dementia (WHO 2012; Prince et al. 2015); therefore, nursing care is a very important aspect of its management (Alzheimer's Society 2014).

Internationally, most people with dementia receive (nursing) care and support at home (OECD 2015). When dementia progresses, however, increasingly complex care needs arise, making in-home care no longer possible and causing many people with dementia to move into a nursing home (Braunseis et al. 2012, Morley et al. 2013; OECD 2015; Prince et al. 2015). In developed countries, often more than 50% of nursing home residents have dementia (Alzheimer's Association

S. Schüssler, MSc, BSc (✉) • C. Lohrmann
Institute of Nursing Science, Medical University of Graz, Billrothgasse 6, 8010 Graz, Austria
e-mail: sandra.schuessler@medunigraz.at

© Springer International Publishing AG 2017
S. Schüssler, C. Lohrmann (eds.), *Dementia in Nursing Homes*,
DOI 10.1007/978-3-319-49832-4_1

2013; Hoffmann et al. 2014; Lohrmann et al. 2015; Matthews et al. 2013). This shows that dementia is a very important disease for investigation in a nursing home setting.

Nursing home residents with dementia have a high prevalence of care dependency (28–83%) and various nursing care problems, like incontinence (urinary, 39–88%; fecal, 43–87%; double, 49–65%) or physical restraints (8–60%) (Schüssler et al. 2014a, b, 2015). These problems also increase over time (Schüssler and Lohrmann 2015), possibly leading to such negative consequences as reduced quality of life, high care and treatment cost, as well as a higher mortality risk (Gustavsson et al. 2011; Lohrmann et al. 2015; OECD 2013; Reid 2008). Therefore, in-depth knowledge about dementia is essential for nursing and other health-care staff in order to support dementia-specific care in nursing homes (Schüssler 2015).

This book provides information on the most important current topics in the field of dementia in nursing homes, sourced from a literature search and subsequent online survey. In March 2015, a database search was performed in PubMed and CINAHL with the keywords *dementia*, *nursing home*, *(geriatric) nursing*, *priorities*, *problems*, and *needs*. In total, 31 priority topics for dementia in nursing homes were identified (see Figure 1.1). After the identification of the topics, an online questionnaire was generated using Google Forms with a five-point Likert scale ranking for each topic with the purpose of identifying its importance for dementia residents in nursing homes. After this, experts in dementia were ascertained through Internet search, as well as scans of dementia organizations and university websites. The online questionnaires were sent via email to 52 dementia experts in March 2015 who were given 2 weeks to fill out the questionnaire. A total of 56% of the experts participated in the survey. The results of the survey can be seen in Figure 1.1. Based on the results, 16 (half of all topics) of the most important topics identified by the experts were included in this book and written about by international experts on dementia.

The content of the book is dedicated to all (academic) nursing professionals, nursing scientists, nursing students, and other health-care professionals. It will be a valuable resource for nursing home practice and nursing home research.

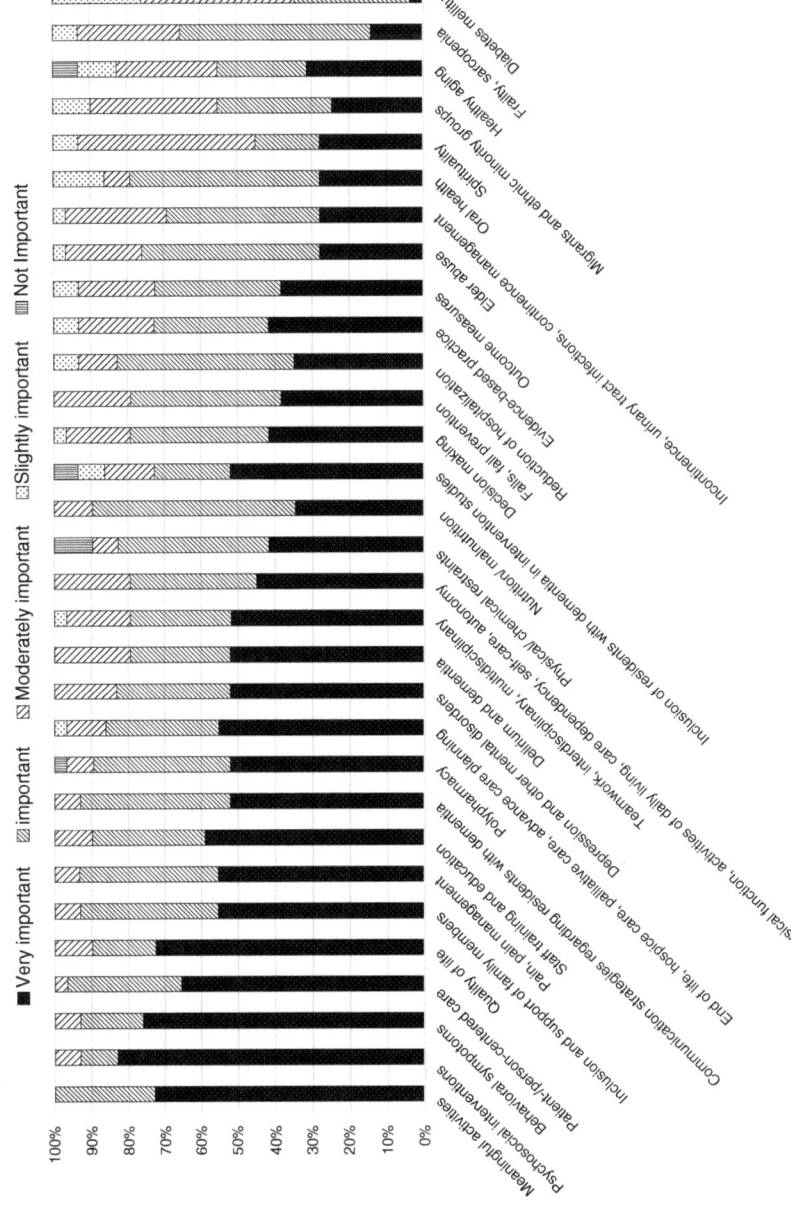

Fig. 1.1 Most important topics for dementia in nursing home

References

Alzheimer's Association (2013) 2013 Alzheimer's disease facts and figures. Alzheimers Dement 9:208–245

Alzheimer's S (2014) Formal care of people with dementia. Alzheimer's Society, London

Braunseis F, Deutsch T, Frese T, Sandholzer H (2012) The risk for nursing home admission (NHA) did not change in ten years – a prospective cohort study with five-year follow-up. Arch Gerontol Geriatr 54(2):e63–e67

Gustavsson A, Brinck P, Bergvall N, Kolasa K, Wimo A, Winblad B, Jönsson L (2011) Predictors of costs of care in Alzheimer's disease: a multinational sample of 1222 patients. Alzheimers Dement 7:318–327

Hoffmann F, Kaduszkiewicz H, Glaeske G, van den Bussche H, Koller D (2014) Prevalence of dementia in nursing home and community-dwelling older adults in Germany. Aging Clin Exp Res 26(5):555–559

Lohrmann C, Bauer S, Mandl M (2015) Pflegequalitätserhebung 14 (Quality of care survey 14). Institute of Nursing Science/Medical University of Graz, Austria

Matthews FE, Arthur A, Barnes LE, Bond J, Jagger C, Robinson L, Brayne C (2013) A two-decade comparison of prevalence of dementia in individuals aged 65 years and older from three geographical areas of England: Results of the Cognitive Function and Ageing Study I and II. Lancet 382(9902):1405–1412

Morley JE, Ouslander JG, Tolson D, Vellas B (2013) Nursing home care. USA, McGraw-Hill Education

OECD (2015) Adressing Dementia - the OECD response. OECD publishing, Paris

OECD (Organisation for economic co-operation and development) (2013) A good life in old age? Monitoring and improving quality in long-term care. OECD, France

Prince M, Prina M, Guerchet M (2013) World Alzheimer report 2013, Journey of caring – an analysis of long-term care for dementia. Alzheimer's Disease International, London

Prince M, Wimo A, Guerchet M, Ali G-C, Wu Y-T, Prina M (2015) World Alzheimer report 2015, The global impact of dementia – an analysis of prevalence, incidence, cost and trends. London, Alzheimer's Disease International

Reid C (2008) Quality of care and mortality among long-term care residents with dementia. Can Stud Popul 35:49–71

Schüssler S, Dassen T, Lohrmann C (2014a) Prevalence of care dependency and nursing care problems in nursing home residents with dementia: a literature review. Int J Caring Sci 7:333–337

Schüssler S, Dassen T, Lohrmann C (2014b) Care dependency and nursing care problems in nursing home residents with and without dementia: a cross-sectional study. Aging Clin Exp Res 28(5):973–982. doi:10.1007/s40520-014-0298-8

Schüssler S, Dassen T, Lohrmann C (2015) Comparison of care dependency and related nursing care problems between Austrian nursing home residents with and without dementia. Eur Geriatr Med 6(1):46–52

Schüssler S, Lohrmann C (2015) Change in care dependency and nursing care problems in nursing home residents with and without dementia: a 2-year panel study. PLoS One 10(10):e0141653. doi:10.1371/journal.pone.0141653

Schüssler S (2015) Care dependency and nursing care problems in nursing home residents with and without dementia. Dissertation, Medical University of Graz, Austria.

WHO (World Health Organization) (2012) Dementia a public health priority. WHO, Geneva

2

Jennifer Wenborn

Abstract
We all need to engage in personally meaningful occupation to maintain our physical and mental health and well-being. People with dementia are no different, but need increasing assistance from others to enable their participation. Despite evidence that activity participation enhances quality of life for people with dementia by reducing challenging behaviour and depression, the quantity and quality of activity provision within care homes are often unacceptably low, especially for those with more advanced dementia. Activity provision is often viewed as the domain of specialist practitioners such as occupational therapists or dedicated activity staff, to be provided at set times, within a formal programme. However, for it to be optimally effective, it needs to be integrated into day-to-day practice by all staff. All staff need to be trained how to provide personally meaningful activity, but training alone is not enough as the manager's leadership is crucial to successfully developing an activity-based culture of care.

This chapter discusses the key components to be considered when providing occupational opportunities for care home residents who have dementia. Activity provision is complex and, as such, links with the content of several of the other chapters, in particular: person-centred care, psychosocial interventions, challenging behaviour, family carers, staff training and education, quality of life and depression.

For human reality, to be is to act, and to cease to act is to cease to be. Sartre (1943)

J. Wenborn
Division of Psychiatry, University College London, London, UK
e-mail: j.wenborn@ucl.ac.uk

© Springer International Publishing AG 2017
S. Schüssler, C. Lohrmann (eds.), *Dementia in Nursing Homes*,
DOI 10.1007/978-3-319-49832-4_2

5

2.1   Introduction

The need to engage in purposeful and meaningful activity is a basic human drive that is essential to maintain physical and mental health and well-being, regardless of age or impairment. Our individual personality, life story, interests, values and beliefs influence our choice of activity, and what we do partly defines who we are, for example, teacher, pianist, walking the dog, and baking.

The need to engage in personally meaningful activity does not diminish for people with dementia, whatever the stage or setting. Tom Kitwood (1997) outlined five main psychological needs of people with dementia that overlap into a central need for love, namely, comfort, attachment, inclusion, identity and occupation. However, the impact of dementia is that it becomes increasingly difficult to perform even the most basic and familiar everyday tasks, and so progressively more and more assistance from family and professional carers is needed to tailor and adapt the activity to match the individual's needs and abilities.

Kitwood saw the provision of appropriate activity opportunities as an integral aspect of person-centred care and a key contributor to quality of life. Activity participation in care homes has been shown to improve residents' quality of life (Zimmerman et al. 2005) and reduce levels of challenging behaviour and improve mood and function (Cohen-Mansfield 2005). As such, the provision of meaningful activities is a critical component when assessing the quality of care in homes. However all too frequently, the level of activity is inadequate, as inactivity has a detrimental effect on residents' physical and mental health and well-being and consequently quality of life.

2.2   Impact of Inactivity

Physiological consequences of inactivity include restricted blood circulation and respiration; raised blood pressure; diminished appetite, gastrointestinal movement and bowel function; and increased risk of urinary infection and incontinence, tissue damage, and chest infection. Mobility can be impaired due to muscles wasting, contractures developing and decreasing bone density that can then increase the risk of falls and fractures. Hence, lack of activity can increase the level of dependency of care home residents. Psychological effects can include decreased alertness, concentration and ability to solve problems, which leads to reduced awareness of oneself and one's surroundings, resulting in disorientation and confusion. This in turn can induce anxiety as residents struggle to make sense of what is happening to and around them, often culminating in displays of agitation and challenging behaviour in an attempt to communicate their anxiety and frustration to caregivers (Brooker et al. 2016). Boredom can also trigger challenging behaviour, including wandering, as an individual attempts to seek stimulation. So, lack of activity increases the frequency and severity of challenging behaviour, and residents who exhibit disruptive behaviour are least likely to engage in activities; but such behaviour reduces whilst residents are engaged in activity.

2.3   Life in a Care Home

The experience of living in a care home has been examined over the years, and the high level of inactivity and subsequent impact on residents' quality of life are a common theme. Townsend (1962) painted a grim picture of life in care homes, concluding that they do 'not adequately meet the physical, psychological and social needs of the elderly people living in them' (p 430). Organised social activities were poorly attended, and in between meals residents just sat in the day room, usually in the same chair, with no activity available. Godlove et al.'s (1982) observational study found that residents were sitting or lying down without engaging in any observable activity at all for 61.9% of the time period and participating in exercise and recreational activities for 4.4%. Wilcocks et al.'s (1987) cross-sectional study of 100 care homes noted that priority was given to providing visible aspects of care, particularly related to hygiene, such as bathing residents or cleaning the amenities, above attending to social needs, which were addressed only after other practical tasks were completed. This study highlights how the organisational culture can perpetuate practice rooted in risk avoidance, for example, task allocation and staff surveillance that effectively removes residents' rights to engage in low-risk activities, thus further reducing their level of independence and privacy.

Nolan et al.'s observational study (1995) found that residents were passive for 87% of the time with the remaining 13% taken up with basic care needs. Although nursing staff were aware of, and concerned by, the lack of activity, this was attributed to a lack of therapy staff. Nolan et al. therefore recommended that ensuring the availability of such stimulation and meaningful activities should be an integral aspect of the continuing care nursing role. Schneider et al.'s (1997) study of 17 UK care homes found that many residents spent their day sitting in a chair, with little opportunity for physical exercise or activity, tending only to socialise within the privacy of their own room. Mozley et al. (2004) reported that 51% of the residents observed were sitting on a chair, possibly dozing, but otherwise inactive.

Ballard et al. (2001) used Dementia Care Mapping (Brooker and Surr 2005) to evaluate the quality of care across 12 UK care homes. The 218 residents spent 17% of their time asleep; 30% socially withdrawn or not actively engaged in any activity; communication with others took up 14%; and just 3% of their time spent engaged in everyday constructive activities other than watching the television which accounted for another 3%. The remaining 33% of time was spent in basic care activities such as eating and toileting.

Martin et al. (2002) identified daytime activities as an unmet need for 53% of residents in residential care, but only 8% of residents in nursing homes, and suggested that the latter group have a decreased need for such input due to the stage of decline reached. This reflects a common perception that people at the more advanced stage of dementia can no longer engage in or enjoy activity. A subsequent study (Hancock et al. 2006) concluded that daytime activities were an unmet need for 76% of 238 residents, rising to 84% for residents with dementia and depression and 90% for those with dementia and anxiety. Unmet needs were associated with increased behavioural problems but not with severity of dementia.

The 'My Home Life' programme highlighted the benefits of meaningful activity to health and well-being, the range of potential activities that can be offered and the need to ensure that activities are personally meaningful and provided at a level appropriate to the severity of dementia. It also discussed residents' reported need to engage in productive roles so as to 'feel useful' and the dilemma this poses in terms of risk assessment and the potential to enhance mealtimes to become a much more enjoyable experience (Reed 2007).

The UK Alzheimer's Society (2008) conducted a survey to establish family carers' perceptions of the quality of dementia care provided within care homes and identified three key problem areas: provision of activities and occupation, treating residents with dignity and respect and the relationship between the care home and family and friends. When the UK Alzheimer's Society (2013) again surveyed family carers, they found that just 41% ($n = 1139$) felt their relative's quality of life was good and 24% thought that opportunities to be involved in activities were poor or very poor. Whilst this is a significant improvement on the 54% who previously stated that their relative did not have enough to do (Alzheimer's Society 2008), there is obviously still much to be done to ensure adequate activity provision across the sector. Care home staff were also surveyed, and whilst 92% ($n = 647$) considered the provision of activities as being important, only 58% felt that adequate opportunities were available within their own care home.

A review of findings from 100 care home inspections (Commission for Social Care Inspection 2008), which included observing 424 residents, all of whom had moderate or severe dementia, ascertained that half of those observed (53%) were doing something (alone or with someone else) for between 76% and 100% of the period observed – usually lunchtime – which is an improvement on previous studies. However, 14% spent less than 25% of their time engaged with anything or anybody, and it was noted that those who spent the least time engaged were usually those with more severe dementia. A later review of unannounced inspections across 500 care homes (Care Quality Commission 2013) found that almost two thirds met all the required standards. However, a recurring theme across those homes that did not meet the standards related to the lack of activities – particularly for people with dementia.

These studies make uncomfortable reading with the consistent message that residents have little opportunity to engage with their environment, with others or in activity, other than when receiving basic personal care. The need for staff to be appropriately trained to provide appropriate activities has been consistently highlighted. Residents with more advanced dementia, who are therefore more dependent, are least likely to participate in activities not only due to a common misperception that they are no longer able to benefit but also a lack of caregivers' knowledge and skill as to how to remedy the situation. Perrin (1997) had previously noted that 'marked occupational poverty exists' for this group of residents (p.938). Whiteford (2000) then defined occupational deprivation as 'a state in which a person or group of people are unable to do what is necessary and meaningful in their lives due to external restrictions. It is a state in which the opportunity to perform those occupations that have social, cultural and personal relevance is rendered difficult if not impossible' (p.200). The potential impacts of occupational deprivation: lack of meaningful time use, maladaptive responses and a barrier to community reintegration, are reflected throughout the accounts summarised above.

2.4   What Makes Activity Meaningful?

Kitwood highlighted the continuing need for people with dementia to 'be occupied … involved in the process of life in a way that is personally significant, whether this consists of action, reflection or relaxation' but acknowledged the increasing challenge of doing so, as memory and other cognitive functions deteriorate.

Focus groups conducted with care home residents with dementia, staff and family carers in three care homes aimed to establish 'What is meaningful activity?' (Harmer and Orrell 2008). Four activity themes were identified: 'reminiscence therapy', 'family and social', 'musical' and 'individual'. Residents most valued activities for their psychosocial characteristics, whilst staff and family carers prioritised activities to maintain skills. Residents saw lack of opportunity and motivation as the main barrier to engagement, whilst staff and family carers highlighted the lack of resources. Two related themes regarding the lack of meaningful activity and what makes activity meaningful were also explored and highlight the need to identify each resident's individual preferences, skills and abilities and to adapt activities to their capabilities, thus facilitating engagement in activities and contributing to well-being.

Popham (2007) ran focus groups with residents, staff and family members and interviewed managers across five care homes to explore what really matters in the care home environment for people with dementia. Twelve themes were identified, and whilst the different groups' priorities varied, the overall most significant factor was 'activities and outings'. Some care staff saw activity provision as the sole responsibility of the activity organiser; residents wanted opportunity to do more day-to-day tasks such as what they used to do at home, and many described the degree of boredom regularly experienced, whilst family members felt the stimulation provided through activity was preferable to their relative sleeping all day.

A recent synthesis of the qualitative evidence arising from 34 studies across 11 countries (Han et al. 2016) identified three themes, connection with: self, with others and with the environment; concluding that being connected is a prime motivation for engaging in everyday activities and so is a vital component to explore in order to identify personally meaningful activities for individuals.

2.5   Providing Meaningful Activity

Enabling meaningful activity for people with dementia in care homes is a complex business. Kitwood's Enriched Model of dementia describes the experience of living with dementia as a combination of five factors: $D = NI + H + B + P + SP$, where D = dementia, NI = neurological impairment, H = health and physical fitness, B = biography/life history, P = personality and SP = social psychology (Brooker 2007). This equation is a useful framework to consider the complexity of activity provision. Four elements are intrinsic to the individual and need to be considered in order to provide activities that meet residents' preferences and capacities, NI = neurological impairment, H = health and physical fitness, B = biography/life history and P = personality, and are discussed here. The fifth, SP = social psychology, is discussed later.

Although the pattern and progression of neurological impairment (NI) that occurs in dementia varies from individual to individual, it inevitably affects the ability to 'do', as the person finds it increasingly difficult to remember, know where they are and who other people are, keep track of time, organise themselves, understand what is being said to them, communicate with other people, make decisions, and learn new things. Activities therefore need to be provided at the right level of challenge or 'fit' to match the individual's abilities. If activities are pitched at too low a level, they can be at best boring and, at worst, demeaning or patronising. Conversely, if activities are pitched at too high a level, they can provoke anxiety and frustration, thus lowering well-being. Staff must therefore have the knowledge, skills and easy-to-use tools to enable them to adapt and present activities at an appropriate level to 'match' the person's current abilities.

Monitoring and maintaining health and physical fitness (H) has been shown to enhance quality of life for care home residents, and evidence supports the physical, cognitive and psychological benefits of physical activity. Residents also experience a wide range of medical conditions common in older age, such as arthritis, which can also affect functional ability. As hearing and visual changes are a normal aspect of the ageing process, most residents will have some degree of hearing and/or visual impairment. All these aspects also need to be considered when selecting and grading activities.

Kitwood highlighted the relevance of utilising knowledge of an individual's biography (B) and personality (P) in order to deliver person-centred care. Knowledge of what someone has done in the past (B), and their beliefs and values and how they dealt with life (P), can help caregivers make sense of their current behaviour and individualise their own approach to maximise resident's well-being. Activities that reflect past preferences have been shown to enhance engagement (Cohen-Mansfield et al. 2010).

Therefore, the key to providing personally meaningful activity is getting to know the individual person in terms of their life story (B), interests and values (P), health and physical capacity (H) and cognitive ability to engage in activity (NI). This enables personally meaningful activities to be selected, adapted and presented at the correct level of challenge or 'fit' to the person's abilities. This enables optimal participation whilst also providing the necessary level of support. Two of these factors are now discussed in more detail: obtaining the individual's life story and assessing the person's capacity to engage in activity.

2.5.1 The Individual's Life Story

Staff need to obtain, record and utilise residents' biographical information when planning care and activity provision. A number of formats are commonly used: a written/pictorial record or timeline presented in a folder or displayed in the residents' bedroom or collecting together relevant objects into a memory box or container. It is a good idea to include a family tree, a list of significant dates, photographs and a frontispiece of current information about their home, family, likes and dislikes, emphasising the more positive aspects. A memory box can also be created to contain objects of significance to represent the person's life. Increasingly creative presentations and innovative practice are now possible utilising technology such as digital picture frames (www.lifestorynetwork.org.uk).

The person can be involved in producing this themselves following a life review process, but in the later stages, carers are often dependent on the knowledge of family and friends and their own experience of working with the resident. Both approaches have been shown to have benefits (Subramaniam et al. 2014; Gridley et al. 2016) such as enabling staff to know and better understand the individual person and their behaviour, informing the care planning process, providing personalised care, ensuring continuity of care, encouraging life review, and reminiscence. The process of collating a life story in collaboration with a member of staff is often valued by family members as it provides an opportunity to remember and portray the person they know and love, and establish rapport with someone now involved in providing their relative's day-to-day care. However, it can also be an emotional activity that needs sensitive handling, and so staff must be appropriately trained. Ensuring confidentiality is important as stories may contain personal information which the person or their relative does not want to share with others.

2.5.2 Measuring Capacity for Activity: The Pool Activity Level (PAL) Instrument

As discussed earlier, it is important to match the demands of the activity to the individual's capacity, both physical and cognitive. A useful tool to assess the level of cognitive ability an individual has to engage in activity is the Pool Activity Level (PAL) Instrument (Pool 2012). The PAL Instrument comprises a number of sections: a Life History Profile, the Checklist, Activity Profiles for each of the Activity Levels and an Individual Action Plan that covers personal care activities. The PAL Checklist covers nine everyday activities, and the results indicate the level of cognitive ability that an individual has reached in terms of being able to engage in activity, be that Planned, Exploratory, Sensory or Reflex Level. The PAL Activity Profiles outline the likely abilities and limitations of a person at that Level and provide guidance on how best to engage and enable an individual, for example, the optimal positioning of tools and provision of verbal instructions and non-verbal directions. This information guides carers to select and present appropriate occupational opportunities to people with dementia, thus matching the person's ability with personally meaningful activity of an appropriate level of challenge or 'fit'. The PAL Checklist has validity and reliability when used to assess older people with dementia (Wenborn et al. 2008), and the Instrument is recommended to assist staff in selecting appropriate daily living and leisure activities (NICE/SCIE 2006; Reed 2007). Once the level of cognitive ability is known, then an activity can be adapted to match. Strategies to adapt activity demands can include changing the objects and tools, use of language and non-verbal communication, and the timing and location (Trahan et al. 2014).

2.6   Impact of the Environment on Activity Provision

The fifth component of Kitwood's enriched model of dementia, SP = social psychology, relates to the extrinsic factors, namely, the environment within which the person with dementia lives. The environment can be viewed as comprising three elements: physical, social and organisational (Calkins 2001). These elements can all potentially impact – positively or negatively – on activity provision and engagement.

2.6.1   Physical Environment

There is an association between the design and/or adaptation of the physical environment with the behaviour and well-being of people with dementia (Kings Fund 2013). Certain design and décor features of the physical environment that have the potential to enhance or impede engagement and activity provision include environmental cues, such as clocks and clear text/pictorial notices to assist orientation to time, place and person. Poor design and layout can result in: wandering, as residents search to make sense of where they are; isolation, if easily accessible communal areas are lacking; incontinence and falls, if toilets and other facilities are not clearly visible. Lack of appropriate walking aids and/or inadequate seating (incorrect height, width, depth, shape) can impede or prevent mobilisation throughout the home, thus lowering levels of physical activity and the potential for stimulation and social interaction. A lack of colour contrast between different levels and surfaces and poor lighting makes it difficult for residents with visual or perceptual impairment to find their way around or carry out everyday activities, for example, white handrails installed on white-tiled walls in toilets and bathrooms are not easily distinguished. The environment (indoor and outdoor) should provide optimal multisensory stimulation (smell, movement, touch, vision, hearing and taste), but avoid sensory overload, for example, excessive noise, as this can have a negative impact on well-being. The potential benefits of incorporating nature into care settings, either through access to outdoor spaces or bringing nature indoors, for example, plants, natural materials, animals and birds, have also been recognised.

The need to risk assess potential activity participation can lead to conflict between providing a homely, stimulating, individualised environment and ensuring the health and safety of residents and staff. One example is residents having to remain seated in the day room so as to enable their constant surveillance by staff. As a result, many residents do not have the opportunity to carry out the simple, daily activities that they frequently say they would like to do, for example, not being 'allowed' into kitchen areas to wash up in case they fall, plus food hygiene regulations that require crockery to be cleaned in a dishwasher.

However, it has been suggested that as dementia progresses, so a person's physical environment shrinks leaving them in a 'bubble' approximatley one metre in diameter, and so the effect of the built environment becomes less important than the capacity of caregivers to enter into the individual's bubble, using appropriate verbal and non-verbal communication and sensory stimulation in order to engage the person (Perrin et al. 2008). Hence, we need also to consider the social and organisational environment.

2.6.2   Social and Organisational Environment

However, the most 'perfect' physical environment does not automatically produce optimum care or increase residents' level of engagement and activity. Skill and expertise is required to communicate with, engage and motivate residents and to select, adapt and present appropriate and meaningful activities to people with a complex combination of disabilities and needs. Even if staff fully acknowledge the importance of activity and have the time and commitment, they often lack the necessary knowledge, skills or tools to put this into action. Many of the studies reviewed earlier in this chapter cite the lack of staff knowledge and skills in a range of topics, including the provision of appropriate activity, and so the need for a well- trained care home workforce, able to meet the complex needs of residents with dementia, is a recurring policy theme.

Staff training can utilise a range of learning strategies including: didactic sessions, one-to-one mentoring, coaching or supervision, role modelling; and the completion of work-based learning tasks. Numerous studies have sought to evaluate their effectiveness but on balance have concluded that whilst training courses increase carer confidence and knowledge in the short term, there is not necessarily any impact on clients in the long term unless the necessary organisational changes are also implemented. Direct care staff may be keen to engage in activities, but they themselves can be disempowered by the environment within which they work, for example, by the management style and organisational factors. So, training in isolation is not enough; the manager is absolutely key to encouraging an activity based culture within the home, facilitating and empowering staff to make the necessary organisational changes required (Lawrence et al. 2012, 2016; Wenborn et al. 2013).

The development of such a culture requires ownership at all levels, led from the top but with an open and inclusive management style (Killett et al. 2016). Just as staff are expected to provide person-centred care, so organisations need to be person-centred towards their staff. Staff often state that there is not the time to provide more activity, but it has been shown that integration of activity into day-to-day care does not need to take additional time to be effective (Volicer et al. 2006), and the staff time saved from dealing with reduced incidence of neuropsychiatric symptoms can be reinvested in activity provision.

2.7   Successful Activity Provision

As highlighted previously, activity provision in care homes is a complex business. Brooker et al.'s action research (2007a, b) developed a multi-level intervention for providing activity opportunities to people with moderate to severe dementia in long-term care settings. The Enriching Opportunities Programme consisted of five key elements: specialist expertise; individualised assessment and case work; an activity and occupation programme; staff training; and management and leadership. The 'Locksmith' – a staff member whose prime role was to discover and develop 'keys' that could unlock the potential for well-being in people with dementia – had a central role in training, mentoring and motivating care staff. So, whilst one individual was clearly responsible for leading activity provision, the whole staff group were key for its day-to-day implementation. The focus was on assessing the individual in terms of their level of cognitive ability and engagement capacity, life history, personality and current interests; in order to produce 'magic moments key cards' which identified a particular activity or trigger to enhance that individual's well-being. Using a repeated measures within-subjects design and Dementia Care Mapping at four points over 18–24 months in three nursing homes providing specialist dementia care, they found a statistically significant improvement in well-being and range of activity; an increase in positive interactions, but no decrease in personal detractions; and a significant decrease in levels of depression, but no change in levels of anxiety. It was a small sample with much variation across the three homes and so the overall effect was small for some measures, but the study indicated that implementation of an activity-based, person-centred intervention is feasible – but dependent on management support at the highest level as well as a highly motivated staff group to ensure its success.

2.7.1   Reducing Challenging Behaviour

The use of antipsychotic medication to 'manage' challenging behaviour, sometimes administered covertly, is fundamentally a form of restraint. In contrast, there is evidence that non-pharmacological interventions such as person-centred care planning can reduce patterns of challenging behaviour (Richter et al. 2012), and so good practice guidelines now recommend this as the first line of management (Alzheimer's Society 2011). The CALM-AD trial (Ballard et al. 2009) found that residents who received a brief psychological intervention, comprising either social interaction or personalised music or removing environmental triggers, achieved a 30% reduction in residents' level of agitation. A systematic review (Testad et al. 2014) found good evidence to support the provision of personalised psychosocial interventions with and without social interaction to improve agitation and for reminiscence therapy to improve mood. A randomised controlled trial of staff training and support focussed on providing individualised care planning resulted in a significant drop in antipsychotic medication usage in the intervention homes (Fossey et al. 2006). A subsequent study sought to evaluate the acceptability and effectiveness of this intervention in practice (Brooker et al. 2016) and found that providing psychosocial interventions such as strengths-based care planning, life story work, supportive environments, meaningful activity and personalised music resulted in a 31% reduction in antipsychotic prescribing, with the biggest decrease in homes with initially the highest rates. A factorial cluster randomised controlled trial evaluated the impact of providing person-centred care in combination with antipsychotic review, social interaction and exercise interventions on health-related quality of life (Ballard et al. 2016). The results indicated a worsening in health-related quality of life following withdrawal of antipsychotic medication in the absence of providing non-pharmacological interventions instead. Hence, it is important not to consider just one approach in isolation but take a whole care home approach in developing person-centred care and providing personally meaningful activities.

2.8   Interventions

A range of activity-based interventions have been demonstrated to be effective for people with dementia and are recommended as good practice (NICE/SCIE 2006), including cognitive stimulation therapy for cognitive symptoms; 'interventions tailored to the person's preferences, skills and abilities' for non cognitive symptoms or behaviour that challenges; and sensory stimulation therapies for people with dementia who are depressed and/or anxious. A review of the effectiveness of all these interventions is beyond the remit of this chapter, and indeed some are presented in detail in other chapters, so the evidence supporting some that are relevant to people residing in care homes is summarised very briefly here.

Cognitive stimulation therapy (CST) incorporates principles of reality orientation, reminiscence, validation and person-centred care. The 7-week programme comprises fourteen 45 min sessions, each related to a theme, for example, sound, childhood, using money. The emphasis is on information processing, and props are used to provide multisensory stimulation. CST is designed to be run by anyone who works with people who have dementia; and a comprehensive manual (Spector et al. 2006) and certified training are available. CST has been shown to improve cognition and quality of life (Spector et al. 2003) and be cost-effective (Knapp et al. 2006); and maintenance CST also improves quality of life (Orrell et al. 2014).

A sensory approach aims to maintain interaction with the environment and other people by providing a range of experiences to stimulate all the senses – smell, movement, touch, vision, hearing and taste – even if verbal communication is no longer possible. We all need sensory stimulation to interpret and interact with our environment, and sensory impairment or deprivation eventually results in physical and/or social disengagement. Sensory impairment can occur as part of normal ageing or due to conditions such as dementia and alters our sensory experience. People in institutional care may experience sensory deprivation through lack of environmental stimulation and sensory opportunities.

The concept of multisensory stimulation originated in The Netherlands with the development of Snoezelen© (literal translation, 'to sniff and doze') for people with learning disabilities which was then extended to people with other conditions, including dementia, brain injury and terminal illness. Now more commonly referred to as multisensory environments or sensory rooms, these facilities provide a non threatening space to gently stimulate the senses. Unpatterned stimuli are used to arouse the senses of smell, movement, touch, vision, hearing and taste. Participants are not required to perform any specific activity but just enjoy the sensation and experience; hence, it is failure-free. Evidence of long-term effectiveness is mixed but consistently supports positive effects on neuropsychiatric symptoms and mood immediately after using the sensory room (Sanchez et al. 2012) and in particular for those with more advanced dementia (Sanchez et al. 2016a, b). Staff must be trained, users assessed and an intervention plan agreed, to ensure provision of an appropriate level and type of stimulation and to avoid the dangers of sensory overload.

However, many of the principles and equipment can be moved and used elsewhere, if a multisensory environment is not available or it is not feasible to get the person to/into the room. For example, using scented bath oils, background music and environmental props can turn a functional bath into a sensory experience. A range of sensory stimuli can be incorporated into any number of activities, as well as the care home environment itself, or used as an activity, such as rummage bags, sensory cushions and aprons.

Animal-assisted therapy has been shown to have a positive effect on the symptoms of depression and quality of life, especially for those with more advanced dementia (Olsen et al. 2016), as well as reducing agitation and anxiety (Majic et al. 2013). Hence, the psychological and physical benefits outweigh the perceived health and safety risks of accommodating animals within the care home environment. Using dolls has gained in popularity over the past decade, despite initial resistance by some who felt it was potentially infantile and demeaning to older people, and so a number of studies have been conducted to evaluate its effectiveness. A recent review identified 11 eligible studies and concluded that the use of dolls could be therapeutic by increasing levels of engagement, communication and dietary intake and reducing episodes of distress, but also noted the potential challenges of putting it into practice due to lack of practitioner knowledge and/or preconceived ideas regarding its use (Mitchell et al. 2016).

Although there is some evidence of effectiveness for these and other interventions, the conclusions and recommendations of most studies and systematic reviews consistently highlight the need for more research. However, the methodological challenge is how to provide interventions which by their very nature need to be personally meaningful and tailored to the individual whilst adhering to the robust nature of a protocol required within a randomised controlled trial. It must also be noted that lack of evidence of effectiveness does not equate to evidence of non effectiveness. Indeed, one of the most important aspects is the selection, adaptation and provision of personally meaningful activities for the individual, so even if an intervention is shown to be effective in the general population it may not appeal to everyone. This is where the skill of care staff, coupled with their knowledge of the person's life story, comes into play. Providing activities that match both interests and capacity is likely to be more effective (Kolanowski et al. 2005).

Conclusion

The need for people with dementia to engage in personally meaningful activity has been demonstrated, as well as the paucity of opportunity for care home residents to do so, with the subsequent detrimental effect on their quality of life due to increased levels of depression and challenging behaviour. Using non pharmacological interventions to reduce challenging behaviour is often a key focus, not surprisingly as it has a detrimental effect on residents' quality of life and uses a disproportionate amount of staff time and service resources. Educational models that aim to equip care staff with enhanced knowledge and understanding of dementia, how it affects behaviour and how individualised care plans can enhance the provision of person-centred care have been evaluated, but a recurring conclusion is how key the manager's role and leadership style are to enable change within the care home setting, in order for service development and improvement to occur and be maintained.

Useful Resources

Life story resources and practice	www.lifestorynetwork.org.uk
Living Well through Activity in Care Homes: The guide for residents, their family and friends (free download, College of Occupational Therapists)	www.cot.org.uk/living-well-care-homes
National Association for Providers of Activities for Older People (NAPA)	www.napa-activities.com/
Pool Activity Level (PAL) Instrument (electronic version)	www.dementia-pal.com

References

Alzheimer's Society (2008) Home from home: a report highlighting opportunities for improving standards of dementia care in care homes. Alzheimer's Society, London

Alzheimer's Society (2011) Optimising treatment and care for behavioural and psychological symptoms of dementia. A best practice guide for health and social care professionals Alzheimer's Society, London. www.alzheimers.org.uk/bpsdguide. Accessed 18 Oct 2016

Alzheimer's Society (2013) Low expectations: Attitudes on choice, care and community for people with dementia in care homes. Alzheimer's Society, London

Ballard C, Fossey J, Chithramohan R, Howard R, Burns A, Thompson P, Tadros G, Fairbairn A (2001) Quality of care in private sector and NHS facilities for people with dementia: cross sectional survey. Br Med J 323(7310):426–427

Ballard C, Brown R, Fossey J, Douglas S, Bradley P, Hancock J, James I, Juszczak E, Bentham P, Burns A, Lindesay J, Jacoby R, O'Brien J, Bullock R, Johnson R, Homes C, Howard R (2009) Brief psychological therapy for the treatment of agitation in Alzheimer disease (The CALM-AD Trial). Am J Geriatr Psychiatry 17(9):726–733

Ballard C, Orrell M, Sun Y, Moniz-Cook E, Stafford J, Whitaker R, Woods B, Corbett A, Banerjee S, Testad I, Garrod L, Khan Z, Woodward-Carlton B, Wenborn J, Fossey J (2016) Impact of antipsychotic review and non-pharmacological intervention on health-related quality of life in people with dementia living in care homes: WHELD–a factorial cluster randomised controlled trial. Int J Geriatr Psychiatry. doi:10.1002/gps.4572

Brooker D (2007) Person-centred dementia care: making services better. Jessica Kingsley Publishers, London

Brooker DJ, Woolley RJ (2007a) Enriching opportunities for people living with dementia: the development of a blueprint for a sustainable activity-based model. Aging Ment Health 11(4):371–383

Brooker DJ, Woolley RJ, Lee D (2007b) Enriching opportunities for people living with dementia in nursing homes: an evaluation of a multi-level activity-based model of care. Aging Ment Health 11(4):361–370

Brooker D, Latham I, Evans S, Jacobson N, Perry W, Bray J, Ballard C, Fossey J, Pickett J (2016) FITS into practice: translating research into practice in reducing the use of anti-psychotic medication for people living with dementia in care homes. Aging Ment Health 20(7):709–718

Brooker D, Surr C (2005) Dementia care mapping: principles and practice. University of Bradford, Baltimore

Calkin M (2001) The physical and social environment of the person with Alzheimer's disease. Aging Ment Health 5(S1):S74–78

Care Quality Commission (2013) Time to listen in care homes: dignity and nutrition inspection programme 2012. Care Quality Commission, London

Cohen-Mansfield J (2005) Nonpharmacological interventions for persons with dementia. Alzheim Care Q 6(2):129–145

Cohen-Mansfield J, Marx M, Thein K, Dakheel-Ali M (2010) The impact of past and present preferences on stimulus engagement in nursing home residents with dementia. Aging Ment Health 14(1):67–73

Commission for Social Care Inspection (2008) See me, not just the dementia: understanding peoples' experiences of living in a care home. CSCI, London

Fossey J, Ballard C, Juszczak E, James I, Alder N, Jacoby R, Howard R (2006) Effect of enhanced psychosocial care on antipsychotic use in nursing home residents with severe dementia: cluster randomised trial. Br Med J 332(7544):756–758

Godlove C, Richard L, Rodwell G (1982) Time for action. University of Sheffield, Oxford

Gridley K, Brooks J, Birks Y, Baxter K, Parker G (2016) Improving care for people with dementia: development and initial feasibility study for evaluation of life story work in dementia care. Health Serv Deliv Res 4(23):4–5

Han A, Radel J, McDowd J, Sabata D (2016) Perspectives of people with dementia about meaningful activities: a synthesis. Am J Alzheimers Dis Other Demen 31(2):115–123. 34

Hancock GA, Woods B, Challis D, Orrell M (2006) The needs of older people with dementia in residential care. Int J Geriatr Psychopharmacol 21(1):43–49

Harmer B, Orrell M (2008) What is meaningful activity for people with dementia living in care homes? A comparison of the views of older people with dementia, staff and family carers. Aging Ment Health 12(5):548–558

Killett A, Burns D, Kelly F, Brooker D, Bowes A, La Fontaine J, Latham I, Wilson M, O'Neill M (2016) Digging deep: how organisational culture affects care home residents' experiences. Ageing Soc 36(1):160–188

Fund K (2013) Improving the patient experience: developing supportive design for people with dementia. In: The king's fund's enhancing the healing environment programme 2009–2012. The King's Fund, London

Kitwood T (1997) Dementia reconsidered: the person comes first. Open University Press, Buckingham

Knapp M, Thorgrimsen L, Patel A, Hallam A, Woods B, Orrell M (2006) Cognitive stimulation therapy for people with dementia: cost effectiveness analysis. Br J Psychiatry 188(6):574–580

Kolanowski A, Litaker M, Buettner L (2005) Efficacy of theory-based activities for behavioral symptoms of dementia. Nurs Res 54(4):219–228

Lawrence V, Fossey J, Ballard C, Moniz-Cook E, Murray J (2012) Making psychosocial interventions work: improving quality of life for people with dementia in care homes. Br J Psychiatry 201:344–351

Lawrence V, Fossey J, Ballard C, Ferreira N, Murray J (2016) Helping staff to implement psychosocial interventions in care homes: augmenting existing practices and meeting needs for support. Int Psychogeriatr 31(3):284–293

Majic T, Gutzmann H, Heinz A, Lang U, Rapp M (2013) Animal-assisted therapy and agitation and depression in nursing home residents with dementia: a matched case control trial. Am J Geriatr Psychiatry 21(11):1052–1059

Martin MD, Hancock GA, Richardson B, Simmons P, Katona C, Mullan E, Orrell M (2002) An evaluation of needs in elderly continuing care settings. Int Psychogeriatr 14(4):379–388

Mitchell G, McCormack B, McCance T (2016) Therapeutic use of dolls for people living with dementia: a critical review of the literature. Dementia 15(5):976–1001

Mozley C, Sutcliffe C, Bagley H, Cordingley L, Challis D, Huxley P, Burns A (2004) Towards quality care: outcomes for older people in care homes. Aldershot: Ashgate in conjunction with Personal Social Service Research Unit (PSSRU), England

National Institute for Health and Clinical Excellence & Social Care Institute for Excellence (NICE/SCIE) (2006) Dementia: supporting people with dementia and their carers in health and social care. National Clinical Practice Guideline Number CG 042. NICE, London

Nolan M, Grant G, Nolan J (1995) Busy doing nothing: activity and interaction levels amongst differing populations of elderly patients. J Adv Nurs 22:528–538

Olsen C, Pedersen I, Bergland A, Enders-Slegers M, Patil G, Ihlebæk C (2016) Effect of animal-assisted interventions on depression, agitation and quality of life in nursing home residents suffering from cognitive impairment or dementia: a cluster randomized controlled trial. Int J Geriatr Psychiatry 31(12):1312–1321. doi:10.1002/gps.4436

Orrell M, Aguirre E, Spector A, Hoare Z, Woods B, Streater A, Donovan H, Hoe J, Knapp M, Whitaker C, Russell I (2014) Maintenance cognitive stimulation therapy for dementia: single-blind, multicentre, pragmatic randomised controlled trial. Br J Psychiatry 204:454–461

Perrin T (1997) Occupational need in severe dementia: a descriptive study. J Adv Nurs 25(5):934–941

Perrin T, May H, Anderson E (2008) Wellbeing in dementia: an occupational approach for therapists and carers, 2nd edn. Churchill Livingstone, Edinburgh

Pool J (2012) The Pool Activity Level (PAL) Instrument for occupational profiling: a practical resource for carers of people with cognitive impairment, 4th edn. Jessica Kingsley Publishers, London

Popham C (2007) What really matters in the care home environment for people with dementia? MSc (in Ageing & Mental Health) Dissertation. University College, London

Reed J (2007) Quality of life. In: Help the aged (2007) my home life: quality of life in care homes: a review of the literature. Help the Aged, London

Richter T, Meyer G, Möhler R, Köpke S (2012) Psychosocial interventions for reducing antipsychotic medication in care home residents. Cochrane Database Syst Rev (12);CD008634

Sánchez A, Millán-Calenti J, Lorenzo-López L, Maseda A (2012) Multisensory stimulation for people with dementia: a review of the literature. Am J Alzheimers Dis Other Demen 28(1):7–14

Sánchez A, Marante-Moar M, Sarabia C, Lorenzo T, Maseda A, Millán-Calenti J (2016a) Multisensory stimulation as an intervention strategy for elderly patients with severe dementia: a pilot randomized controlled trial. Am J Alzheimers Dis Other Demen 31(4):41–350

Sánchez A, Masedaa A, Marante-Moarb M, de Labrab C, Lorenzo-López L, Millán-Calentia J (2016b) Comparing the effects of multisensory stimulation and individualised music sessions on elderly people with severe dementia: a randomized controlled trial. J Alzheimers Dis 51:303–315

Sartre JP (1943) L'Être et le néant. Translated from French by Barnes HE (2003) Being and nothingness: an essay on phenomenological ontology. Routledge, Abingdon

Schneider J, Mann AH, Levin E, Netten A, Mozley CG, Abbey A, Egelstaff R, Kharicha K, Todd C, Blizard B, Topan C (1997) Quality of care: testing some measures in homes for elderly people. Discussion Paper 1245, Personal Social Services Research Unit (PSSRU), University of Kent at Canterbury

Spector A, Thorgrimsen L, Woods B, Royan L, Davies S, Butterworth M, Orrell M (2003) Efficacy of an evidence-based cognitive stimulation therapy programme for people with dementia: randomised controlled trial. Br J Psychiatry 183(3):248–254

Spector A, Thorgrimsen L, Woods B, Orrell M (2006) Making a difference: an evidence-based group programme to offer cognitive stimulation therapy (CST) to people with dementia. The manual for group leaders. Hawker Publications, London

Subramaniam P, Woods B, Whitaker C (2014) Life review and life story books for people with mild to moderate dementia: a randomised controlled trial. Aging Ment Health 18(3):363–375. doi:10.1080/13607863.2013.837144

Testad I, Corbett A, Aarsland D, Osland Lexow K, Fossey J, Woods B, Ballard C (2014) The value of personalized psychosocial interventions to address behavioral and psychological symptoms in people with dementia living in care home settings: a systematic review. Int Psychogeriatr 26(7):1083–1098

Townsend P (1962) The last refuge. Routledge & Keegan Paul, London

Trahan M, Kuo J, Carlson M, Gitlin L (2014) A systematic review of strategies to foster activity engagement in persons with dementia. Health Educ Behav 41(5):70S–83S

Volicer L, Simard J, Heartquist J, Medrek R, Riordan M (2006) Effects of continuous activity programming on behavioral symptoms of dementia. J Am Med Dir Assoc 7:426–431

Wenborn J, Challis D, Pool J, Burgess J, Elliott N, Orrell M (2008) Assessing the validity and reliability of the Pool Activity Level (PAL) Checklist for use with older people with dementia. Aging Ment Health 12(2):202–211

Wenborn J, Challis D, Head J, Miranda-Castillo C, Popham C, Thakur R, Illes J, Orrell M (2013) Providing activity for older people with dementia in care homes: a cluster randomised controlled trial. Int J Geriatr Psychopharmacol 28:1296–1304

Whiteford G (2000) Occupational deprivation: global challenge in the new millennium. Br J Occup Ther 63(5):200–204

Wilcocks D, Peace S, Kellaher L (1987) Private lives in public places. Tavistock, London

Zimmerman S, Sloane PD, Williams CS, Reed PS, Preisser JS, Eckert JK, Boustani M, Dobbs D (2005) Dementia care and quality of life in assisted living and nursing homes. Gerontologist 45(S1):133–146

Patient-/Person-Centered Care

3

Kathryn A. Weigel

Abstract

Person-centered care (PCC) for persons with dementia is based on the belief that personhood can be maintained despite cognitive impairment, and it is considered the gold standard for caring for persons with dementia in long-term care settings. PCC values the individual and honors and facilitates the expression of his/her autonomy. PCC in dementia care is not to be confused with patient-centered care, which is the term used to refer to the engagement of the patient in his/her healthcare in a more general sense. Informal and formal PCC has been utilized in dementia care since the 1990s, with noted differences among countries in implementation, initiatives, progress, and success. This chapter offers an overview of the concept, background, implementation concerns, example PCC models and frameworks, current research evidence, and a list of some useful resources.

Keywords

Person-centered care • Dementia • Dementia care

3.1 Introduction

The term "patient-/person-centered care" is currently used in healthcare to denote the focus on involving the patient in his/her care following initiatives by organizations, such as the Institute of Medicine (IOM) in the United States, to increase the

K.A. Weigel, MS, RN, GCNS
University of St. Francis Cecily and John Leach College of Nursing, Joliet, IL, USA
e-mail: KWeigel@stfrancis.edu

© Springer International Publishing AG 2017   21
S. Schüssler, C. Lohrmann (eds.), *Dementia in Nursing Homes*,
DOI 10.1007/978-3-319-49832-4_3

quality and effectiveness of care. However, person-centered care (PCC) has been used as an approach in the design and delivery of care for individuals with dementia since the late 1990s to enhance the quality of care and the quality of life for individuals with dementia. The term person-centered, rather than patient-centered, care is used in this context due to its widespread acceptability and its holistic and personalized ethos (Love and Pinkowitz 2013). Pioneered by Tom Kitwood and Kathleen Bredin in the late 1980s and early 1990s in the United Kingdom (UK), PCC values the individual and honors and facilitates the expression of his/her autonomy. PCC is more than simply individualized care; it is ensuring that all interpersonal interactions between the person and the staff are understood in relation to how the person feels and how they enhance the person's sense of well-being. As noted by Barbosa et al. (2015), forms of PCC approaches include the following: behavior-oriented approaches, such as simplified tasks and simple one-step instructions; emotion-oriented approaches, such as reminiscence and validation therapy; cognition-oriented approaches, such as reality orientation; and stimulation-oriented approaches, such as recreational, art, and music therapies and multisensory stimulation.

3.2   Background

Beginning with the work of Kitwood and Bredin, experts in the UK have successfully proposed many policy initiatives leading to the successful application of PCC across the entire trajectory from diagnosis to death. Members of the Bradford University Dementia Group developed Dementia Care Mapping (DCM) from Kitwood's model as a method to map out care for individuals and for the setting as a whole; and this method has been used to plan, deliver, and evaluate care, indicating positive outcomes as well as areas in need of change and/or improvement (Brooker 2015). The group also developed a training program for primary care practitioners, and there has been movement to incorporate PCC in hospitals as well. Brooker advanced DCM in 2007 with her person-centered dementia care (PCDC) model known as the VIPS framework. This model focuses on valuing the person, individualization of care, the perspective of the person, and a supportive social environment (Brooker 2015).

In the UK, the National Institute for Health and Clinical Excellence (NICE) and the Social Care Institute for Excellence (SCIE) collaborated to develop guidelines and standards for quality care, and the first evidence-based guideline on dementia was published in 2007 (NICE and SCIE 2007). The guideline pointed to the need for training of both health and social staff in order to provide this quality care, such as that developed by the Bradford Dementia Group, and the collaborative has continued to work on the articulation of standards and the measurement of outcomes. In the United States (US), the Dementia Initiative, formed in 2012, issued the white paper titled "Dementia Care: The Quality Chasm," which laid out a four-part framework for person-centered dementia care. These four parts included the core values and philosophy of the person, the structure of the long-term care service and support settings in which the person lives (note that this does not include those persons receiving care by family members or friends), the operational practices of the structure that support person-centered care, and the individualized practices that are used in interacting with the person (Dementia Initiative 2013). In response to worldwide requests by governments and Alzheimer's associations for more efforts focused on improving the quality of dementia care services, the World Health Organization (WHO) held its first conference on dementia in 2015. WHO's Global Action on Dementia report (World Health Organization 2015), which calls for greater emphasis on quality care of persons with dementia at the global level, resulted from this meeting of experts across the globe.

3.3   Implementation

When moving from a concept into daily practice, questions arise about how to put PCC into action, beginning with the question of how care providers can know the preferences, needs, and values of a person with dementia. This is followed by the questions: How can they ensure that the person's values guide all decisions about his/her care? How and to what extent can they involve family members without compromising the fundamental focus on individual autonomy and choice? How can person-centered care be measured if the person is unable to complete the questionnaires being used to evaluate patient experience? (Maslow 2013). Thus, the implementation of PCC requires careful and thorough consideration of many factors.

Since valuing the person is the fundamental principle of PCC, it is vital for the caregiver to listen, observe, and use multiple sources to learn about the person's history, values, and preferences, and what brings them joy, and then use that knowledge to plan and provide care in a trusting relationship (Molony and Bouma 2013). Care is built around the person's strengths and honoring the person's personhood and autonomy, which implies the necessity of offering and not denying opportunities for the person to make choices. These opportunities can be modified according to the person's cognitive/emotional/communication/physical abilities. The organization must be supportive of the care initiative from the top down. In order to provide PCC, the focus of the organization must shift from the completion of tasks within set time frames to that of prioritizing the understanding of the person's experience in the planning and provision of care (Kitwood 1997). Among other issues, this requires that the organization be willing and able to provide and support appropriate training and modify staffing patterns, programs, and the environment.

3.4   PCC Models/Frameworks

Several frameworks/models of PCC have been developed. One of these is the VIPS framework originally designed by Brooker in 2007. This framework consists of: V, for valuing people with dementia and those who care for them; I, for treating people as individuals; P, for looking at the world from the perspective of the person with dementia; and S, for a positive social environment in which the person living with dementia can experience relative well-being (Brooker 2015). Guidance on the implementation of PCC in the long-term care setting is outlined in the framework, with an emphasis on the necessity of staff education on how to practice PCC. Another is the ABLE model of PCC, which was first conceived as a quality improvement project. This model incorporates Montessori principles and has four areas of focus: A, for abilities and capabilities of the person; B, for the background of the resident; L, for leadership, culture change, and education of staff; and E, for physical environment changes (Roberts et al. 2015).

The physical environment must also be considered in the delivery of PCC, and individual work by several recognized dementia experts can be summarized by a set of eight key environmental design ideas. These include exit control, walking paths, common spaces, privacy and personalization, garden access, residentialness, sensory comprehension, and support for capacity. Controlled exits allow for independence, clear walking paths clarify destinations, common spaces offer rooms with indicators of purpose and related expected socially appropriate behaviors, bedrooms need to be personalized and provide privacy, and any outdoor/garden areas must be safe and easily accessible. The residence has to maintain a sense of feeling at home; what the individuals see, hear, smell, and touch needs to be understandable to them; and the physical environment needs to support the individuals' highest levels of independence (Zeisel 2013).

3.5   Current Research Evidence About PCC

Many investigators in many countries have conducted research on the implementation and effects of PCC on persons with dementia and their formal and informal caregivers. Of course, in the case of PCC in nursing homes, those studies exploring persons in residential setting and their formal caregivers are most applicable.

3.5.1   Effects of PCC on Persons with Dementia

Several recent studies explored the effect of PCC on problematic behaviors of persons with dementia and related outcomes. Chenoweth et al. (2009) conducted the Caring for Aged Dementia Care Resident Study (CADRES), a cluster randomized trial that demonstrated that PCC resulted in significant decreases in agitation that was also cost-effective. Burack et al. (2012) conducted a two-year study exploring the effect of PCC on resident behavior, comparing seven long-term care communities utilizing PCC with six matched communities that did not. The results indicated a significant decrease in agitated behaviors in the groups utilizing PCC and a significant increase in agitated behaviors in the groups that did not utilize PCC. Li and Porock (2014) conducted a systematic review of resident outcomes of PCC in long-term care. They found 24 studies from three countries and that PCC resulted in significant decreases in the use of psychotropic medications and depression and lower levels of helplessness, boredom, and loneliness. As part of the Well-Being and

Health for People with Dementia (WHELD) program, Ballard et al. (2016) conducted a randomized control trial using a PCC intervention in 16 nursing homes in London area that resulted in decreases in problematic behavior and significant reductions in the use of antipsychotic medications and in mortality.

3.5.2   Effects of PCC on Formal/Professional Caregivers of Persons with Dementia

Some studies explored the effect of PCC on the formal/professional caregivers of persons with dementia. Jeon et al. (2011) explored the effects of PCC and DCM on staff in a cluster randomized trial in 15 residential aged care sites in Sydney, Australia, and found significant decreases in emotional exhaustion over time in the DCM group. Passalacqua and Harwood (2012) developed a communication skills intervention for caregivers based on the VIPS framework (see Sect. 3.4) and tested it with 26 paraprofessional caregivers in a for-profit memory care facility in the Southwest US. The results indicated a significant decrease in caregivers' depersonalization of residents, a significant increase in caregivers' hope for persons with Alzheimer's, and an increase in caregivers' empathy. A systematic review by Barbosa et al. (2015) focused on the impact of PCC on staff caring for persons with dementia in residential care settings and found that five of the seven qualifying experimental and quasi-experimental studies suggested that PCC had positive effects on staff stress, burnout, and job dissatisfaction. A study by Roberts et al. (2015) included an examination of the effect on family members as well in an 18-month mixed methods pilot study of the effect of implementation of the ABLE model (see Sect. 3.4) of PCC on the residents, care staff, and family members of a 15-bed dementia care unit. The results of that study indicated statistically significant reductions in the use of antipsychotic and sedative medications and resident agitation that was accompanied by significant changes in staff perceptions of the care environment, knowledge of dementia care, the organization, and the content of care.

3.5.3   Effects of the Physical Environment on the Provision of PCC

Other studies explored the effect of the physical environment in the provision of PCC on the persons with dementia and their formal/professional caregivers. The Person-Centered Dementia Care and Environment (PerCEN) study, for instance, a randomized controlled trial implementing PCC and person-centered environments (PCEs) for persons with dementia, was conducted from 2009 to 2013 in 38 units in 38 different residential facilities for the aged. Using the data obtained in this study, Chenoweth et al. (2014) examined the effect of PCC and PCEs on resident agitation, emotional responses to care, quality of life, and depression, as well as the quality of care interaction. Although the results indicated statistically significant improvements in quality of life and decreases in agitation for both the PCC and PCE groups, there was no significant difference in either variable for the PCC + PCE group. There were significant improvements in the quality of care interactions and resident care responses observed in the PCC + PCE group, but no group resulted in improvement in resident depression scores.

3.6   Conclusion

PCC has been shown to result in positive effects on persons with dementia, their formal/professional caregivers, and the organizations in which they receive care. The recent calls for patient-/person-centered care in healthcare reinforce the central focus of PCC that the person needs to be valued and their autonomy be honored and facilitated. There are several well-developed frameworks/models and related training and implementation materials and support available that can make this possible for more settings, facilities, and organizations.

3.7   Resources

The following are useful resources in developing and implementing PCC:

- *ABLE model*: http://www.able-differently.org/about-us/able-health-model/
- *The Alzheimer's Voice*: Person-Centered and Person-Directed Dementia Care: https://nadrc.acl.gov/node/26
- *Bradford University School of Dementia Studies*: http://www.bradford.ac.uk/health/dementia/
- *Eden Alternative*: http://www.edenalt.org/
- *Green House Project*: http:/www.aplaceformom.com/blog/green-house-project-next-big-think-in-long-term-care/
- *Montessori for Dementia*: http://montessorifordementia.com.au/
- *National Alzheimer's and Dementia Resource Center*: https://nadrc.acl.gov/
- *Pioneer Network*: http://pioneernetwork.net/
- *STAR training*: http://www.startraining.eu/index.php?lang=en
- *VIPS Framework*: http://www.worcester.ac.uk/discover/9980.html

References

Ballard C, Orrell M, YngShon S et al (2016) Impact of antipsychotic review and nonpharmacological intervention on antipsychotic use, neuropsychiatric symptoms, and mortality in people with dementia living in nursing homes: A factorial cluster-randomized controlled trial by the Well-Being and Health for People with Dementia (WHELD) Program. Am J Psychiatry 173:252–262

Barbosa A, Sousa L, Nolan M et al (2015) Effects of person-centered care approaches to dementia care on staff: a systematic review. Am J Alzheimers Dis Other Demen 30(8):713–722

Brooker D (2015) Person-centered dementia care: making services better, 2nd edn. Bradford Dementia Group Good Practice Guides. Jessica Kingsley Publishers, London

Burack OR, Weiner AS, Reinhardt JP (2012) The impact of culture change on elders' behavioral symptoms: a longitudinal study. JAMDA 13:522–528

Chenoweth L, Forbes J, Fleming R et al (2014) PerCEN: a cluster randomized controlled trial of person-centered residential care and environment for people with dementia. Int Psychogeriatr 26(7):1147–1160

Chenoweth L, King M, Jeon Y et al (2009) Care for Aged Dementia Care Residents Study (CADRES) of person centred care, dementia-care mapping, and usual care in dementia: a cluster-randomised trial. Lancet Neurol 8:317–325

Dementia Initiative (2013) Dementia care: the quality chasm. Accessed at http://www.leadingage.org/uploadedFiles/Content/Members/Nursing_Homes/Quality/DementiaCare TheQualityChasm.pdf

Jeon YH, Luscome G, Chenoweth L et al (2011) Staff outcomes form caring for aged dementia care resident study (CADRES): a cluster randomized trial. Int J Nurs Stud 49(5):508–518

Kitwood T (1997) Dementia reconsidered: the person comes first. Oxford Univ Press, Buckingham

Li J, Porock D (2014) Resident outcomes of person-centered care in long-term care: a narrative review of interventional research. Int J Nurs Stud 51:1395–1415

Love K, Pinkowitz J (2013) Person-centered care for people with dementia: a theoretical and conceptual framework. J Amer Soc Aging 37(3):23–29

Maslow K (2013) Person-centered care for people with dementia: opportunities and challenges. J Amer Soc Aging 37(3):8–15

Molony SL, Bouma R (2013) The care manager role in person-centered care for people with dementia. J Amer Soc Aging 37(3):79–82

National Institute for Health and Clinical Excellence (NICE) and the Social Care Institute for Excellence (SCIE) (2007) Dementia: supporting people with dementia and their carers in health and social care. National Collaborating Centre for Mental Health, London. Accessed at https://www.nice.org.uk/guidance/cg42?unlid=539472848201646613

Passaloacqua SA, Harwood J (2012) VIPS communication skills training for paraprofessional dementia caregivers: an intervention to increase person-centered dementia care. Clin Gerontol 35:425–445

Roberts G, Morley C, Walters W et al (2015) Caring for people with dementia in residential aged care: successes with a composite person-centered care model featuring Montessori-based activities. Geriatr Nurs 36:106–110

World Health Organization (WHO) (2015) Global Action on dementia, WHO Ministerial Conference, Geneva, Switzerland, 16–17 March. Accessed at http://apps.who.int/iris/bitstr eam/10665/179537/1/9789241509114_eng.pdf

Zeisel J (2013) Improving person-centered care through effective design. Generations J Am Soc Aging 37(3):45–52

Psychosocial Interventions

Evelyn Finnema, Cora van der Kooij, Rose-Marie Dröes, and Linda Wolter

Abstract

In section A, we focus on the use of the adaptation-coping model as a theoretical and practical framework in the care for persons with dementia in combination with integrated emotion-oriented care in the different phases of dementia. First of all, we address the adaptation-coping model and the main principles and method of integrated emotion-oriented care. We subsequently discuss a number of adaptive tasks that elderly people with dementia can be confronted with. We describe how these adaptive tasks can cause disruptions in the functioning or in behavior and mood. We then examine to what extent integrated emotion-oriented care attempts to prevent, reduce, or eliminate these disruptions and what the expected effect is on the behavior and mood of the person with dementia.

In section B we will look at the implementation of psychosocial interventions to residents with dementia in nursing homes. We begin by looking at theory that aids in furthering our insights into the importance of building a trusting relationship with nursing home residents. Building on trust, we will explore Erickson's theory as it relates to aging. Here, we will discuss several types of interventions and mediums that have shown significant and enduring success with older adults.

E. Finnema, PhD, RN (✉) • C. van der Kooij, PhD, RN
NHL University of Applied Sciences, Leeuwarden, The Netherlands
e-mail: evelyn.finnema@nhl.nl

R.-M. Dröes
VU University Medical Center, Amsterdam, The Netherlands

L. Wolter, PhD, LCSW (✉)
University of St Francis, Joliet, IL, USA
e-mail: lwolter@stfrancis.edu

© Springer International Publishing AG 2017
S. Schüssler, C. Lohrmann (eds.), *Dementia in Nursing Homes*,
DOI 10.1007/978-3-319-49832-4_4

Keywords
Dementia • Adaptation-coping • Psychosocial care • Emotion-oriented care •
Psychosocial intervention • Group work with dementia residents

4.1   Section A: Coping with Dementia – Integrated Emotion-Oriented Care for Nursing Home Residents[1]

Evelyn Finnema, Cora van der Kooij, and Rose-Marie Dröes

4.1.1   The Adaptation-Coping Model

Elderly people with dementia who have been institutionalized in a psychogeriatric nursing home may experience the consequences of their disease and their changed living conditions (stay at the nursing home, loss of independence, etc.) as stressful. The adaptation-coping model (Dröes 1991) provides a framework from which the problems of the person with dementia can be viewed. It offers aids for diagnosis, for the treatment and evaluation of the psychosocial problems of elderly people with dementia.

The adaptation-coping model is based on the coping theory formulated by Lazarus and Folkman (1984) and the adaptive tasks distinguished by Moos and Tsu (1977) for chronic illness. Dröes (1991) operationalized the model for psychosocial care for elderly people with dementia. One of the most important starting points of the adaptation-coping model is people's constant striving for balance. When people are confronted with changes in their existence, this unavoidably leads to a disruption of the existing balance. By coping with these changes consciously, but even more often unconsciously, they try to regain a balance. Moos and Tsu (1977) indicate that in general seven adaptive tasks are important for the restoration of the disrupted balance. The difficulty the individual patient experiences with the various adaptive tasks is determined in part by his personality and life history. Furthermore, illness-related problems and social and material circumstances also have an effect. According to Dröes (1991), the adaptive tasks distinguished by Moos and Tsu, the adaptation process they describe, and the factors that influence this process also apply to people with dementia. Dröes (1991) describes in detail which coping strategies people with dementia appear to use when they are coping with the different adaptive tasks. She indicates how various behavior and mood problems, such as aggressive, depressed, and anxious behavior, inactivity, and socially isolated

---

[1] This chapter is adapted from Finnema EJ, Van der Kooij CH, Dröes RM (2015) Omgaan met dementie: belevingsgerichte begeleiding en zorg in de verschillende stadia van dementie. In: Dröes RM, Schols J, Scheltens Ph (ed) Meer Kwaliteit van Leven. Integratieve Persoonsgerichte Dementiezorg. Leusden: Diagnosis Uitgevers, p 163–185.

Table 4.1 Adaptive tasks related to nursing home residents with dementia

Adaptive tasks	Adaptive domains
Coping with own invalidity	Cognitive adaptation
Developing an adequate relationship with the staff	
Maintaining an emotional balance	Emotional adaptation
Maintaining a positive self-image	
Preparing for an uncertain future	
Coping with the nursing home environment	Social adaptation
Developing and maintaining social relationships	

behavior, should perhaps be interpreted as (in some cases not quite adequate) coping behavior. In her opinion, a reduction of these behavior and mood problems indicate a reduction of experienced stress and psychosocial problems, and that would be proof of better adaptation. Depending on the adaptive tasks on which improvement is observed, one can say there has been cognitive or mental, emotional, or social adaptation (see Table 4.1).

Dröes' description of coping strategies is based on Verwoerdt (1976) and Lazarus and Folkman (1984). Verwoerdt described various defense mechanisms in people with dementia, namely, strategies aimed at management and control such as intellectualization; separation of reason and emotion; certain obsessive-compulsive mechanisms; overcompensation and counterphobic behavior; strategies to keep the threat outside consciousness, such as suppression, denial, rationalization, projection, and introjection; and regressive strategies, such as regressive behavior, giving up, and withdrawal.

Lazarus and Folkman (1984) made a distinction between problem-oriented and emotion-oriented coping strategies. Problem-oriented strategies focus on resolving the problems that have caused tension and on restoring a sense of control. Examples are analytical strategies, such as searching for relevant information and thinking up solutions, "(...) but also strategies that focus on the individual in question, such as motivational or cognitive changes, changing the level of aspiration, mental preparation for the consequences of the disease, finding alternative ways of fulfillment and learning new skills (...)" (Dröes 1991, p. 43). Emotion-oriented strategies focus primarily on reducing the emotional tension that is caused by the consequences of the disease. Examples are "avoiding behavior, selective attention, reinterpretation of the situation and behavior strategies, such as (...) meditation, alcohol consumption, expressing anger and looking for emotional support and reassurance" (Dröes 1991, p. 43).

In most situations, people use a combination of problem-oriented and emotion-oriented strategies according to Lazarus and Folkman (1984). However, when the stress situation is appraised as impossible to control or influence (as may happen in the case of serious illness), people generally tend more toward emotion-oriented ways of coping.

Although there is a clear distinction between the various adaptive tasks in theory, it is not always possible in everyday practice to infer from the way in which he behaves with which adaptive task the elderly person with dementia has a problem.

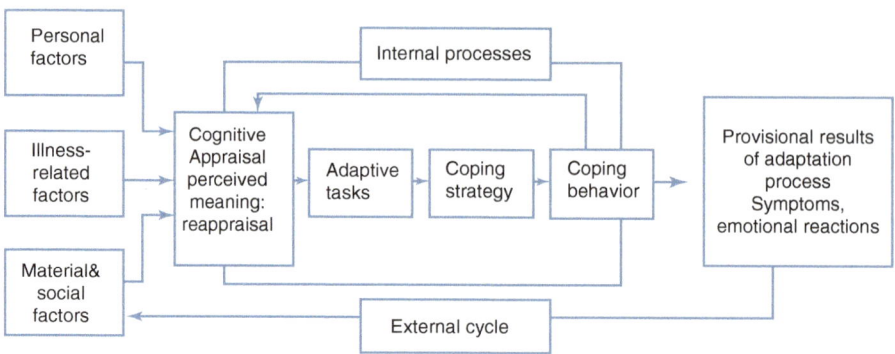

Fig. 4.1 The Adaptation-coping model (Dröes 1991)

A correct interpretation of the behavior (Dröes refers to this as "psychosocial diagnosis") is therefore always based on a combination of knowledge about the person, his life history, his personal experience of the situation and his functional abilities, an analysis of the social and material circumstances in which the behavior occurs, and an understanding of the coping strategy (strategies) he uses.

In view of all this, it is obvious that the adaptation process is complex and dynamic, and also interactional, i.e., the continuous interaction with the environment affects the coping behavior (external cycle). This creates an opening for the environment to influence disruptions in behavior and mood by means of, among other things, emotion-oriented care and other treatment and support methods. Several studies confirm the "stress-coping" notion (Moore 1997). The problems indicated by people with dementia were related first of all to their own cognitive deterioration and the disabling effects this had on their everyday functioning. In addition, the problems referred to the emotional burden and social consequences of the disease for themselves as well as their environment. People with dementia indicated, for example, that it is difficult to become dependent on others and to stay in touch with friends and acquaintances (Cohen 1991; Dröes 1991; Kiyak and Borson 1992; Cotrell and Schulz 1993; Cotrell and Lein 1993). An indication for the experience of stress in dementia from neurobiological research is that several stress-regulating systems in our body prove to be highly activated in Alzheimer's disease (Hoogendijk 1998) (Fig. 4.1).

4.1.2 Integrated Emotion-Oriented Care

In practice, the term emotion-oriented care is used as a collective name for approaches that try to link up with the experiences and perceptions of the person with dementia (Finnema et al. 2000a, b). Emotion-oriented care approaches include:

- The validation approach (Feil 1989a, b), which aims at empathizing with the emotions and perceptions of the people with dementia and validating their feelings

- Reminiscence, which uses objects, old photographs, and utensils (Rossaert 1989; Thornton and Brotchie 1987)
- Sensory activation, i.e., attempting to make contact through various senses by means of sounds, smells, and hugs (Achterberg and Kok 1992)
- Reality orientation, which aims to support the cognitive functioning of the person with dementia and therefore his sense of control, through training, offering structure, clear timetables, and aids, such as a photograph on the bedroom door and other reference points in the environment (Spector et al. 2012)
- Passivities of daily life (PDL), which pays attention to comfortable sitting or lying positions and passive relaxation exercises and which is based in part on haptonomic principles (Eijle and Van der Wulp 1988; Rabe 1993)

The integrated emotion-oriented care approach strives for an application of (suitable elements from) the emotion-oriented approaches mentioned, integrated in the daily care. Our starting point is the definition of integrated emotion-oriented care as formulated by Van der Kooij (2003, 2013, 2016):

"Integrated emotion-oriented care is the integrated application of emotion oriented approaches and communicative skills, customized to the individual person with dementia, taking into account his needs and physical and mental disabilities, for the purpose of offering feelings of security and trust to the person with dementia and helping him to adjust to the consequences of his illness."

Nowadays, it is generally accepted that there are no standard prescriptions for the way caregivers should communicate with people with dementia. In every situation, it is necessary to tune into the unique personality of the person with dementia, his particular personality, his situation, his life history, his needs, and his way of coping with the disease. The most important question for the caregiver is not whether a particular method was applied as described, but whether there was a situation or a moment of mutual understanding and contact (Halek and Bartholomeyzcik 2006). Integrated emotion-oriented care focuses on the awareness of and reflection on the "moments of contact" and on building up an emotional relationship with the person with dementia (Van der Kooij 2003, 2016).

4.1.2.1 Phases of Ego-Experience and Perceptions

Little is known about how people perceive themselves during the dementia process. Integrated emotion-oriented care starts from four subsequent phases of "Ego-experience": threatened Ego-experience, wandering Ego-experience, hidden Ego-experience, and sunken Ego-experience (Van der Kooij 2003, 2016). These phases are based on the phases of dementia as described earlier by Verdult (1993) and on Feil's (1989a, b) four stages of disorientation: orientation problems, confusion in time, repetitive movement, and vegetation.

During the phase of *threatened Ego-experience*, people lose their grip on themselves and their environment. They start having trouble remembering and thinking. People they know appear to be strangers, familiar spaces are unknown, and the secure feeling about self in the continuity of past, present, and future is uprooted. The degree in which people are aware of the problems as a result of their dementia varies.

During the phase of *wandering Ego-experience*, the person with dementia gets lost, as it were, in an individual reality. The chronology of his past erombles, and he loses the ability to arrange and name his perceptions.

The *hidden Ego-experience* is characterized by apparent isolation and inaccessibility. It seems like the person with dementia resides in a personal, inner, timeless world where he doesn't need anyone and won't allow anyone in. Making contact is still, however, possible.

In the *sunken Ego-experience*, the person with dementia no longer responds to his environment; there seems to be no more interaction of feelings.

To gain some understanding of the experiences and perceptions of the person with dementia, an assessment is made of the Ego-experience phase, as well as how he experiences his current situation and how his life history influences his experience of the present. Experiencing the current situation refers to how the dementing person copes with, and experiences, the consequences of his illness and his institutionalization in the nursing home (cf. Dröes 1991).

4.1.2.2 Care Needs and Care Objectives

The different phases of Ego-experience in integrated emotion-oriented care are distinguished to provide caregivers with a frame of reference to help assess the individual care needs of people with dementia. Five general care needs are distinguished (Van der Kooij 2003), which are derived from Maslov's (1972) hierarchy of needs and which have been modified for dementia on the basis of descriptions by, among others, Feil (1984), and Kitwood and Bredin (1992). The care needs concern being able to meet basic physical needs, security, trust and structure, contact and connectedness, self-respect, and self-realization. The general care objectives are in line with these care needs and are described as accepting dependence, experiencing security, experiencing connectedness, experiencing appreciation, and experiencing affirmation or even validation.

4.1.2.3 Methods in the Different Phases of Dementia and Phases of Ego-Experience

Although the care needs and care objectives are, to a greater or smaller extent, relevant to every phase of Ego-experience, they require different methods during different phases. Starting point for action and making contact is always the perception and experience of the person with dementia. Van der Kooij has distinguished six areas of experience: sensory, rational, emotional, physical, social, and spiritual experience. This classification of areas of experience is based in part on the stimulation of the general psychological functions "perception, thinking, and feeling," as they are given shape in sensory activation, the reality orientation

Table 4.2 Integrated emotion-oriented care in relation to adaptive tasks

Adaptive task	Integrated emotion-oriented care
Coping with own invalidity	Help the person with dementia to cope with the constraints. Support him and encourage him to do the things he still can
Developing an adequate care relationship with the staff	Behave empathetic and make use of knowledge of the life history of the person with dementia. Accept the resident as the person he was and is today
Maintaining an emotional balance	Respect emotions and confirm or weak them off. Offer pleasant sensory stimuli (music, good food, etc.)
Maintaining a positive self-image	Promote the dignity of the person with dementia to let him remember positive events and encourage him to do activities that he can
Preparing for an uncertain future	Show understanding for the feelings of the person with dementia about present and future and offer activities that make it here and now makes sense
Coping with the nursing home environment	Let the person with dementia feel at home and continue to maintain his habits to prevent hospitalization. Involve the person with dementia in recreational activities
Developing and maintaining social relationships	Match the needs of individual contacts and encourage the person with dementia to fulfill several social roles

approach, and the validation approach, respectively. As the body of the person with dementia is frequently "touched" in caring and nursing contact, Van der Kooij made experience of the own body a separate field of attention in care. One approach that integrated emotion-oriented care derives techniques from in this area is the method passivities of daily life (PDL), a method that was developed by Dutch physiotherapists (Eijle and Van der Wulp 1988). In the German-speaking Europe, this is known as Basale Stimulation (Fröhlich 1991). Van der Kooij derived the experience areas social and spiritual experience from Maslov's hierarchy of needs (Maslov 1972). Social experience refers to making contact. In this context techniques from the validation approach and reminiscence are used. Spiritual experience refers to self-realization, signification, and achieving or not achieving ego integrity. Techniques from reminiscence and the validation approach are used here (Table 4.2).

4.1.2.4 Care in the Phase of Threatened Ego-Experience
Acceptance of Dependency People in the phase of the threatened Ego-experience are generally quite able, in their own way, to take care of themselves. For that reason, caregivers take over actions, very tactfully, only when necessary. They also look for opportunities to offer options.

Experiencing Security and Trust An important goal during this phase is to make the person with dementia experience control. Someone who feels threatened looks for security. There are various ways of helping the person with dementia in this respect: offering clearly organized options, a warm (small-scale) living environment, a fixed schedule, maintaining familiar rules of conduct, a place of one's own, supporting the dementing person's norms and values, developing and/or maintaining rituals and common practices (e.g., drinking coffee or reading the newspaper in a small group every morning), and making sure there are plenty of reference points, such as photographs and objects around someone's bed, personal toiletries, and a personal chair in the living room. These are ways of creating an organized and structured environment.

Experiencing Connectedness People in the threatened Ego-experience appear to keep others at a distance. This is often caused by fear, anger, or feelings of loneliness. Emotion-oriented care is based on the notion that these people need others to feel safe and to make contact. This can be done in many ways, for example, by radiating security and closeness. The caregiver can furthermore mirror the attitude of the person with dementia. His body language, eyes, and voice manifest tension, anger, or anxiety. By showing security, interest, and respect during the mirroring, the chances that the person feels understood are increased. This provides a basis for contact.

Experiencing Appreciation The sense of self-worth is enhanced by appealing to personal qualities in a day program or week program, by activating familiar actions and social roles, and by asking people to do things like read to others, help with domestic or household activities, and advise or console another resident.

Experiencing Affirmation and Validation In this phase, the person with dementia experiences himself as before and makes frenetic efforts to keep it that way. Caregivers can support the person with dementia by behaving "normally," not correcting or confronting, and providing support only when necessary.

4.1.2.5 Care in the Phase of Wandering Ego-Experience

Accepting Dependence Lost abilities require a prothetic approach and environment, a gradual taking over of actions that lead to fear of failure and a reduction of complexity. Supporting the memory of the person with dementia requires tact on the part of the caregiver. Sometimes the person with dementia will appreciate this; other times, he will hold onto his own reality. In this phase, it is pointless to enter into discussion about facts or words. This makes the person with dementia feel corrected and patronized.

Experiencing Security and Trust The person with dementia derives control from structure, familiar faces, spaces, rituals, objects, reference points on the ward (Holden 1983; Hanley 1981; Hanley et al. 1981), and support of the ability to make one's own choices and decisions.

Experiencing Connectedness Making contact with people in the wandering Ego-experience phase is often still possible. People in this phase take the initiative to make contact. If the reaction is positive, a reciprocity and interaction of feelings develop. During this phase, the person can make very apt remarks and does not let conventions limit him anymore. Word finding problems do not stop him from having conversations. The discussion partner only helps to keep the conversation on track and offers words, draws conclusions, or summarizes what has been discussed (Feil 1989a, b, 1992). In this, the partner needs to be both empathic and prothetic.

Experiencing Appreciation For people in this phase, life themes and losses play an important part in their experience of reality. These themes are discussed individually as well as in groups. This may bring about a sense of (delayed) validation, understanding, compensation, or satisfaction. Whether the person experiences his reality positively or negatively depends to a great extent on the person and his life history. If someone has not built up a positive self-perception during his life and has known few good relationships, the behavior in this phase can be difficult to manage.

Experiencing Affirmation and Validation The perception of the own identity becomes fragmented due to gaps in the memory. Caregivers can validate the feeling of identity of the person with dementia by addressing him in his identity and by incorporating, whenever possible, satisfying activities from the past into his current life in the nursing home (e.g., helping with the dishes, folding the laundry, polishing the silver or brass). In general, this will make the dementing person feel appreciated. Some caution is required, however. An excessive appeal on who one used to be, what one was able to do, or what brought pleasure in the past can also be very confrontational in the current situation.

4.1.2.6 Care in the Phase of Hidden Ego-Experience
Accepting Dependence During this phase, the person is totally dependent on others. The person with dementia is likely to accept this more easily if he trusts those others. Caregivers need to build up this trust, e.g., by always carrying out care actions in the same way and by making themselves recognizable by means of the tone of voice, type of greeting, and physical contact. Despite the fact that one is dependent, experiencing the freedom to choose is still very important. Selecting the moments and ways in which choices are offered to the person with dementia requires creativity and tact.

Experiencing Connectedness In this phase, the person depends on the initiatives of others for contact. Many people in this stage of dementia are, however, still open to liveliness, cheerfulness, humor, music, and movement (Buckwalter et al. 1995). Caregivers need to be alert to this in their contacts and in offering activities. Mirroring body posture and movements may help to tune oneself to the feelings of the person with dementia and invite him to share those feelings. Sometimes, eye contact helps to make the person with dementia experience closeness and intimacy; sometimes, sitting with him for a moment is enough. To the person with dementia, the person who is so close to him may symbolize someone from his life history. Who this is exactly is irrelevant. The verbal technique used is the technique of ambiguity (Feil 1992): "Isn't that nice?" "Is it that bad?." The person with dementia feels understood. Experiencing appreciation: contact opportunities should be sought in the physical and sensory experience. The caregiver needs to show respect, warmth, and understanding.

Experiencing Affirmation and Validation Although their sense of who they are is vague for people in the hidden Ego-experience, they do prove sensitive to an appeal to their identity, for example, by reminiscing together with the person with dementia with the aid of old photographs or familiar objects about positive events in his past. Awareness of the life history of the resident with dementia is therefore important.

4.1.2.7 Care in the Phase of Sunken Ego-Experience

Accepting Dependence and Control People in the phase of sunken Ego-experience were once thought to be in a vegetative stage. The care would therefore be limited to the body. In the integrated emotion-oriented care, the daily care is also used to nourish the person with dementia and provide him with pleasant sensations. People with high muscle tone and contractures are easier to help with principles from, e.g., the PDL approach and basal stimulation, and they respond well to relaxing massage. The person with dementia responds primarily to physical and sensory stimuli. These can be offered, for example, through bodily experiences like massage and warm bathing, sensory stimulation, aroma therapy, and music.

4.1.3   How Integrated Emotion-Oriented Care Can Influence Adaptation

In the adaptation-coping model, the seven adaptive tasks are considered as important aspects of cognitive, emotional, and social adaptation in dementia. Starting from the "coping" perspective, we examine for each of the adaptive tasks how they can cause behavior and mood problems or disruptions in the daily functioning of people with dementia. Subsequently, we describe how integrated emotion-oriented care attempts to prevent, reduce, or eliminate these disruptions and problems.

4.1.3.1 Integrated Emotion-Oriented Care and Cognitive Adaptation

Coping with the Own Invalidity

A dementia syndrome, as stated before, is characterized primarily by cognitive disabilities. Accepting and coping with these disabilities in daily life requires constant adaptation from the person with dementia.

Adaptation may take place, for example, by developing skills that compensate for the disabilities. Due to the presence of cognitive impairments and the ongoing deterioration, a general assumption is that people with dementia are able to adapt or, as Sacks (2012) puts it, "to reassemble their world," only to a very limited extent.

Various authors point out that the behavior of people with dementia proves that they find ways of coping with the consequences of their illness (Dröes 1991; Cotrell and Lein 1993; Clare 2009; Dirkse et al. 2011; de Werd et al. 2013). Dröes (1991) mentions four coping strategies that appear to be used with regard to "coping with the own invalidity": obsessive and compulsive behavior, taking the shape of, e.g., extreme neatness and the urge to walk; denial, as manifested in confabulation and the denial of cognitive disabilities; avoidance, which refers to avoiding test situations; and regression (reduction of interests and initiative, increased egocentricity, dependent behavior, and motor passivity) (Dröes 1991; Clare 2002, 2003; De Boer 2011; Steeman 2013).

According to Dröes, the regressive coping strategy in particular has negative side effects for the person with dementia and his environment. If taken to extremes, this coping strategy can be accompanied by insecurity, suspicion, disruptive behavior, and "excess disabilities" (this refers to the fact that the person with dementia exhibits more disability in his daily life function than one would expect on the basis of his abilities; Cohen 1986; Dröes 1991). She feels that activating and supporting these people may contribute to a reduction of these accompanying symptoms, partly because the person with dementia experiences which possibilities and skills he still has through activities and partly because he learns to trust people in his environment who will help out when necessary.

What does integrated emotion-oriented care do? Integrated emotion-oriented care offers support, in the context of the care objective "accepting dependence," with regard to the problems that elderly people with dementia can experience with coping with the disabilities that may come with old age and dementia.

In the different phases of Ego-experience, the following strategies are central:

1. Care "with hands behind your back"
2. Offering prothetic support and gradual taking over of actions
3. Building up trust in case of (total) taking over of actions, continuing to respect free choice
4. Offering physical and sensory stimuli

By always customizing the care to what is pleasant for the resident and what he is still able to do, the elderly person is validated in his individual being and possibilities.

Developing an Adequate Care Relationship with the Staff

In the nursing home, the resident with dementia depends on the nursing staff in terms of getting the required help and assistance. It is therefore important that an adequate care relationship with the staff is developed. One of the preconditions for this, from the perspective of the person with dementia, is to trust the caregivers. As a rule, this trust will develop if the elderly person regularly experiences that the caregivers sense what he can do himself and what he cannot and that they are willing to help him with the actions and activities he wants to be helped with and keep their distance when he chooses. Based on this trust, the person with dementia usually will not have a problem accepting the offered help. He feels respected in his autonomy and independence.

One of the problems, however, that elderly nursing home residents with dementia may have to face is the daily changing of the staff. This complicates the development of a trust relationship, especially for people who have trouble telling the different staff members apart. Two coping strategies that dementing elderly people seem to use to cope with this situation are regression and resistance (Dröes 1991; De Lange 2004). In this case, regression is characterized by a compliant, helpless, and passive attitude: to placate to their mind anonymous caregivers and to be ensured of care, the elderly person adopts a submissive and helpless attitude toward every caregiver. He exhibits so-called good patient behavior. One of the negative side effects of this strategy is the so-called acquired helplessness (Nelson and Farberow 1980). If the person with dementia fails to develop a sound care relationship with the staff, it can furthermore lead to depression (Flannery 2002; Miesen 2012). The nondevelopment of an adequate care relationship can also result in resistance in order to get some control over the situation. This can be expressed in, for example, agitated, aggressive, rebellious, and uncooperative behavior toward the staff. This is also referred to as bad patient behavior. This behavior should be viewed as an expression of dissatisfaction with the existing relationship with the staff.

What does integrated emotion-oriented care do? In the context of the care objective "experiencing control," integrated emotion-oriented care explicitly offers attention to the development of a sound care relationship between residents and caregivers. In the first three phases of Ego-experience, the following strategies are central:

1. Offering security, e.g., in the shape of a warm living environment, and developing and maintaining rituals
2. Offering structure by means of familiar faces, familiar rooms, and reference points on the ward
3. Inspiring trust by assigning the same caregiver to particular residents as much as possible (resident assignment) and by carrying out care actions and procedures along established lines

In all phases, the caregiver must delve into the life history of residents and try to empathize as much as possible with their experiences and perceptions, so that they can tune to the person more adequately in the care relationship.

The techniques used are derived from, among other approaches, reminiscence (talking with the resident about the past based on old photographs or objects) and validation (empathic communication): listening closely to the words the person uses, trying to verbalize unspoken needs that are expressed in behavior, mirroring actions and posture of the person with dementia, and going along in the movement rhythm of the person with dementia.

4.1.3.2 Integrated Emotion-Oriented Care and Emotional Adaptation

Maintaining an Emotional Balance

The changes that the dementia brings to the life of the elderly person, such as cognitive impairments, the forced move to the nursing home, and being separated from family and friends, can cause a considerable disruption of the emotional balance. Dröes (1991) mentions coping strategies that elderly people with dementia appear to be using to maintain control over the grief, anxiety, and uncertainty that come with these changes: overcompensation and counterphobic behavior, as expressed in agitated, aggressive, and hostile behavior; suppression, e.g., in wandering behavior (during the day and during the night) and manic behavior; depression with projective traits (whining, agitated, accusing); and depression with regressive traits (withdrawing, apathetic and excessively dependent behavior). If there is not enough activity and distraction for the person with dementia, the "suppression" strategy can easily lead to (night time) restlessness. Accompanying symptoms of the "regressive and projective depression," respectively, are sad and aggressive behavior. Important determinants for maintaining an emotional balance are having fun regularly, being able to freely express positive and negative feelings, and a sense of control (Dröes 1991).

The general principle is validation of feelings of anxiety, happiness, sadness, and anger by naming them, so that residents may feel understood. This method is taken from the validation approach. In some cases, caregivers also help to control or guide emotions, e.g., by using humor, putting things in perspective or using confrontation, or leaving the resident alone.

To have the person with dementia experience he is appreciated, the following strategies are among those used in the successive phases of Ego-experience: (1) appeal to personal qualities, (2) talk about life themes and losses individually and in groups, (3) show respect and warmth, and (4) nourish the resident in the daily care and have him experience pleasant sensations. In all phases of dementia, the staff examines what the resident enjoys, and this is taken into account in the care. Examples are playing specific music, offering nice foods, and letting them smell pleasant fragrances. This method is based on the principles of sensory activation/snoezelen.

What does integrated emotion-oriented care do? The attention that integrated emotion-oriented care pays to the affective functioning of residents with dementia may be expected to actually help them to maintain an emotional balance with less agitated, restless, dependent, depressive, and anxious behavior.

Maintaining a Positive Self-Image

Illnesses that are accompanied by permanent functional disabilities require an adjustment of the self-image that takes into account the invalidity. According to Van der Wulp (1986), this is a precondition for experiencing continuity in past, present, and future. If there is no revision of the self-image, the patient may experience this as a conflict with continuity and a disruption of his identity. This, obviously, has negative consequences for the satisfaction with the current life situation and on mood in general.

Based on this line of reasoning, Dröes (1991) indicates that it is not inconceivable that some people with dementia, i.e., those who withdraw frequently into the past and deny the present, do this because they have a problem with their self-image, which has been affected by the consequences of their illness. But perhaps other behaviors can also be explained from this perspective. She names five coping strategies that people with dementia appear to use to maintain an acceptable self-image: denial, as manifested in confabulation and living in the (active) past in one's mind; avoidance (avoiding situations where one is confronted with one's inability); projection, as exhibited in paranoid delusions; withdrawing into one's own phantasy world, as manifested in, e.g., positive delusions; and depression, as a problem-oriented strategy to obtain attention and validation from others in the environment. If these strategies do not lead to the desired result, the balance may yet be disrupted, and the person with dementia may fall into a real depression. On the other hand, reduction of the coping behaviors mentioned (confabulation, living in the past, avoiding behavior, delusions, and depressive behavior) and an increase of satisfaction with the current situation indicate acceptance and adjustment of the self-image.

According to Dröes (1991), the regular experience of success (experiencing what one is still able to do) and validation of the sense of identity are important conditions for maintaining a positive self-image.

What does integrated emotion-oriented care do? In the context of the care objective "experiencing validation," integrated emotion-oriented care attempts to stimulate the sense of self-worth and in this way have a positive influence on the self-image of the person with dementia.

In the first three phases of Ego-experience, the following strategies are used: (1) Approaching the person with dementia in a "normal" way, by accepting what he is and not correcting or confronting him (all the time), only supporting him when necessary with memory facts or words; (2) Validating the person with dementia, if this is not confronting or asking too much of him, in his (current) identity by fitting in satisfactory activities from the past in his current life in the nursing home whenever possible; (3) Appealing to his identity by reminiscing together with the person with dementia, for example, with old photographs or familiar objects, about positive events in his past

In the final phase of Ego-experience, the method is limited to having the person with dementia experience pleasant sensations, because it is assumed that he no longer has a sense of identity.

The techniques used in the different phases are derived from the reality orientation approach, the validation approach, reminiscence, sensory stimulation, and PDL. The attention that integrated emotion-oriented care pays to the identity feelings of the person with dementia (in the past and the present) and the actions that are undertaken to have the person with dementia experience success in his daily functioning are expected to contribute to a modified self-image and preservation of the sense of self-worth on the one hand. On the other hand, they are expected to lead to the person with dementia having to attempt less actively to keep his self-image positive. In terms of behavior and mood, this means that we expect the person with dementia will exhibit less of the coping behaviors mentioned (confabulation, living in the past, delusions, and depressive behavior) and will be less dissatisfied with his current situation.

Preparing for an Uncertain Future

The negative prognosis of dementia and the progressiveness of the disease with its increasing disabilities make the future for people with dementia extremely uncertain: it is unclear to what extent and how quickly they will become dependent on others, whether or not these others are willing and able to take on this care, whether or not they can stay in their own home, etc. This uncertainty can furthermore be compounded by fear of the approaching death. In this context also, withdrawing into the past and denial appear to be frequently used strategies to maintain a balance (Dröes 1991). There is no confrontation with the present and the future. If the person with dementia does confront them, it is possible he will gradually accept the loss. If this takes place at an early stage, the necessary arrangements can be made, in consultation with the partner or family, for the time when the person enters a more serious stage and is no longer able to make his own decisions. However, experiencing one's own deterioration and the awareness that one suffers from a progressive disease can also lead to the person losing heart, because he no longer feels his life has meaning. Verwoerdt (Dröes 1991) considers refusing to eat and preferring to lie down signals that the person is giving up.

The support people experience from their faith or from others in their immediate environment may contribute to their being less anxious and more able to accept the losses they go through.

What does integrated emotion-oriented care do? Although "preparing for an uncertain future" is not a separate care objective within integrated emotion-oriented care, attention is given to "the spiritual experience and signification" of residents.

Integrated emotion-oriented care offers support with regard to accepting the losses that people with dementia go through and in preparing for the end of life.To help accept the losses, caregivers discuss with the residents, especially in the first two phases of Ego-experience, how he experiences his current situation and show understanding and compassion when the resident is anxious or no longer sees a meaning to life.

To inventory which activities or religious beliefs the resident derives meaning from, the caregivers approach the resident himself and his family. Apart from reading or listening to music, integrated emotion-oriented care applies activities like going to church, attending bible study group, or singing together, to give the residents support and new energy. Preserving fixed habits, such as praying before meals and sleep, has the same function. This method of integrated emotion-oriented care is expected to have a positive effect on the acceptance of the losses the person goes through. It therefore is expected to lead to a reduction of anxiety and feelings of insecurity. This might reduce the necessity to withdraw into the past and deny the current situation, and the chance that the person gives up in an early stage, because he no longer sees any purpose to his life, may become smaller.

4.1.3.3 Integrated Emotion-Oriented Care and Social Adaptation

Coping with the Nursing Home Environment
The forced move to a nursing home brings about a number of drastic changes in the life of the elderly person with dementia: he loses his familiar surroundings and a large part of his freedom of movement and privacy; the role of nursing home resident requires adaptation to the nursing home values, norms, and rules; and the person with dementia is expected to undergo various treatments, such as physiotherapy, movement therapy, and/or activity therapy.

Elderly people appear to use different coping strategies to handle the stress that the institutionalization may cause (Dröes 1991): denial, as shown in confabulation, living in the past, and convincing oneself that one is only visiting the nursing home; suppression, identified by euphoric and relieved behavior; command and control of the new environment, as shown by expectant or explorative behavior and active participation in organized activities; and expression of feelings (rebellious, agitated, and aggressive behavior).

The closed world of the nursing home furthermore carries the risk that residents will hospitalize with time. Hospitalization can be understood as a type of regressive coping with an environment one (believes one) cannot influence. The person submits to the norms and rules, the organization, and the representatives of this organization (staff). This regression enhances the dementia syndrome and is characterized by, among other things, passivity, dependent and subservient behavior, apathy, and socially isolated behavior. By creating a domestic environment, regularly organizing recreational/creative activities and emphasizing the resident role and the say of the person with dementia, the adjustment in the nursing home can be furthered, and hospitalization phenomena may perhaps be prevented to some extent.

What does integrated emotion-oriented care do? In the context of the care objectives "experiencing control, appreciation, and validation" and the "social experience" field, integrated emotion-oriented care also offers the elderly person with dementia support in coping with the nursing home environment. The underlying reasoning is that residents will feel more at home in the nursing home if they feel safe, if their values and norms are respected and they have satisfying activities and contacts that link up with their own experiences and perceptions, and that this simultaneously counters, or prevents, hospitalization phenomena.

In the first three phases of Ego-experience, the following strategies are used to accomplish the mentioned objectives: (1) activating residents to take on social roles and stimulating them to participate in domestic and recreational/creative activities, helping them preserve old habits and rhythms by adjusting the care, helping them develop new habits in the new living environment, and making sure there are sufficient reference points; (2) discussing feelings regarding losses (e.g., of the own home) and stimulating them to participate in satisfying recreational/creative activities which are tuned to the abilities of residents and their experiences/perceptions; and (3) offering warmth and showing understanding and respect in direct contacts with a resident. People in the phase of sunken Ego-experience are scarcely aware of their environment. Still, people who are in this phase sometimes are placed in the living room lying on bed. Sometimes their rooms are given a warm and vivid atmosphere with mobiles, pictures, dolls, and so on.

The methods described are derived in part from ideas regarding normalization of the living environment and in part from the validation approach (discussing life themes, social roles) and the reality orientation approach (reading the paper, structuring activities, reference points).

The resident and his family are asked to supply the information needed to determine which activities are experienced as significant by the residents.

In integrated emotion-oriented care, the nursing assistant is assigned an important role as the person who creates the atmosphere in the nursing home. To further the homy atmosphere, she will, e.g., wash the dishes in the living room, iron, make coffee, or sow on buttons, and she will actively involve residents by asking them to help drying the dishes, folding the laundry, pouring the coffee, or distributing biscuits. Nursing assistants also guide relaxation activities, such as playing cards and singing.

In view of the individualized methods used in integrated emotion-oriented care to help familiarize dementing people in the nursing home with their new living environment and create a home there, one can expect that they will initiate activities more frequently and will participate in organized activities in the nursing home. Furthermore, one can expect that manifestations of hospitalization, such as passivity, dependent and subservient behavior, apathy, and socially isolated behavior, will be reduced or prevented.

Developing and Maintaining Social Relationships

In the long run, suffering from dementia unavoidably brings changes to the social life. Existing social contacts change, fade, or are lost. Communication breaks down. Not only because the person with dementia becomes cognitively impaired, which hinders the maintenance of relationships, but also because friends and acquaintances often don't know how to deal with the (changed) person with dementia. The move to the nursing home furthermore implies a physical separation from family, friends, and acquaintances. To prevent isolation after admittance to the nursing home, it is important that the person with dementia makes new contacts. Elias indicates that loneliness is partly related to the significance that people have to others. Important preventative aspects of loneliness are participating in activities and feeling that one means something to others (Linnemann et al. 1990). Behaviors that indicate that the person with dementia tries to build up a new social network include active participation in social activities inside and outside the nursing home and actively functioning in different social roles, such as conversation partner, kitchen help, table setter, coffee pourer, table companion, etc. (Hanson et al. 1986; Dröes 1991). In actual reality, however, we see a lot of social passivity (sleeping, sitting, little initiative, and social contact) among nursing home residents with dementia (Hiatt 1987). According to Dröes (1991), this social passivity can perhaps be partly explained as regressive coping (withdrawing) with the socially depriving environment (institutional rules, patient role, high social density). The person with dementia runs the risk, however, of becoming lonely and isolated within the nursing home.

What does integrated emotion-oriented care do? In the context of the care objective "experiencing connectedness," integrated emotion-oriented care responds to the need of the resident with dementia for social contact. This response uses not only information about their current social functioning but also about how they functioned in the past. Did a person like to be by himself before, or was he more of a sociable person? What is that like now? Is it easy for the resident to make contact with other residents and staff? Does the resident like to sit in a circle or does he prefer the isolation of his own little corner? This information may be helpful to find, for example, a suitable place in the living room, the potential new friends, the offer of group activities, the role of the resident in those activities, etc. Proposals made to the person with dementia to participate in activities are aimed at continuing old and/or developing new contacts. For example, the resident can be stimulated to fulfill particular roles (such as coffee pourer, card playing partner, dance partner, member of the singing club) in order to expand his contacts. This method is partly based on the validation approach. Furthermore, in the successive phases of Ego-experience, the following strategies are used in the personal life to make residents experience a sense of connectedness:

• Phase 1: showing understanding for the feelings (tension, anger, anxiety) that the resident experiences in his situation, radiating security, interest, respect, and closeness
• Phase 2: responding to social initiatives from residents, helping to keep the conversation on track, and empathic communication
• Phase 3: offering activities that will invite the resident to make contact with his environment (including music and movement), mirroring the resident's posture and movement, and eye contact help to tune to his feelings and invite him to share feelings
• Phase 4: contact by means of physical and sensory stimuli

In view of the method of integrated emotion-oriented care to preserve contact with the residents and give them the opportunity to fulfill social roles – whenever possible – we may expect that residents will withdraw (regressive coping) less frequently after institutionalization in the nursing home and that they will make more contact with fellow residents and caregivers.

4.1.4 Finally

In this chapter we have seen how integrated emotion-oriented care provides guidance and support to people with dementia in different areas of adaptation. We described which strategies integrated emotion-oriented care implies in different stages or phases of Ego-experience in dementia. We have tried to make clear how you can recognize as a care professional when someone has problems with the cognitive, emotional, and/or social adaptation and how you can support the person with dementia using the integrated emotion-oriented care approach. People with dementia will therefore experience less stress, and there will be fewer behavioral and mood disturbances.

4.2 Section B: Implementing Psychosocial Interventions

Linda Wolter

4.2.1 Introduction

Psychosocial intervention (PSI) is defined as "A non-pharmacologic intervention intended to alter a person's environment or reaction to lessen the impact of a mental disorder" (McGraw-Hill 2002). The intent of PSI is to maintain and improve the quality of life for the residents. For residents with dementia, the uses of psychosocial interventions address both the environment and the residents' perceptions and reactions (Kasl-Godley and Gatz 2000). Psychosocial interventions are grounded in many different theories; despite the fact that psych-dynamic theories have much in common, ego psychology puts relatively more emphasis on how the ego successfully copes with conflict and adapts to the environment (Wolitzky 1995). Dementia results in weakened ego functioning diminished mastery over the environment and increased dependency (Kasl-Godley et al. 2000). Psychosocial interventions assist the residents in developing new coping and adaption skills.

Watts et al. (2013) state that psychosocial interventions intended to help people maintain a good quality of life. Interventions include:

- Adjustment to a dementia diagnosis
- Communication
- Stress, anxiety, and depression
- Memory and cognitive functioning
- Living independently, quality of life
- Support for partners and families

As mentioned earlier in this chapter, Finnema et al. (2000) stated that building trust with the residents and nursing staff's attunement to their moods and behaviors are key to building trust and considered the first step in successfully implementing psychosocial intervention with dementia residents. For trust to be established, it is important for the nursing staff to understand how trust initially is experienced and internalized.

4.2.2 Building Trust

McLeod (2013) states Erick Erickson's life-span developmental theory speaks to psychosocial tasks each individual must resolve. According to Erickson, the first stage of development, trust versus mistrust, occurs at birth to age three. When the infant experiences hunger, pain, fear, etc., they communicate their distress by crying. It is through the caregiver's attunement and timely response that the infant's distress and discomfort are alleviated and trust is established. In working and caring for dementia residents, attunement, timely responsiveness, and consistency create the foundation for building trust. When the facility or nursing home staff fails to provide an attuned, timely, and consistent environment, residents will display challenging behaviors, such as agitation and aggressiveness, or become withdrawn and depressed. Building trust and secure environment with residents is both the nursing staff's and facilities' responsibility.

Sutor et al. (2001) noted that dementia residents who referred from long-term care facilities to the Mayo clinic psychiatric wards were docile and pleasant when they were on the ward but exhibited challenging behaviors when they returned to their care facilities. Smith states, "What we realized then is that the problems didn't reside in the residents but in the setting". Environmental settings influence both moods and behaviors. Research has found that higher nursing home staffing leads to higher quality of care (Harrington et al. 2000). The level of individual care should be considered when scheduling of care staff and patience ratio. In addition, training for care providers will assist staff ability to provide consistency when implementing psychosocial interventions. With dementia residents, timely response to requests for assistance or addressing physical discomfort not only builds trust but also may limit the residents' agitation and aggressive behaviors. In addition, consistency among multiple care providers will enhance and maintain a sense of trust and predictability for the residents.

It is with the establishment of a secure environment and consistent staff responses the focus for implementing psychosocial intervention shifts from the residence's external world to their internal world and through reminiscence and self-reflection, thus enhancing the residents' dignity and sense of worth. "Given the considerable impact the social environment has on the personal dignity of people with mild to moderate dementia, it is important in caregiving not to confine attention to health-related or even any individual aspects alone, but also to take interpersonal aspects into consideration" (Gennip et al. 2016).

4.2.3 Enhancing Integrity Through Reminisces and Self-Reflection

Erickson's (1959) eighth stage in the life-span is ego integrity versus despair. It is during this time that the individual will contemplate their accomplishments and are able to develop integrity if they view themselves as leading a successful life (McLeod et al. 2013). Characteristics of integrity include honesty, reliability, and honor. It is through reflection and reminisces the residents will examine their past. Reflections as a psychosocial intervention include careful thoughts about one's behavior and values. Implementing this intervention is best done through verbal or written communication. Reflection of meaning refers to the deeply held thoughts and meanings underlying life experiences. Care providers assist reflection by encouraging the residents through questions about what they thought and how they felt during the experiences. In some cases, the care provider may hear different residents reflect on similar life experiences, marriage, parenthood, and careers and find the same event can have a different meaning to the different individuals (Hill 2009). For residents in nursing homes, self- reflections and reminiscent interventions done individually provide a safe and supportive environment to look inward and remember.

Activities done in group settings, be it other family members, residents, or community visitors, provide both social and psycho skill building. According to Kennard (2016), reminisce activities vary in mediums and include:

- Visually: photographs and slides. Painting pictures, looking at objects of auto-biographical meaning
- Music: using familiar tunes from the radio, CDs, or making music using various instruments
- Smell or taste: using smell kits, different foods
- Tactile: touching objects, feeling textures, painting, and pottery

Reminisce activities such as mentioned above all aid in and enhance social skills of dementia residents in nursing homes. Group work or group activities have always been seen as powerful interventions in working with people who feel isolated, lonely, and fearful. These emotions are common among dementia residents in nursing homes. In addition to social skills building, reminisce groups have shown other health benefits such as decreasing depression and pain, improving mood, decreasing stress, and calming challenging behaviors (Cohen-Mansfield et al. 2005).

Traditional barriers to providing psychosocial groups to the aging population such as location, accessibility, and transportation are nonexistent for nursing home residents. Many nursing home residents establish new friendships and relationships with others. The relationships that exist among nursing home residents are potent and, however, should not be viewed as the culmination for social interaction. The "social" aspect of psychosocial interventions is achieved through groups. Building a broader perspective of the residents' world should include diversity that extends beyond the facility's staff and other residents.

4.2.4   Multigenerational Programs

As important as the activities are, so too is the group membership. One medium of intervention that has shown consistent success for older adults is intergenerational programs. Intergenerational programs began in 1963 as part of the war on poverty in the United States. Intergenerational programs are social vehicles that offer younger and older generations the opportunities to interact and become engaged in issues concerning our society (Generations United 2002). Benefits for older adults include enhanced socialization, stimulated learning, increased emotional support, and improved health.

Carlson et al. (2000) found in their study that older adults want to remain productive and engaged in the community. A way to prevent isolation in their later years is to increase interaction with children and youth through intergenerational programs. Learning is life-long experience. One study showed that older adult quality of life is enhanced through learning and sharing what they know with others. Glass (2003) found older adults show an increase in emotional support and improved health and through structured and social activities. In another study, adults with dementia or other cognitive impairments experience more positive effect during interactions with children than they did during non-intergenerational activities (Jarrott and Bruno 2003).

Galbraith et al. (2015) found in their literature review of 27 research projects looking at intergenerational programs for dementia residents that music, art-based, and narrative programs were most common in intergenerational programs. Outcomes include effects on perceptions of aging and dementia, behavior, mood, engagement, and sense of self. Activities that were meaningful for participants and supported shared opportunities for relationship building and growth saw outcomes that are more positive.

Creating multigenerational programming is relatively easy. Extending invitations to local elementary, high schools, and universities can provide a rich pool of younger people who can benefit from one-on-one time with older adults. For residents in nursing homes, children and adolescents may be viewed a "breath of fresh air" and provide a sense of happiness that comes from giving something to another.

4.2.5   Summary

In this section, we have discussed psychosocial interventions. How nursing home staff provides attunement, knowledge, and consistent and timely responses to residents is significant to building a trusting, safe environment. Psychosocial interventions for dementia residents, such as sensory stimulation and reminiscence activities, are fundamental to long-term health and well-being. In addition, the mediums, individual, group, or multi-generational in which reflective and reminisce activities occur, are crucial to residents' ability to adapt and grow in new environments.

References

Section A: Coping with Dementia: Integrated Emotion-Oriented Care for Nursing Home Residents

Achterberg I, Kok W (1992) Snoezelen met psychogeriatrische bewoners, Denkbeeld Tijdschrift voor Psychogeriatrie 5:12–13

Boer ME de (2011). Advance directives in dementia care. Perspectives of people with Alzheimer's disease, elderly care physicians and relatives. Thesis. Amsterdam. Vrije Universiteit

Buckwalter KC, Faan LA, Gerdner MA, Richards Hall G et al (1995) Shining through: the humor and individuality of persons with Alzheimer's disease. J Gerontol Nurs 3:11–15

Clare L (2002) We'll fight it as long as we can: coping with the onset of Alzheimer's disease. Aging Ment Health 6:139–148

Clare L (2003) Managing threats to self: awareness in early stage Alzheimer's disease. Soc Sci Med 57:1017–1029

Clare L (2009) Working with memory problems: cognitive rehabilitation in early dementia. In: Moniz-Cook E, Manthorpe J (eds) Psychosocial interventions in early stage dementia; a European evidence-based text. Jessica Kingsley Publishers, London

Cohen D (1986) Psychopathological perspectives: differential diagnosis of Alzheimer's disease and related disorders. In: Poon LW (ed) Handbook of clinical memory assessment of older adults American Psychological Association, Washington D.C., pp 81–88

Cohen D (1991) The subjective experience of Alzheimer's disease: the anatomy of an illness as perceived by patients and families. American Journal of Alzheimer's Care and Related Disorders & Research 6:6–11

Cotrell V, Lein L (1993) Awareness and denial in the Alzheimer's disease victim. J Gerontol Soc Work 19:115–132

Cotrell V, Schultz R (1993) The perspective of the patient with Alzheimer's disease: a neglected dimension of dementia research. Gerontologist 33:205–211

De Lange J (2004) Omgaan met dementie het effect van geïntegreerde belevingsgerichte zorg op adaptatie en coping van mensen met dementie in verpleeghuizen; een kwalitatief onderzoek binnen een gerandomiseerd experiment. Academisch Proefschrift Vrije Universiteit, Amsterdam

de Werd M, Boelen D, Kessels R (2013) Foutloos Leren bij dementie Een praktische handleiding. Boom/Lemma

Dirkse R, van Dixhoorn I, Hoogeveen F, Kessels R (2011) (Op)nieuw geleerd, oud gedaan. Kosmos uitgeverij

Dröes RM (1991) In beweging: over psychosociale hulpverlening aan demente ouderen. De Tijdstroom, Utrecht

Feil N (1984) Communicating with the confused elderly patient. Geriatrics 39:131–132

Feil N (1989a) The Feil method. How to help the disoriented old-old. Edward Feil productions, Cleveland

Feil N (1989b) Validation: an empathic approach to the care of dementia. Clin Gerontol 8:89–94

Feil N (1992) Validation therapy with late-onset dementia populations. In: Jones GMM, Miesen BML (eds) Care-giving in dementia, research and applications. Tavistock/ Routledge, London/ New York

Finnema EJ, Dröes RM, Kooij CH, Ribbe MW, Tilburg W van (2000a) The adaptation-coping model as theoretical framework for research on emotion-oriented care among nursing home residents with dementia. In: Finnema E Emotion-oriented care in dementia; a psychosocial approach. Dissertation,Vrije Universiteit Amsterdam

Finnema EJ, Dröes RM, Ribbe MW, van Tilburg W (2000b) The effects of emotion-oriented approaches in the care for persons suffering from dementia: a review of the literature. Int J Geriatr Psychiatry 15:141–161

Flannery RB (2002) Treating learned helplessness in the elderly dementia patient: preliminary inquiry. Am J Alzheimers Dis Other Demen 17(6):345–349

Fröhlich A (1991) Basale stimulation. Verlag Selbstbestimmtes Leben, Düsseldorf

Halek M, Bartholomeyczik S (2006) Verstehen und Handeln. Forschungsergebnisse zur Pflege von menschen mit Demenz und herausforderndesd Verhalten. Universität Witten/Herdecke

Hanley IG (1981) The use of signposts and active training to modify ward disorientation in elderly patients. J Behav Ther Exp Psychiatry 12:41–247

Hanley IG, McGuire RJ, Boyd WD (1981) Reality orientation and dementia: a controlled trial of two approaches. Br J Psychiatry 138:10–14

Hansson RO, Jones WH, Carpenter BN, Remondet JH (1986) Loneliness and adjustment to old age. Int J Aging Hum Dev 23:41–53

Hiatt LG (1987) Environmental design and mentally impaired older people. In: Altman HJ (ed) Alzheimer's disease: problems, prospects, and perspectives. Plenum Press, New York/London, pp 321–328

Holden UP (1983) Thinking it through. In: A handbook for those, working with the elderly. Winslow Press, London

Hoogendijk WJG (1998) Brain changes in depression: a combined clinical and post-mortem study in depressed patients with or without Alzheimer's or Parkinson's disease. Vrije Universiteit, Amsterdam, Dissertation

Kitwood T, Bredin K (1992) A new approach to the evaluation of dementia care. J Adv Health Nurs Care 1:41–60

Kiyak HA, Borson S (1992) Coping with chronic illness and disability. In: Ory MG, Abeles RP, Lipman PD (eds) Aging, health and behavior. Sage Publications, London

Lazarus RS, Folkman S (1984) Stress, appraisal and coping. Springer Publishing Company, New York

Linnemann M, Leene G, Bettink K, Schram M, Voermans J (1990) Uit eenzaamheid: over hulpverlening bij ouderen. Bohn Stafleu VanLoghum, Houten/Antwerpen

Maslov A (1972) Psychologie van het menselijk zijn. Lemniscaat, Utrecht

Miesen B (2012) Zorg om mensen met dementie. Springer

Moore I (1997) Living with Alzheimer's: understanding the family's and patient's perspective. Geriatrics 52:33–36

Moos RH, Tsu VD (1977) The crisis of physical illness: an overview. In: Moos RH (ed) Coping with physical illness. Plenum Medical Book Company, New York/London, pp 3–21

Nelson FL, Farberow NL (1980) Indirect self-destructive behavior in the elderly nursing home patient. J Gerontol 35:949–957

Rabe W (1993) Passiviteiten van het Dagelijks Leven. Zorg voor diep demente ouderen. Denkbeeld, Tijdschrift voor Psychogeriatrie:14–15

Rossaert I (1989) Reminiscentie: leven en werken met herinneringen. Tijdschr Gerontol Geriatr 20:167–168

Sacks O (2012) An anthropologist on Mars. Knopf Doubleday Publishing Group, New York

Spector A, Thorgrimsen L, Woods B, Orrell M, Brock E (2012) Kognitive Anregung (CST) für Menschen mit Demenz. Huber Verlag, Bern

Steeman E (2013) The lived experience of older people living with early-stage dementia. Thesis, Katholieke Universiteit Leuven

Thornton S, Brotchie J (1987) Reminiscence: a critical review of the empirical literature. Br J Clin Psychol 26:93–111

van der Kooij CH (2003) Gewoon lief zijn? Het Maieutisch zorgconcept en het invoeren van geïntegreerde belevingsgerichte zorg op psychogeriatrische verpleeghuisafdelingen. Academisch proefschrift Vrije universiteit Amsterdam, Lemma, Utrecht

van der Kooij CH (2016) Das mäeutische Plfege- und Betreuungsmodell. Darstellung und Dokumentation. Hogrefe, Bern

van der Kooij CH, Dröes RM, De Lange J, Ettema TP, Cools HJM, van Tilburg W (2013) The implementation of integrated emotion-oriented care: did it actually change the attitude, skills and time-spent of trained caregivers? Int J Soc Res Pract 12:536–550

van Eijle J, van der Wulp JC (1988) Passiviteiten van het Dagelijks Leven. Tijdschrift voor Verzorgenden:280–283

Verdult R (1993) Dement worden: een kindertijd in beeld, belevingsgerichte begeleiding van dementerende ouderen. Intro, Baarn

Verwoerdt A (1976) Clinical geropsychiatry. The Williams & WilkinsCo, Baltimore

Verwoerdt A (1981) Individual psychotherapy in senile dementia. In: Miller NE, Cohen GD (eds), Aging, vol 15. Raven Press, New York

Section B: Implementing Psychosocial Interventions

Carlson M, Seeman T, Fried LP (2000) Importance of generativity for healthy aging in older women. Aging 12(2):132–140

Cohen-Mansfield J, Lipson S, Patel D et al. (2005) Wisdom from the front lines: clinicians' descriptions of treating agitation in the nursing home: a pilot study. J Am Med Dir Assoc 6:257–264. https://www.ncbi.mln.nih.gov/pubmed. Accessed May 2016

Erickson E (1959) Identity and the life cycle. In: Levy T, Orlans M (eds) Attachment, trauma, and healing: understanding and treating attachment disorder in children and families. CWLA Press, Washington, DC

Finnema EJ, Dröes RM, Ribbe MW, van Tilburg W (2000c) The effects of emotion-oriented approaches in the care for persons suffering from dementia: a review of the literature. Int J Geriatr Psychiatry 15:141–161

Galbraith B, Larkin H, Moorhouse A, Oomen T (2015) Intergenerational programs for persons with dementia: a scoping review. J Gerontol Soc Work 58(4):357–378. doi:10.1080/01634372.2015.1008166

Generations United (2002) Young and old serving together: meeting community needs through intergenerational partnerships. Generations United, Washington, DC

Gennip Isis E, Roeline H, Pasman W, Oosterveld-Vung M, Wilems DL, Onwuteaka-Philipsen BD (2016) "How dementia affects personal dignity: a qualitative study on the perspective of individuals with mild to moderate dementia" pub. Oxford University Press on behalf of The Gerontological Society of America

Glass TA (2003) Successful aging. Brocklehurst's textbook of geriatric medicine and gerontology, 6th edn. Harcourt Health Sciences, London

Harrington C, Kovner C, Mezey M, Kayser-Jones J, Burger S, Mohler M, Burke R, Zimmerman D (2000) Experts recommend minimum nurse staffing standards for nursing facilities in the. Gerontologist 40(1):5–16

Hill CE (2009) Helping skills: facilitating exploration, insight, and action, 3rd edn. American Psychology Association Pub, Arlington County

Jarrott S, Bruno K (2003) Intergenerational activities involving persons with dementia: an observational assessment. Am J Alzheimers Dis Other Demen 18(1):31–37

Kasl-Godley J, Gatz M (2000) Psychosocial interventions for individuals with dementia: an integration of theory, therapy, and a clinical understanding of dementia. Clin Psychol Rev 20(6):755–782

Kennard C (2016) Reminisce as activity and therapy. https://www.verywell.com/reminiscence-as-activity-and-therapy-97499. Accessed June 2016

McGraw-Hill (2002) Concise dictionary of modern medicine. http://medical dictionary.thefreedictionary.com/psychosocial+intervention. Accessed 17 June 2016

McLeod (2013) Erik Erikson E-publication by simply psychology. http://www.simplypsychology.org/Erik-Erikson.html. Accessed May 2016

Sutor B, Rummans TA, Smith GE (2001) Assessment and management of behavioral disturbances in nursing home residents with dementia. Mayo Clin Proc 76(5):540–550

Watts S, Moniz-Cook E, Guss R, Middleton J, Bone A, Slade L (2013) Early psychosocial interventions in dementia: a compendium 2013. www.dementiaaction.org.uk/assets/0000/5804/BPS_FPOP_DAA. Accessed 6 June 2016

Wolitzky DL (1995) The theory and practice of traditional psychoanalytic psychotherapy. In: Gurman AS, Messer SB (eds) Essential psychotherapies: theory and practice. The Guildford Press, New York, pp 12–54

Martin Smalbrugge, Sandra A. Zwijsen,
Raymond C.T.M. Koopmans, and Debby L. Gerritsen

Abstract

Challenging behavior is highly prevalent in nursing home residents with dementia. For many of the residents, the challenging behavior was also the main reason of admission to the nursing home. The challenging behavior leads to loss of quality of life and stress and burden for caregivers, both informal and formal. Especially agitation and aggression are a challenge. Managing challenging behavior in residents with dementia asks for a systematic and multidisciplinary approach, focusing on finding and treating the underlying problems. Psychoactive drugs should be used on strict indication; psychosocial interventions are first-choice treatment. In this chapter, professionals are given guidance for a systematic, multidisciplinary, and timely detection, analysis, treatment, and evaluation of challenging behavior in nursing home residents with dementia.

Keywords

Challenging behavior • Dementia • Nursing home • Care program

M. Smalbrugge, MD, PhD (✉) • S.A. Zwijsen
Department of General Practice and Elderly Care Medicine/EMGO+ Institute for Health and Care Research, VU Medical Centre, P.O. Box 7057, 1007 MB, Amsterdam, The Netherlands
e-mail: m.smalbrugge@vumc.nl

R.C.T.M. Koopmans • D.L. Gerritsen
Department of Primary and Community Care, Centre for Family Medicine, Geriatric Care and Public Health, Radboud University Medical Centre, Nijmegen, The Netherlands

© Springer International Publishing AG 2017

55

S. Schüssler, C. Lohrmann (eds.), *Dementia in Nursing Homes*,
DOI 10.1007/978-3-319-49832-4_5

5.1   Introduction

Over the course of the disease, the behavior of people with dementia changes. Over 90% of people with dementia show behavior that is challenging to themselves and/ or the people surrounding them (Brodaty et al. 2015; Borsje et al. 2015). Eventually, this challenging behavior often is a reason for admittance to a nursing home. Not surprisingly, the prevalence of challenging behavior in nursing home units for people with dementia is high, up to 80% (Selbaek et al. 2013).

Challenging behavior is associated with a diminished quality of life of people with dementia and higher burden for both care staff and family members (Van de Ven- Vakhteeva et al. 2012; Zwijsen et al. 2012; Ornstein and Gaugler 2012). For family members, apathetic behavior is the most burdensome as it seriously affects the relationship between the persons with dementia and their relatives (Covinsky et al. 2003; De Vugt et al. 2003). For care staff, agitation is the most distressing form of challenging behavior (Zwijsen et al. 2012).

Guidelines emphasize the use of psychosocial interventions as a first-order treatment. Although there seems to be a trend toward diminishing the use of psychoactive drugs, the odds of being prescribed such medication for people with dementia and challenging behavior are high (Gustafsson et al. 2016; Maust et al. 2016). These drugs have serious side effects, and in a report of Banjaree (2009), it is estimated that the use of psychoactive drugs adds 1800 deaths of people with dementia in Britain per year. Experts agree that psychoactive medication should be a last resort option, but many practitioners struggle to find another way to approach challenging behavior.

In the treatment of challenging behavior, it is very important to acknowledge that behavior is a symptom of underlying problems. The key to improving the approach to challenging behavior and to diminishing the use of psychoactive drugs is therefore to find and treat the underlying problems.

This asks for a systematical approach, in which multiple disciplines, and also informal caregivers, are involved. This chapter gives guidance to professionals in the process of timely detection, analysis, and treatment of challenging behavior in dementia.

5.2   Getting Grips on Challenging Behavior

5.2.1   Definition

To be able to come to grips with challenging behavior, a clear description and definition of behavior is needed. In the glossary of psychological terms of the American Psychological Association, behavior is defined as "The actions by which an organism adjusts to its environment." This definition has several implications. First, behavior is a reaction to something, an internal or external stimulus. Secondly, behavior is in some way meaningful; a person is coping with a situation (although this can be a subconscious process). Finally, behavior does not exist in a vacuum, but it is dependent on the environment.

> **Definition of Challenging Behavior**
> Behavior is considered challenging, when this meaningful reaction leads to distress or direct harm for the person with dementia or for persons living with or caring for him or her.

Following the definition above, behavior, and challenging behavior in particular, is much more than it seems at first sight. When aiming to understand and treat behavior that is challenging, it is therefore important to work methodically and multidisciplinary (NICE 2006; IPA 2002).

5.2.2 Detection

The first step in a good approach to challenging behavior in dementia is a timely detection of behavioral changes of residents. Nursing staff is often so overbusy with care tasks that subtle behavioral changes are not noticed. Only when behavior becomes unbearable for the residents and/or staff, a point is made of managing the behavior. This is a pity, for timely detection and treatment might prevent escalation of the behavior. It is therefore important to frequently discuss the behavior of all residents among coworkers. It can be helpful to regularly use detection tools to monitor behavior (Table 5.1).

5.2.3 Analysis

The analysis of challenging behavior starts with a clear description of behavior. For clarity in discussing the behavior among coworkers and other disciplines, it is important to differentiate between observations and interpretations. Interpretations are often personal and colored by our own judgment, experience, and knowledge of a situation. Observations, in contrast, are straightforward and allow others to make their own interpretations of the behavior. Although this seems obvious, it is often hard to give a description that is free of judgment or interpretation. Often, behavior is described as

Table 5.1 Tools that can be helpful for monitoring behavior

Detection tools	Description
Neuropsychiatric inventory (NPI)	A questionnaire on 12 neuropsychiatric symptoms that can either be administered by interview (NPI-NH) or by filling in a score sheet (NPI-Q)
Behavioral symptoms in Alzheimer's disease (Behave-AD)	Clinical rating scale on six behavioral symptoms, administered by interview
Resident assessment instrument (RAI)	A structural assessment on various domains of nursing home care, used for care planning
Cohen-Mansfield agitation inventory (CMAI)	A questionnaire containing 29 items on agitated behavior that can be scored on a 7-point Likert scale

"anxious" or "angry," while the actual observation is "rapid breathing" or "raising her voice." It is helpful to use the mnemonic: "I see ….[observation] and therefore I think …[interpretation]. For example, "I see mrs. X pacing up and down the corridor and asking bystanders passers-by in a high pitched voice 'where am I? Help me!', therefore I think she is anxious and disoriented." A clear description of the behavior also contains information about the place, time, duration, and environment during the behavior. All this information facilitates the analysis of the behavior.

After having made a clear description of the behavior, it is time to start the analysis. There are several explanatory models for behavior, which overlap and do not exclude one another. When analyzing behavior, it is helpful to keep the explanatory models in mind.

5.2.3.1 Unmet Needs

When dementia progresses, communication becomes increasingly difficult. The ability to translate thoughts and needs to meaningful language deteriorates, for example, because of word finding problems. Also, people may have difficulty to translate their feelings and bodily sensations (e.g., hunger or pain) into concrete needs. The unmet needs model (Cohen-Mansfield et al. 2015) states that because of these communication problems and because of a decreased ability to be self-supporting in fulfilling one's own needs, many needs of people with dementia are unmet. Challenging behavior subsequently arises as an outcome of frustration, as a means of fulfilling needs or as a means of communicating needs.

The unmet needs that lead to the challenging behavior may have various causes. In the unmet needs model, needs are categorized as "environmental," "current condition," and "lifelong habits and personality." Environmental needs can refer to physical or psychosocial environment. The physical environment may create an unmet need for a person who wants to wander around, when there is no space to do so. The psychosocial environment can be the interaction with other people, for example, caregivers may create an unmet need when a person with dementia wants to be independent and autonomous while all tasks are taken over by nursing staff. The current physical or mental condition of a person with dementia may create an unmet need, for example, pain that arises when he or she is unable to communicate pain. Lastly, lifelong habits and personality may not attune with the current way that one's life is arranged, which can result in an unmet need (Cohen-Mansfield et al. 2015).

When a person exhibits challenging behavior, it is therefore very important to make an objective description and to analyze which needs this person may have and which of those needs may be unmet. Together with disciplines like a physician, dietician, and/or occupational therapist, nursing staff can examine physical needs such as the possibility of a person being hungry, in pain, or sitting uncomfortably. The psychologist may help with analyzing psychological and psychosocial needs. It can be helpful to use the Camberwell Assessment of Needs for the Elderly (CANE) to structure the process of analyzing unmet needs (Cohen-Mansfield et al. 2015).

5.2.3.2 Progressively Lowered Stress Threshold

The progressively lowered stress threshold (PLST) model (Hall and Buckwalter 1987; Smith et al. 2004) starts with the assumption that every person had a threshold for the amount of stress he can cope with before he becomes upset. This threshold is more or less stable once it is set in adulthood, although it can be temporarily lowered by circumstances such as feeling ill or going through a major life event. The basic principle of the PLST model is that due to brain damage, the stress threshold of people with dementia lowers during the disease. Also because of brain damage, people with dementia experience stimulants that are not particularly distressing for healthy people as stressors (e.g., the noise of a television or people walking by), and due to cognitive impairment, many stressful situations arise (e.g., not knowing where you are or not recognizing family or friends). Because of these disadvantages, the chance of a person with dementia to cross the stress threshold and become upset is heightened. The third disadvantage a person with dementia has to deal with is that he or she is often unable to recognize the feeling of crossing the threshold and/or is unable to independently undertake action to lower the stress. The behavior that follows is a result of coping with stress, for example, by shouting out or becoming agitated.

The model helps caregivers in analyzing behavior and adapting the environment so that it becomes less stressful. It also explains the pattern of behavior that is often seen in residential settings. Often, in the afternoon or the early evening, challenging behavior is most apparent. The PLST model might explain this phenomenon, because stressors accumulate during the day while the stress threshold decreases during the day because of the lowered amount of energy most people with dementia have. When a clear behavioral pattern is recognizable throughout the day, it is thus helpful to analyze the amount of stressors and the possibility of adapting the environment and the daily activity plans.

5.2.3.3 Model of Functional Analysis

With functional analysis, factors that cause behavior or that cause behavior to continue are analyzed (Moniz et al. 2012). Usually, the ABC approach is used in which A stands for "antecedent," B for "behavior," and C for "consequences." Antecedents of behavior can be found by observing the situation before the challenging behavior starts. For example, you can observe a person sitting quietly in a chair while nurses are passing by ("A"). In "B," the behavior is described objectively and detailed, for example, "Mr. Smith begins to move in his chair and makes a clicking sound with is tongue. After 2 min, he stands up and calls out 'help help' to the nurses." Finally, the consequences following the behavior are described. Often, immediate and prolonged consequences are described, for the immediate consequences can cause behavior to continue while prolonged consequences are often the reason for consulting a physician or psychologist. An immediate consequence could be that a nurse speaks with Mr. Smith, calms him down, and helps him back into his chair. A prolonged consequence could be that nurses become frustrated, avoid or ignore Mr. Smith. Preferably, the interventions that are drawn up after making a functional analysis aim at the antecedent, for this might prevent the behavior from happening. However, this is not always possible, for example, when encountering a specific fellow resident is an antecedent. Also, an antecedent might also be a consequence, for example, when calling out of one resident (A) leads to another resident shouting back (C) which triggers (A) agitation (B) in the first resident. If, for whatever reason, treating the antecedent is not possible, treatment will focus on diminishing the consequences that cause the behavior to continue.

5.2.3.4 Combining Several Views: The Biopsychosocial Model

The models that are described above do not exclude each other and can be used together when analyzing challenging behavior. The models overlap in that they are based on the principle that challenging behavior is a symptom that something is upsetting the person with dementia. Because the reason why a person with dementia becomes upset can lie on different levels and on different areas of expertise, multi-disciplinary collaboration is crucial for the analysis and treatment of challenging behavior. It is important to combine the analysis of biological factors, psychological factors, and social factors into one biopsychosocial model in which all aspects of the behavior are joined together (Cohen-Mansfield 2000; Zwijsen et al. 2016).

Biological Factors

The physician does a thorough physical examination, medication review, psychiatric examination, and when appropriate further tests: blood testing, cultures, X-ray, etc. Physical problems (infections, pain, constipation), side effects of medication, delirium, and depression are all known to be associated with challenging behavior. These factors should be ruled out as attributing factor or be treated appropriately.

Psychological Factors

The psychologist makes a functional analysis of the behavior to determine what causes the behavior and what causes the behavior to continue. It is possible that the behavior is caused by psychological issues like a mood disorder or a personality disorder. To analyze these causes, the psychologist might do a neuropsychological assessment, an assessment of personality, a hetero anamnestic interview, or an assessment of mood or anxiety issues.

Social Factors

Assessing the social factors contributing to the behavior is also part of a functional analysis. For this, a psychologist or a nurse might observe the person with dementia in different situations and on different locations. In the observation, there is specific attention for the physical environment, the interaction between residents and between nursing staff and resident, and the amount of stimuli present (both auditory, visual, smell and touch).

After the physician, the psychologist, and the nurse make their analysis, they discuss their findings to draw up a hypothesis about the cause of the challenging behavior.

5.3   Treatment

The analysis of the challenging behavior ends with a hypothesis about the cause of the behavior and/or about the factors that lead to the continuation of the behavior. This hypothesis is the starting point for the treatment plan.

Table 5.2 Using a goal attainment scale (GAS)

The GAS can be used in making treatment goals individual while also standardizing the outcome measures of the treatment. When using GAS, at least three treatment goals are established and prioritized. For each goal, the expected outcome is set. After that, possible other outcomes are noted down from "much less than expected" up onto "much better than expected".

Goal 1: restless behavior

Much less than expected = −2 points	Mr. G. does not stop moving and walking around for more than 10 min all day
Less than expected = −1 point	Mr. G. sits down during one of the meals
Expected =0 point	Mr. G. sits down during meals
More than expected =1 point	Mr. G. sits down during meals and for half an hour during the rest of the day
Much more than expected =2 points	Mr. G. does not walk around for over half an hour

The first step of the treatment plan is to establish a treatment goal and to measure the current situation for evaluation purposes. The goal attainment scale can be helpful in clarifying the expected outcome of the treatment (Bouwens et al. 2008) (Table 5.2).

Defining a treatment goal can be done on two levels. The first level stems from the definition of challenging behavior: diminishing the emotional stress and the danger imposed by the behavior on the person with dementia or on persons living with or caring for him or her. The second level focusses on the outcomes of the analysis of factors attributing to the challenging behavior, for example, pain, electrolyte disturbances, depression, and interaction problems between staff and person with dementia.

There are several treatment options from which can be chosen:

5.3.1 Treatment of Physical Factors

Treatment of physical factors attributes to the challenging behavior: infections, pain, constipation, electrolyte disturbances, and side effects of medications. This asks for a physician with expertise in geriatrics. Treatment of these problems may in some cases need referral to a hospital setting, which may not be in accordance with patients' wishes and also may have other negative consequences (more stress, unfamiliar care personnel): this requires communication with the residents' representatives using shared decision-making rules.

5.3.2 Functional Analysis-Based Interventions

The treatment of factors that cause the behavior (antecedent) or cause the behavior to continue (consequences) is part of the functional analysis-based approach (Moniz et al. 2012). Each of the interventions described underneath might be appropriate, as long as they are aimed at the antecedent or consequences that were found in the analysis.

5.3.3   Music Therapy

Music therapy (Chang et al. 2015) can be individual or group based. A therapist examines the personal preferences and the abilities of the person with dementia to determine which musical activities are appropriate. A person might engage in making music him- or herself, or he or she might only listen to music that calms down or cheers up. In individual music therapy, the music and activities are very personalized which can confirm the feeling of personhood and identity. When music therapy is group based, the focus is less on personal preferences and more on interaction with each other and sharing experiences through music.

5.3.4   Training Staff

Communication skills and person-centered care can be improved by educational programs (Spector et al. 2016). There are educational programs for family members and care staff. Psychoeducation on dementia and challenging behavior are often part of such programs. Tools and tips are provided to make care more person centered (e.g., using biographical information in daily care for the resident) and to communicate in a way that is more appropriate for people with dementia (e.g., adapting the speed of communication, using gestures and touch).

5.3.5   Sensory Interventions

Sensory interventions aim at stimulating the senses to bring comfort and reduce restlessness and agitation (Padilla 2011). Some sensory interventions aim at a single sense, such as touch or smell; others are multisensory, such as Snoezelen (Chung et al. 2002). Sensory interventions can be used specifically for people with dementia who have lost their verbal communication skills, for it taps into the senses to make contact and bring comfort.

5.3.6   Pharmacological Interventions for Challenging Behavior[1]

When viewing challenging behavior as a symptom of underlying problems, the first step is always analyzing the possible underlying problems. The first choice of treatment is to treat the underlying problems with the appropriate non-pharmacological interventions (Livingston et al. 2005). However, sometimes, psychoactive

---

[1] The recommendations in this paragraph are based on the NICE guideline Dementia, last revision May 2016 (https://www.nice.org.uk/guidance/cg42/evidence/full-guideline-including-appendices-17-195,023,341).

medications may be part of the treatment. For example, when a person suffers from psychotic symptoms or when all other non-pharmacological options have not yielded satisfactory results.

5.3.6.1 Symptoms of Psychosis (Hallucinations/Delusions); Agitation/Aggression

Residents with dementia and symptoms of psychosis or with agitation/aggression should only be offered pharmacological treatment (antipsychotics or benzodiazepines) in the first instance if they are severely distressed/agitated or there is an immediate risk of harm to the person or others. If distress and/or agitation are less severe, the interventions described in 3.1–3.5 should be used before a pharmacological intervention is considered. The main reason for this is the high risk of serious side effects: death, stroke, decline in cognition, somnolence, falls, and severe extrapyramidal effects. Haloperidol or risperidone can be chosen for residents with Alzheimer's disease, vascular dementia, and mixed dementias with symptoms of psychosis or agitation/aggression. For residents with DLB (dementia with Lewy bodies)/Parkinson's dementia and agitation/aggression, clozapine can be used. Clozapine can also be used when signs of Parkinsonism are present or appear after starting of haloperidol or risperidone in residents with Alzheimer's disease, vascular dementia, and mixed dementias. There is some evidence that sertraline and citalopram can be used as an alternative for antipsychotics for agitation/aggression in residents with Alzheimer's disease, vascular dementia, and mixed dementias and trazodone in residents with DLB.

In case of DLB and *psychotic symptoms*, the use of an acetylcholinesterase inhibitor is recommended as first-choice medication. An acetylcholinesterase inhibitor can further be used as an alternative to antipsychotics for residents with Alzheimer's disease and *agitation/aggression* if a non-pharmacological approach is inappropriate or has been ineffective *and* antipsychotic drugs are inappropriate or have been ineffective.

Haloperidol as well as short-acting benzodiazepines can be used in situations of acute severe agitation/aggression with severe distress and risk of harm. If oral use is impossible, intramuscular use is advised in the lowest dose possible. Careful monitoring of vital signs by nursing staff is necessary in these instances.

Good monitoring of effects and side effects (especially extrapyramidal features) is mandatory, and tapering/stopping of all of the medication described above is recommended after 3 months of use.

5.3.6.2 Depression or Depressive Symptoms

There is no evidence for effect of antidepressants in patients with dementia and depressive symptoms. Even in dementia patients with a comorbid major depressive disorder, the evidence for a positive effect of antidepressants is inconclusive. However, in case of comorbid major depression use of a selective serotonin reuptake inhibitor is recommended, combined with a non-pharmacological approach (see chapter about depression in dementia). Antidepressants with anticholinergic side effects should be avoided. In severe depression, electroconvulsive therapy can be considered.

5.3.6.3 Anxiety or Anxiety Symptoms

There is some evidence for the effectiveness of short-acting benzodiazepines (lorazepam, oxazepam) for anxiety in residents with dementia, only for short-term periods with a maximum of 4 weeks.

For other forms of challenging behavior in residents with dementia such as vocally disruptive behavior, wandering, resistance against care, and sexual inappropriate behavior, there is no evidence for effectiveness of psychotropic drugs.

5.4   Evaluation

Each treatment plan should include an evaluation date. During this evaluation, it is determined whether or not all treatment was performed as planned and whether or not the treatment goal is achieved (which can be determined by remeasuring the situation or using the goal attainment scale). After evaluation, it can be decided whether the treatment was effective, reanalysis is needed, and/or treatment should be continued.

5.5   Requirements to Get Grips on Challenging Behavior in the NH

This chapter has been about the importance of analyzing challenging behavior and about possible interventions. There are certain requirements for being able to manage challenging behavior in the way that is described in this chapter.

When analyzing the possible causes of challenging behavior or when aiming to adapt care to personal preferences of a resident, biographical knowledge of the resident is essential. Therefore, it is very helpful to note down the life course and personal history of a resident upon admittance to a nursing home, and it may even prevent some challenging behaviors. Also, it is very important that the professionals who provide care and treatment to people with dementia have been properly educated in observing and analyzing behavior of people with dementia. A physician specialized in older people with dementia and a (geronto)psychologist should ideally be part of the care team, but should at a minimum be available for consultation on a regular basis. Time and planning should allow for frequent multidisciplinary deliberation. For appropriate use of psychoactive medication, a pharmacist should be involved, and medication reviews should be part of usual care. For these requirements to be fulfilled, the management of a residential care facility must be aware of the importance of a thorough structured and multidisciplinary approach of challenging behavior in dementia.

Conclusion

Challenging behavior is highly prevalent in nursing home residents with dementia. It has a negative impact on the quality of life of the resident and may cause considerable stress and even harm to informal and formal caregivers and other residents. In most residents multiple factors contribute to the challenging behavior, and therefore a systematic and multidisciplinary approach using a biopsychosocial framework is needed to come to grips with this behavior. Treatment has to be focused on the detected underlying problems. Psychotropic drugs should be used cautiously in a restricted way and always in combination with non-pharmacological treatment options. Capstone of this systematic approach is evaluation of provided treatment and adjustment of treatment when treatment goals are not reached. For (medical) directors of long-term care facilities for persons with dementia, it is important to realize the basic requirements that enable the use of a systematic and multidisciplinary approach to challenging behavior in residents with dementia.

References

Banjaree S (2009) The use of antipsychotic medication for people with dementia: time for action. Minister of State for Care Services, Report

Borsje P, Wetzels RB, Lucassen PL, Pot AM, Koopmans RT (2015) The course of neuropsychiatric symptoms in community-dwelling patients with dementia: a systematic review. Int Psychogeriatr 27:385–405

Bouwens SF, van Heugten CM, Verhey FR (2008) Review of goal attainment scaling as a useful outcome measure in psychogeriatric patients with cognitive disorders. Dement Geriatr Cogn Disord 26:528–540

Brodaty H, Connors MH, Xu J, Woodward M, Ames D (2015) The course of neuropsychiatric symptoms in dementia: a 3-year longitudinal study. J Am Med Dir Assoc 16:380–387

Chang YS, Chu H, Yang CY, Tsai JC, Chung MH, Liao YM et al (2015) The efficacy of music therapy for people with dementia: a meta-analysis of randomised controlled trials. J Clin Nurs 24:3425–3440

Chung JC, Lai CK, Chung PM, French HP (2002) Snoezelen for dementia. Cochrane Database Syst Rev:CD003152

Cohen-Mansfield J (2000) Heterogeneity in dementia: challenges and opportunities. Alzheimer Dis Assoc Disord 14:60–63

Cohen-Mansfield J, Dakheel-Ali M, Marx MS, Thein K, Regier NG (2015) Which unmet needs contribute to behavior problems in persons with advanced dementia? Psychiatry Res 228:59–64

Covinsky KE, Newcomer R, Fox P, Wood J, Sands L, Dane K et al (2003) Patient and caregiver characteristics associated with depression in caregivers of patients with dementia. J Gen Intern Med 18:1006–1014

De Vugt ME, Stevens F, Aalten P, Lousberg R, Jaspers N, Winkens I et al (2003) Behavioural disturbances in dementia patients and quality of the marital relationship. Int J Geriatr Psychiatry 18:149–154

Gustafsson M, Isaksson U, Karlsson S, Sandman PO, Lovheim H (2016) Behavioral and psychological symptoms and psychotropic drugs among people with cognitive impairment in nursing homes in 2007 and 2013. Eur J Clin Pharmacol. doi:10.1007/s00228-016-2058-5

Hall GR, Buckwalter KC (1987) Progressively lowered stress threshold: a conceptual model for care of adults with Alzheimer's disease. Arch Psychiatr Nurs 1:399–406

IPA (2002) Behavioral and psychological symptoms of dementia (BPSD) educational pack. The International Psychogeriatric Association (IPA), Belgium, Report

Livingston G, Johnston K, Katona C, Paton J, Lyketsos CG (2005) Systematic review of psychological approaches to the management of neuropsychiatric symptoms of dementia. Am J Psychiatry 162:1996–2021

Maust DT, Langa KM, Blow FC, Kales HC (2016) Psychotropic use and associated neuropsychiatric symptoms among patients with dementia in the USA. Int J Geriatr Psychiatry. doi:10.1002/gps.4452

Moniz Cook ED, Swift K, James I, Malouf R, De VM, Verhey F (2012) Functional analysis-based interventions for challenging behaviour in dementia. Cochrane Database Syst Rev (15):CD006929

NICE (2006) Dementia. Supporting people with dementia and their carers in health and social care. National Institute for Health and Clinical Excellence, London, Report

Ornstein K, Gaugler JE (2012) The problem with "problem behaviors": a systematic review of the association between individual patient behavioral and psychological symptoms and caregiver depression and burden within the dementia patient-caregiver dyad. Int Psychogeriatr 24:1536–1552

Padilla R (2011) Effectiveness of environment-based interventions for people with Alzheimer's disease and related dementias. Am J Occup Ther 65:514–522

Selbaek G, Engedal K, Bergh S (2013) The prevalence and course of neuropsychiatric symptoms in nursing home patients with dementia: a systematic review. J Am Med Dir Assoc 14:161–169

Smith M, Gerdner LA, Hall GR, Buckwalter KC (2004) History, development, and future of the progressively lowered stress threshold: a conceptual model for dementia care. J Am Geriatr Soc 52:1755–1760

Spector A, Revolta C, Orrell M (2016) The impact of staff training on staff outcomes in dementia care: a systematic review. Int J Geriatr Psychiatry. doi:10.1002/gps.4488

Van de Ven- Vakhteeva J, Bor H, Wetzels RB, Koopmans RT, Zuidema SU (2012) The impact of antipsychotics and neuropsychiatric symptoms on the quality of life of people with dementia living in nursing homes. Int J Geriatr Psychiatry 8:530–538

Zwijsen SA, Kabboord A, Eefsting JA, Hertogh CM, Pot AM, Gerritsen DL et al (2012) Nurses in distress? An explorative study into the relation between distress and individual neuropsychiatric symptoms of people with dementia in nursing homes. Int J Geriatr Psychiatry 29:384–391

Zwijsen SA, van der Ploeg E, Hertogh CM (2016) Understanding the world of dementia. How do people with dementia experience the world? Int Psychogeriatr 28:1067–1077

Inclusion and Support of Family Members in Nursing Homes

6

Hilde Verbeek

Abstract

The involvement of family members in nursing homes is vital for the well-being of people with dementia residing in nursing homes. They can contribute to maintaining a sense of personhood, assist with care, and are advocates for people with dementia. Despite this wide acknowledgement of the importance of family participation in nursing homes, barriers to the implementation of participatory family care have been identified. This chapter describes common dilemmas in care practice in establishing collaboration and partnership between staff and family in nursing homes. Important barriers relate to attitude and role conflict, communication, and the organization. Furthermore, promising interventions (such as the Partner in Caregiving program) and new care models aimed at small-scale, homelike care environments are presented in building partnerships.

Keywords

Family caregiving • Dementia

6.1 Family Involvement in Nursing Homes

Family caregivers are of great importance in nursing homes, especially for people with dementia. Nowadays, person-centered models of care are prominent in dementia care and emphasize strengthening residents' autonomy and overall well-being (Verbeek et al. 2009). Older people should be enabled to continue their lifestyle as

H. Verbeek, PhD
Department of Health Services Research, Maastricht University, Maastricht, The Netherlands
e-mail: h.verbeek@maastrichtuniversity.nl

© Springer International Publishing AG 2017   67
S. Schüssler, C. Lohrmann (eds.), *Dementia in Nursing Homes*,
DOI 10.1007/978-3-319-49832-4_6

before admission to a nursing home. Program design should ensure that residents are known as people. Family caregivers play an important role to establish this, for example, by providing the historical background for residents, make care decisions, provide personal and social care, and are advocates for people with dementia (Port et al. 2005). Family members aim to maintain a sense of personhood for people with dementia residing in nursing homes, as it is important for family that their loved one is treated as an individual (Sandberg et al. 2001; Bramble et al. 2009). Literature shows that family caregivers remain involved in the lives of their loved ones following admission into nursing homes (Gaugler 2005). This evidence is important to battle against the myth that families abandon their relatives in nursing homes (Rowles et al. 1996). The decision to admit people with dementia into a nursing home is very emotional for family caregivers and triggers feelings of guilt and loss and most relatives want to stay actively involved in the care process (Tornatore and Grant 2004). Family caregivers feel continuing the responsibility for care often after admission, although they are relieved from their round-the-clock care at home (Ross et al. 2001).

Family involvement in long-term care is a multidimensional construct and consists of aspects such as visiting, advocacy, monitoring, and providing socioemotional, instrumental, and personal care (Gaugler 2005). Looking at more quantitative aspects of family involvement, previous studies have investigated the visiting frequency, duration, and type of care tasks family members conduct. A European study showed that family caregivers visited overall approximately 3–4 times a week, with an average duration of over 100 min (Bleijlevens et al. 2015). There were, however, large differences between countries. In northern countries such as Estonia, Finland, and Sweden, visits were less frequent (around 2 times a week), while in other countries such as Spain, visits were more frequent, up to 5 or 6 days a week (Bleijlevens et al. 2015). Other studies suggest that on average, family caregivers visit and/or provide care between 4 and 9 h per week (Gaugler et al. 2004; Port et al. 2005). Tasks that family caregivers conduct include a wide range of personal, instrumental, and socio-emotional tasks, such as grooming, clipping fingernails, doing laundry, shop for the resident, writing letters, maintaining the apartment, and dealing with family guilt feelings (Gaugler 2005). Furthermore, family members felt responsible for new dimensions of assistance not originally engaged in the community, such as promoting family understanding of nursing home policies, initiating actions to ensure good staff/family relations (Gaugler 2005) as well as supervision and monitoring of quality of care (Moss et al. 1993; Max et al. 1995), representing and maintaining residents' continuity and connectivity with other family members and friends (Bern-Klug and Thompson 2008). However, a considerable amount of role ambiguity can be apparent, as staff felt that a particular task was the responsibility of the nursing home, whereas families felt that certain care tasks remained their responsibility (Gaugler 2005). Family members themselves stress the importance that preserving the identity of their relative could only be accomplished through collaborative efforts with staff (Gaugler 2005). They often perceive effective involvement as being a teaching resource to nursing staff, so that staff members would deliver sensitive, person-centered individualized care to the person with dementia living in the nursing home.

The building of a partnership between families and staff is increasingly advocated as a means to ensure high-quality care in nursing homes (Penning and Keating 2000). To enhance the feeling of belonging and dignity for people with dementia, a collaboration between family and nursing home staff should be established. For realizing person-centered care and continuation of own lifestyle for people with dementia living in a nursing home, family should be seen as partners in the care for residents instead of visitors (Holmgren et al. 2013). Goals should include family members of people with dementia in nursing homes as this is important to support residents and also to support family members. Previous research indicates that when nursing staff members become more involved with family caregivers and keep open lines of communication, family caregivers' satisfaction increases, which improves their feeling of confidence that their loved one is well being cared for (Volicer et al. 2008; Piechniczek-Buczek et al. 2007). Family-perceived involvement was significantly and positively correlated with satisfaction and impressions of the facility (Irving 2015). Elements considered as most important by family members were the feeling that residents were well cared for, having trust in the staff of the nursing home and being informed about changes in the residents' care plan.

6.2   Dilemmas in Care Practice

Realizing a partnership in every day care practice can be challenging, as both family caregivers and staff experience barriers. When people with dementia move into a nursing home, they and their family have to adjust and follow nursing home rules and routines (Bauer and Nay 2003). Family members often feel guilty over the decision to place their loved one into a nursing home. During the transition, they express a high need for information about the transition and would like to be recognized as an expert in knowing the loved one (Afram et al. 2015; Abrahamson et al. 2009; Chen et al. 2007; Givens et al. 2012). Staff members discover that the new resident brings family members who both expect continued involvement in care and need information and attention (Hertzberg et al. 2001). Staff-family relationships evolve in a social and physical environment that is familiar to staff, but is foreign to family members, who find themselves in a strange place with new roles to play and complex rules to interpret (Utley-Smith et al. 2009). Establishing and maintaining an effective staff-family relationship can be challenging for both parties. Four main barriers can be identified that hinder collaboration between staff and family: attitude and role conflict, communication, knowledge, and organization.

6.2.1   Attitude and Role Conflict

Although nursing staff recognizes the importance of family members as a helpful resource in getting to know the resident and providing care, they often prefer completing their tasks without their help (Wilson et al. 2009). In this way, the nursing homes' routines and rules are assured. Furthermore, nursing staff may also perceive working and interacting with family members as difficult and challenging (Haesler et al. 2010). They expect family to fit in their work routines, which may cause friction (Bauer and Nay 2003). In order to achieve person-centered care through better collaboration with family caregivers, nursing staff need to recognize that family participation is of major importance and can add value. Moreover, the translation of this perception into clinical practice seems challenging but crucial in the establishment of a good relationship (Bauer and Nay 2003; Haesler et al. 2010).

From the opinion of staff, family members sometimes hold distorted expectations toward the care nursing homes should provide, and these expectations are often conflicting with those of staff (Holmgren et al. 2013). For example, staff and family may have dissimilar thoughts about how care should be provided and the available amount of time for personal attention for their loved one (Haesler et al. 2010; Majerovitz et al. 2009; Utley-Smith et al. 2009). These family members can be described as demanding, challenging or selfish, as they fail to realize that finite resources in a nursing home must be allocated fairly among residents and relatives.

An important factor contributing is the difference in role perception. Nursing staff often regard themselves as the experts in care for people with dementia as they have the professional skills. Family caregivers may feel marginalized by nursing staff, who traditionally perceive the nursing home arena as their professional territory (Holmgren et al. 2013). It was found that nursing staff characterize a good relationship with family members by the readiness of family caregivers to rely on the expert role of staff and to relinquish the responsibility of care (Kellett 2000). Families are expected to value staff's caring efforts. This may cause tension, as at the same time family caregivers envision a certain role for themselves within the nursing home. The sense of losing the caregiver role for family members when relocating a loved one into a nursing home may cause difficulties with staff, especially since most family has provided care at home for a long time. There appears to be a barrier between the preferred role family wants to fulfill and the role they actually fulfill. Disagreement on responsibilities between formal and family caregivers can either cause gaps in patient care or duplication of tasks (Haesler et al. 2007; Ward-Griffin and McKeever 2000) and leads to a general feeling of dissatisfaction in the resident's care. On the other hand, conflict could also be caused by nursing staff trying to meet family's expectations and not succeeding in this (Utley-Smith et al. 2009). Therefore it is extremely important for both formal and family caregivers to determine role division and responsibilities from the onset of placement and to appreciate and see each other as equals in the care for nursing home residents (Corazzini et al. 2015; Haesler et al. 2007)

6.2.2 Communication

Good communication between family caregivers and nursing staff is vital for a partnership in care. It can increase satisfaction and family involvement and reduce complaints (Majerovitz et al. 2009). Sharing personal interests, work, and hobbies between nursing staff and family contributed to a trustful relationship (Haesler et al. 2007). Having a trustful relationship between family caregivers and staff can encourage family to visit and remain involved in the care for residents with dementia. Furthermore, emotional support to residents and family can encourage communication between staff and family (Majerovitz et al. 2009). It is important that communication focuses on the psychological and social needs of the resident and family members, as well as the focus on medical treatment.

Perspectives of family and staff may differ. Families would like to receive better orientation to the nursing home along with guidance and information during the placement procedure. Furthermore, families value clear, complete, and timely information on the resident's condition and treatment. Finally, mutual respect and approaching family in a sensitive manner are highly appreciated by families (Majerovitz et al. 2009). Utley-Smith et al. (2009) highlight several benefits of promoting integration of the family, such as improved information exchange, increased trust, mutual understanding of expectations and goals, decreased dissonance in family-staff relationships, and ultimately improved care results for residents. Family members would potentially have more current information, hold more realistic care expectations, be engaged in productive dialogue with staff members, and have fewer formal complaints when connections are increased and exchange of information would be improved.

Nursing home staff, on the other hand, also value good communication with family caregivers because in many cases the family knows what the resident wants and needs and also expects (Majerovitz et al. 2009). For staff members, improved connections and communication could also be beneficial. Staff may gain valuable family input into care planning, feel appreciated and have more positive encounters with the family, have less time taken away from clinical work, and experience fewer state and regulatory interventions (Utley-Smith et al. 2009). However, family members feel (partly) responsible for the care of the resident and thus want to maintain a level of control over the care. Staff members, on the other hand, experience role conflict in their attempt to manage the often incompatible expectations of employers and family members (Abrahamson et al. 2009). Furthermore, nursing staff feel that family members complain quickly but seldom offer praise for their work and that family does not always recognize their intimate knowledge of the resident (Majerovitz et al. 2009).

Family members perceive a greater sense of safety and security over their loved one when nursing home staff members communicate frequent and timely (Lopez et al. 2013). Communicating about role division is important (Corazzini et al. 2015; Haesler et al. 2007; Majerovitz et al. 2009) and needs to be incorporated from the beginning. Also, mutual respect and letting family know they are doing the right thing in placing their loved one into a nursing home help in establishing good communication. Perceived barriers include a high staff turnover, stress among nursing staff, and irregular work schedules.

Family members of a nursing home resident often find it hard to equally participate in the decision-making process when deciding over treatment, especially in the end of life stage. According to Givens et al. (2012), this is mainly due to the lack of knowledge of the disease trajectory, which makes it hard to engage in decisions regarding treatment. Family caregivers addressed the need for attaining more knowledge regarding the disease in general and the progression. Besides knowledge on the disease, family can also take advantage of constructing the life story of their loved one (Kellett 2007; Kellett et al. 2010). It enables family to get to know their loved one as a whole again, in contrast to seeing their loved one as a person with symptoms of dementia who needs care. Using life stories, constructed by the resident's family, can help nurses letting residents genuinely participate in activities. Setting up a biography opens possibilities and enables staff to really see the patient as a whole within the context of family.

6.2.3 Organization

Organizational barriers are perceived that hinder the building of a partnership between family and nursing staff. The overall care philosophy is of great importance. Nursing homes have tended to reflect a "visitor" philosophy that treats families as outsiders or intruders in the working routines or a "servant" philosophy that dictates the nature of their involvement stating what their tasks are (Caron 1997). A supportive organizational environment, enabling a "client" philosophy that coordinates with family members to meet the needs of the resident, family, and staff, is needed to create a partnership in care.

In practice, a high workload for nursing staff resulting in stress and unclarity about working schedules for family caregivers to know who is working at the unit are seen as barriers (Haesler et al. 2007). Managerial support is necessary to address workloads and staffing issues. Furthermore, the introduction of new care models focusing on collaboration with families is necessary, and providing practical support for staff education is essential to promote constructive family-staff relationships (Majerovitz et al. 2009). Finally, unclarity on rules and regulations may impede involvement of family caregiver in the care process.

6.3 Good Practice Programs Building Partnerships

A few intervention programs have been developed to improve collaboration between family members and staff in nursing homes. The earliest programs were specifically targeted at families only and aimed to improve the quality of the relationship between family and staff (e.g., Peak 2000). Other programs have been developed that provide education and support to both staff and family members.

The Partner in Caregiving program aims to improve communication and collaboration and is designed to intervene not only on the part of family members but also to engage staff and administrators to effectively change facility policies (Pillemer et al. 2003; Robinson et al. 2007). The program consists of two parallel workshops series, one targeted at nursing staff and one targeted at family caregivers. Training is provided on improving communication skills (e.g., active listening, providing constructive feedback, cultural differences), development of skills for conflict resolving, and creating empathy. A dementia-specific version has been developed, building on the same program structure, adding components of understanding behavioral symptoms as well as numerous case studies focused on residents with dementia (Robinson et al. 2007). In a large randomized controlled trial, the program demonstrated positive outcomes. Especially spouses increased their involvement with care and family caregivers experienced improvement in communication and behaviors of staff. Staff reported reduced conflict with families. For residents, agitation decreased and overall the facility implemented more family-focused programs (Robinson et al. 2007).

Family Involvement in Care (FIC) is another dementia-specific program which was designed to negotiate and establish partnerships and cooperative role behaviors between family caregivers and staff (Maas et al. 2004). The FIC program included family orientation and education sessions, as well as the negotiation, formation, and evaluation of written partnership agreements between family and staff. Significant beneficial intervention effects were found primarily on family outcomes, such as improvement of emotional reactions (e.g., less feelings of loss for family), better perceptions of staff relationships, and more positive perceptions of care (Maas et al. 2004). Furthermore, providing physical care and consideration of the relative increased for family members in the FIC (Maas et al. 2000).

A final program is called the Family Matters program, which was designed to help families work with staff and residents to create a role for themselves that would benefit the residents' quality of life and simultaneously improve family-staff relations (Zimmerman et al. 2013). The program encourages families to work with the resident and nursing staff to identify an activity in which they could participate in one or more of four areas: doing things, getting around, looking good, and eating well, aiming to promote the residents' quality of life. These four areas were identified as areas in which families would be willing to be involved. A fifth area of helping the community was later identified for families who could not conceive of a way to improve their resident's quality of life. First results indicate modest effects with merely positive results for nursing staff related to less burnout and more of a sense of working in partnership with families. Staff also perceived that families were more empathic. However, it was suggested that family guilt and sense of conflict increased. Family caregiver burden was indicated to decrease (Zimmerman et al. 2013).

Abovementioned programs all target families and nursing staff in traditional dementia care facilities. However, these nursing homes are often based on a medical model of care, emphasizing illness and treatment of underlying pathology. Usually, rules and routines governing daily life permit little individualization. Nowadays, person-centered models of care are prominent in dementia care and emphasize strengthening residents' autonomy and overall well-being (Verbeek et al. 2012). Older people should be enabled to continue their lifestyle as before admission to a nursing home. Families are therefore an important part of the care process.

The nursing home environment often does not match with these new person-centered therapeutic goals. As a result, new initiatives have been developed worldwide that provide health, social, and nursing care in a small-scale and homelike environment (Verbeek et al. 2009). Radical alterations have been made in comparison with traditional nursing homes, implementing changes in the organizational, physical, and social environment of settings.

One of these small-scale and homelike care concepts is shared housing arrangements (SHA), developed in Germany (e.g., Gräske et al. 2015). The first SHA was established by family caregivers of people with dementia, seeking for alternative concepts of care and support (Fischer et al. 2011). Inclusion of family members is one of the core domains in SHA. Family members are part of the group living in SHA and do not focus only on their own relatives; they also look after other residents in SHA. First results indicate that 45% of the residents receive a weekly visit by their family members (Gräske et al. 2015). The involvement of family members in SHA is common, with estimates of 45% of family members visiting on a weekly basis, but similar compared with other care arrangements. Furthermore, it was found that an active participation of family members in SHA contributed to a better quality of life of residents, especially for the domains of social relationships and social isolation. Interestingly, people with dementia who had a family but who received no visits had a lower quality of life compared with residents without family at all.

Other studies find positive effects of family participation in small-scale, homelike care environments, indicating that family members are more satisfied with care provision compared with traditional nursing homes (Verbeek et al. 2012; de Rooij et al. 2012). Small-scale, homelike care environments may have characteristics that improve family caregiver communication and involvement with nursing staff, such as small caseload, homelike environment, autonomy, and attention for continuation of self-identity for residents. The personal contact with nursing staff and involvement with the everyday care process are important reasons for this (Verbeek et al. 2012). Family members had more contact and were more satisfied with the contact with nursing staff and felt that staff paid more attention to their feelings. Furthermore, nursing staff working in small-scale, homelike care environments showed better listening skills toward the residents (de Rooij et al. 2012).

Conclusion

Family members are of great importance to ensure the well-being of residents with dementia living in nursing homes. The involvement of family caregivers is shaped by changes in their relationship and role, and the process of acceptance and loss is continuously present. In order to create a partnership between family caregivers and nursing staff, interventions are needed that alter the attitude and roles of caregiving, communication, and organizational routines. Changing of the care philosophy is crucial in this process, by focusing on equality, respect, and collaboration between families and nursing staff in order to accomplish high-quality care for people with dementia.

References

Abrahamson K, Suitor J, Pillemer K (2009) Conflict between nursing home staff and residents' families does it increase burnout? J Aging Health 21(6):895–912

Afram B, Verbeek H, Bleijlevens MHC, Hamers JPH (2015) Needs of informal caregivers during transition from home towards institutional care in dementia: a systematic review of qualitative studies. Int Psychogeriatr 27:891–902

Bauer M, Nay R (2003) Family and staff partnerships in long-term care. A review of the literature. J Gerontol Nurs 29:46–53

Bern-Klug M, Thompson S (2008) Responsibilities of family members to nursing home residents: "She's the only mother I got". J Gerontol Nurs 34:43–52

Bleijlevens MHC et al (2015) Changes in caregiver burden and health-related quality of life of informal caregivers of older people with Dementia: evidence from the European RightTimePlaceCare prospective cohort study. J Adv Nurs 71:1378–1391

Bramble M, Moyle W, McAllister M (2009) Seeking connection: family care experiences following long term dementia care placement. J Clin Nurs 18:3118–3125

Caron W (1997) Family systems and nursing home systems: an ecosystemic perspective for the systems practitioner. In: Hargrave T, Hanna S (eds) The aging family: new visions in theory, practice and reality. Brunner/Mazel, New York, pp 235–258

Chen CK, Sabir M, Zimmerman S et al (2007) The importance of family relationships with nursing facility staff for family caregiver burden and depression. J Gerontol B Psychol Sci Soc Sci 62(5):253–260

Corazzini K, Twersky J, White HK et al (2015) Implementing culture change in nursing homes: An adaptive leadership framework. Gerontologist 55:616–627

Fischer T, Worch A, Nordheim J et al (2011) Ambulant betreute Wohngemeinschaften für alte, pflegebedürftige Menschen – Merkmale, Entwicklungen und Einflussfaktoren (Shared-housing arrangements for care-dependent older persons - characteristics, development and drivers). Pflege 23(2):97–109

Gaugler JE (2005) Family Involvement in Residential Long-Term Care: A Synthesis and Critical Review. Aging & Ment Health 9:105–118

Gaugler JE, Anderson KA, Zarit SH, Pearlin LI (2004) Family involvement in nursing homes: Effects on stress and wellbeing. Aging Ment Health. 8:65–75

Givens JL, Lopez RP, Mazor KM, Mitchell SL (2012) Sources of stress for family members of nursing home residents with advanced dementia. Alzheimer Dis Assoc Disord. 26:254–259

Gräske J, Meyer S, Worch A et al (2015) Family visits in shared-housing arrangements for residents with dementia – a cross-sectional study on the impact on residents' quality of life. BMC Geriatr 15:14

Haesler E, Bauer M, Nay R (2007) Staff-family relationships in the care of older people: a report on a systematic review. Res Nurs Health 30(4):385–398

Haesler E, Bauer M, Nay R (2010) Recent evidence on the development and maintenance of constructive stafffamily relationships in the care of older people – a report on a systematic review update. Int J Evidence-based Healthcare 8:45–74

Hertzberg A, Ekman SL, Axellson K (2001) Staff activities and behaviour are the source of many feelings: Relatives' interactions and relationships with staff in nursing homes. Journal of Clinical Nursing 10:380–388

Holmgren J, Emami A, Eriksson LE, Eriksson H (2013) Being perceived as a 'visitor' in the nursing staff's working arena – the involvement of relatives in daily caring activities in nursing homes in an urban community in Sweden. Scand J Caring Sci 27:677–685

Irving J (2015) Beyond family satisfaction: Family-perceived involvement in residential care. Australasian J Ageing 34:166–170

Kellett U (2000) Bound within the limits: facing constraints to family caring in nursing homes. Int J Nurs Pract 6:317–323

Kellett U (2007) Seizing possibilities for positive family caregiving in nursing homes. J Clin Nurs 16:1479–1487

Kellett U, Moyle W, McAllister M, King C, Gallagher F (2010) Life stories and biography: a means of connecting family and staff to people with dementia. J Clin Nurs 19:1707–1715

Lopez RP, Mazor KM, Mitchell SL, Givens JL (2013) What is family-centered care for nursing home residents with advanced dementia? Am J Alzh Dis Other Dementias 28:763–768

Maas ML, Swanson E, Buckwalter KC et al (2000) Nursing interventions for Alzheimer's family role trials: final report (RO1NR01689). University of Iowa, Iowa City

Maas ML, Reed D, Park M et al (2004) Outcomes of family involvement in care intervention for caregivers of individuals with dementia. Nurs Res 53(2):76–86

Majerovitz SD, Mollott RJ, Rudder C (2009) We're on the same side: improving communication between nursing home and family. Health Communication 24:12–20. Social Policy Research Unit, University of York

Max W, Webber P, Fox P (1995) Alzheimer's disease: the unpaid burden of caring. J Aging Health 7:179–199

Moss MS, Lawton MP, Kleban MH et al (1993) Time use of caregivers of impaired elderly before and after institutionalization. J Gerontol 48(3):S102–S111

Peak T (2000) Families and the nursing home environment: adaptation in a group context. J Gerontol Soc Work 33:51–66

Penning MJ, Keating N (2000) Self, informal and formal care: Partnerships in communitybased and residential care settings. Can J Aging 19:75–100

Piechniczek-Buczek J, Riordan ME, Volicer L (2007) Family member perception of quality of their visits with relatives with dementia: a pilot study. J Am Med Dir Assoc 8(3):166–172

Pillemer K, Suitor JJ, Henderson CR et al (2003) A cooperative communication intervention for nursing home staff and family members of residents. Gerontologist 43:96–106

Port CL, Zimmerman S, Williams CS et al (2005) Families filling the gap: Comparing family involvement for assisted living and nursing home residents with dementia. Gerontologist 45:87–95

Robinson J, Curry L, Gruman C, Porter M, Henderson CR, Pillemer K (2007) Partners in caregiving in a special care environment: cooperative communication between staff and families on dementia units. Gerontologist 47:504–515

de Rooij AH, Luijkx KG, Spruytte N et al (2012) Family caregiver perspectives on social relations of elderly residents with dementia in small-scale versus traditional long-term care settings in the Netherlands and Belgium. J Clin Nurs 21(21–22):3106–3116

Ross MM, Carswell A, Dalziel WB (2001) Family caregiving in long-term care facilities. Clin Nurs Res 10:347–363

Rowles GD, Concotelli JA, High DM (1996) Community integration of a rural nursing home. J Appl Gerontol 15:188–201

Sandberg J, Lundh U, Nolan MR (2001) Placing a spouse in a care home: the importance of keeping. J Clin Nurs 10:406–416

Tornatore JB, Grant LA (2004) Family caregiver satisfaction with the nursing home after placement of a relative with dementia. J Gerontol B Psychol Sci Soc Sci 59(2):80–88

Utley-Smith Q, Colón-Emeric CS, Lekan-Ruthledge D et al (2009) The nature of staff-family interactions in nursing homes: staff perceptions. J Aging Stud 23:168–177

Verbeek H, Kane RA, van Rossum E et al (2009) Promoting resilience in small-scale, homelike residential care settings for older people with dementia: experiences from the Netherlands and the United States. In: Resnick B, Gwyther LP, Roberto KA (eds) Resilience in aging: concepts, research and outcomes. Springer, New York, pp 289–304

Verbeek H, Zwakhalen SM, van Rossum E et al (2012) Small-scale, homelike facilities in dementia care: a process evaluation into the experiences of family caregivers and nursing staff. Int J Nurs Stud 49:21–29

Volicer L, DeRuvo L, Hyer K et al (2008) Development of a scale to measure quality of visits with relatives with dementia. J Am Med Dir Assoc 9(5):327–331

Ward-Griffin C, McKeever P (2000) Relationships between nurses and family caregivers: partners in care? Adv Nurs Sci 22:89–103

Wilson CB, Davies S, Nolan M (2009) Developing personal relationships in care homes: realising the contributions of staff, residents and family members. Ageing & Soci 29:1041–1063

Zimmerman S, Cohen LW, Reed D et al (2013) Families matter in long-term care: results of a group-randomized trial. Seniors Housing & Care J 21(1):3–20

Pain in Dementia

7

Sandra M.G. Zwakhalen

Abstract

Pain in dementia is a frequent occurring problem. This chapter provides insight in the challenges and opportunities of assessing and managing pain in older people with dementia. The patient's self-report reflects the older persons' subjective experience of pain the best. However due to the communicative and cognitive problems, the use of self-report is often restricted. Therefore a variety of observational pain assessment tools have been developed to optimize the assessment and registration of pain. The chapter furthermore discusses the use of interventions developed to relieve the pain in older people with dementia.

Keywords

Pain • Tools • Assessment • Management • Behavior

7.1   A Brief Explanation on Pain

Pain is defined by the International Association for the Study of Pain (IASP) as an unpleasant sensory and emotional experience associated with actual or potential tissue damage or described in terms of such damage (International Association for the Study of Pain 1986). McCaffery formulated another frequent used definition; *"Pain is whatever the experiencing person says it is, existing whenever he/she says it does"* (McCaffery and Beebe 1989).

S.M.G. Zwakhalen, PhD, RN
Department of Health Services Research, CAPHRI School for Public Health and Primary Care, Maastricht University, PO BOX 616, 6200 MD Maastricht, The Netherlands
e-mail: S.Zwakhalen@maastrichtuniversity.nl

© Springer International Publishing AG 2017   77
S. Schüssler, C. Lohrmann (eds.), *Dementia in Nursing Homes*,
DOI 10.1007/978-3-319-49832-4_7

By the first definition, it becomes clear that pain is not only physical but also an unpleasant emotional experience of the patient. Moreover, it says that there is no direct tissue damage but that damage can be potential as well. The second definition is very clear on whose authority pain is: the patient. The definition by McCaffery is often used in clinical practice. Unfortunately, some patients are restricted to claim this authority due to the fact that they cannot verbally express their pain by proper words or even won't be able to answer simple yes or no questions (Pasero and McCaffery 2002). This unfortunately accounts for a substantial amount of people with dementia. The cognitive problems they experience together with their functional limitations (e.g., speech impairment) restrict them to express the experienced pain adequately. It is therefore the nurse or other care workers who should be alert to pick up the cues present that may reveal pain.

7.2 Presence of Pain in Dementia

Most studies demonstrate that older people have higher rates of pain prevalence (Elliott et al. 1999).

Prevalence rates of pain in older population are high (Achterberg et al. 2010; Patel et al. 2013; Zwakhalen et al. 2009). A study that estimated prevalence rates of pain in nursing home residents with dementia showed prevalence rates up to 80% (Takai et al. 2010). As the number of persons with dementia continues to rise, all care workers in different care settings will face the same challenge to battle pain in dementia in order to offer excellent patient care and improve the quality of life (QoL) of this vulnerable patient population. It is well known that undertreatment of pain could lead to various additional problems, like cognitive (e.g., concentration problems) and behavioral symptoms (e.g., aggression or depression) at patient level, as well as to greater and heavier demands on caregivers and increased care demands and costs at organization level (AGS Panel on Pharmacological Management of Persistent Pain in Older Persons 2009).

For a long period of time, pain in people with dementia has been a neglected area of research. Patients with dementia have been systematically excluded from scientific research on pain. However in the last decade, a considerable change has occurred resulting in more interest and studies involving older pain patients with and without dementia (Takai et al. 2010; Zwakhalen et al. 2006). Despite this increase of interest, still too many elderly suffer from untreated pain. In older patients this pain is often chronic and persistent over time and affects their daily lives consistently. Chronic pain is defined as pain that occurs for at least 3–6 months (International Association for the Study of Pain 1986). In older adults this pain is often located in the musculoskeletal system causing joint pain (Grimby et al. 1999). The persistence of chronic pain is associated with increased mortality rates (Torrance et al. 2010). Pain can also occur due to a fall or sudden injury. Then, the pain is often acute and may disappear after recovery of the injury usually within 3 months.

7.3 Assessing Pain in Dementia

Illustration of the Problem
"An old man, Mr X. diagnosed with Alzheimer's disease, is agitated. Each morning he starts to resist and fights when nurses assist him getting dressed. At night he is restless and noisy. Nurses think it is the dementia that progresses and decide to restrain the man during night shifts for safety reasons. Eventually it turns out he has a fractured leg, but nobody knew that he had fallen during a walk on his own and experienced pain. Staff wonders how they could have missed the cues on pain displayed by this man."

This case report of an Alzheimer patient suffering as a consequence of inadequate pain diagnosis is one of many reports and reveals just the tip of the iceberg. While it is known that dementia patients without pain are more mobile and autonomous and have a higher QoL (Kalinowski et al. 2015; Kolzsch et al. 2013), too much evidence still reveals that pain is poorly controlled in patients with severe dementia (Achterberg et al. 2013). The main reason for this undertreatment is the underrecognition or misinterpretations of important pain cues by proxies. Often, pain assessment in patients with dementia relies primarily on observing the person's behavior. Although it is one of the main tasks of clinicians and nurses to interpret behavior and respond to the needs of persons with advanced dementia, interpreting these behavioral cues displayed by people with dementia is extremely challenging. However it is the care workers duty to make sure that prompt recognition and treatment is available for all, including people with dementia. Pain should therefore be routinely monitored, assessed, and registered (Gordon et al. 2005). A hierarchy of pain assessment approaches has been recommended by Hadjistavropoulos and colleagues to guide assessment (Hadjistavropoulos et al. 2007) which is in line with (inter)national guidelines on pain in older adults (AGS Panel on Pharmacological Management of Persistent Pain in Older Persons 2009; Royal College of Physicians 2007) (see gray box).

Short Overview Hierarchy of Pain Assessment (Hadjistavropoulos et al. 2007)
- Try to obtain *self-report* of pain from all patients.
- Search for potential causes of pain.
- Observe patient *behaviors*/pain cues.
- Ask proxies (formal and informal caregivers) about behavior changes that may be present due to pain.
- Attempt an analgesic trial and reassess the pain.

7.3.1   Self-Report of Pain

Self-reporting is considered the "gold standard" in pain assessment. Self-report of pain is defined as the ability to indicate presence and/or severity of pain verbally, in writing, or by other means such as finger span, pointing, head movement, or blinking eyes to answer yes or no questions (http://www.geriatricpain.org). Self-report scales can be used to assess and standardize the pain and its intensity. Most scales have been developed for a different setting before being used in older patients with dementia (Herr and Garand 2001). Most often, these scales were developed to assess pain in children. Examples of commonly used self-report scales include the Visual Analogue Scale (VAS) (Huskisson 1974), Verbal Rating Scale (VRS) (Jensen and Karoly 1992), Numeric Rating Scale (NRS) (Farrar et al. 2001), and the Wong-Baker FACES Pain Rating Scale (Wong and Baker 1988). It is often a matter of trial and error to test the scales in older adults. However it is well worth trying since many of the older adults with mild to moderate dementia are able to use one of the scales in a reliable way. Closs and colleagues (2004) tested, for example, five different self-report scales in cognitively impaired older patients (the Verbal Rating Scale, horizontal Numeric Rating Scale, FACES Pictorial Scale, Color Analogue Scale, and mechanical Visual Analogue Scale) and concluded that the verbal rating scale was the most successful with this group. In total 80.5% of the overall sample of cognitively impaired could complete the scale and 36% of those with severe cognitive impairment. Verbal and numeric rating scales are recommended by guidelines on pain for older patients to assess pain intensity. Table 7.1 presents an overview of some most frequently used one-dimensional self-report scales used in older patients with dementia including those who are living in nursing homes. Pain intensity is only one dimension of pain.

Table 7.1 Overview of one-dimensional self-report scales

Name scale	Example of specification of scale	Description of the self-report scale	Recommended in older adults with dementia
Visual Analogue Scale (VAS)	Colored VAS	10 cm line with "no pain" at one anchor and "worst imaginable pain" at the other anchor	No, high failure rates have been reported
Numeric Rating Scale (NRS)	0–10 numeric rating scale	Visual Analogue Scale with numeric ratings presented (0–5 up to 0–20 scale range)	Yes
Verbal Descriptive Scale (VDS)	Pain thermometer (Herr and Mobily 1993)	Scale with verbally labeled boxes	Yes
FACES or Pictorial Pain Scales	FACES Pain Scale (Beiri et al. 1990), Wong-Baker FACES Pain Rating Scale (Wong and Baker 1988)	Scale with expressions of faces representing the feeling of the older person in pain	Yes, however validity and intervals of pictorial scale (items) are questionable

Besides the one-dimensional scales, multidimensional self-reported scales exist that provide a more comprehensive view on pain and include other aspects like pain location. Most well-known multidimensional scales are the McGill Pain Questionnaire (Melzack 1987) and the Brief Pain Inventory (Cleeland and Ryan 1994). Although both are very well known in clinical practice, given the comprehensiveness, the use of both scales is limited in cognitively impaired older people.

7.3.2 Behavioral Assessment of Pain

As the dementia progresses, the ability to self-report decreases (Pesonen et al. 2009), and other methods of pain assessment become necessary. The importance of adequate pain assessment is widely acknowledged and research predominantly focused on the development of behavioral pain assessment tools. Numerous behavioral pain assessment scales have been developed. Over ten reviews have been conducted including over 30 behavioral pain assessment tools for people with dementia (e.g., Herr et al. 2006; Husebo and Corbett 2014; Lichtner et al. 2014; Lobbezoo et al. 2011; Lord 2009; Park et al. 2010; Stolee et al. 2005; van Herk et al. 2007; Zwakhalen et al. 2006). An updated overview of assessment tools to measure pain with older people can be assessed via the City of Hope Pain and Palliative Care Resource Center (http://prc.coh.org/PAIN-NOA.htm). In general all reviews conclude that no single instrument can be recommended for broad use in clinical practice. Several instruments (e.g., PAINAD, MOBID, PACSLAC) show acceptable psychometric qualities. Almost all tools are easy to use but much harder to interpret limiting its clinical usefulness. Therefore it is often a matter of preference and taking the context of the care setting into account when making a choice for a specific scale. Most of the tools have a cutoff score for the presence of pain available, like an onset of pain score. However authors were often unable to determine pain severity scores for the behavioral tools. In itself this is not surprising since people may vary enormously in their expressive behavior. Furthermore it's worth mentioning that most of the tools were developed and tested in nursing home residents who often experience chronic pain. Consequently reliability and validity of the tools in other settings and other pain conditions (e.g., acute pain) are limited. Table 7.2 presents an overview of frequently used observational pain assessment scales for people with dementia. Given the enormous amount of scales available, a selection of tools is presented. Only scales that have been translated in more than one language are included in Table 7.2.

As a result of the research on tool development, it became clear that (1) patients with dementia display heterogeneous and atypical pain behavior (AGS Panel on Pharmacological Management of Persistent Pain in Older Persons 2009), (2) patients with verbal capacity displayed other behavior compared to nonverbal severe dementia patients (Kaasalainen et al. 2013), (3) behaviors associated with pain in this patient population are not unique to pain (e.g., guarding sore area or facial expressions), and (4) less obvious pain cues (e.g., behavioral problems like aggression and agitation) are frequently overlooked (Kaasalainen et al. 2013; Zwakhalen et al. 2007).

Table 7.2 Overview of frequently used observational scales to assess pain in dementia

Scale and developer	Description of the items/ characteristics	Number of items	Scoring method	Languages available
The Abbey Pain Scale (Abbey et al. 2004)	Vocalization; facial expression; change in body language; behavioral change; physiological change; physical change	6	4-point scale Total score ranges from 0 to 18	Original language English Japanese Italian
Checklist of Nonverbal Pain Indicators (Feldt 2000)	Nonverbal vocalizations; facial grimacing or wincing; bracing; rubbing; restlessness; vocal complaints	6	Absent or present Total score range from 0 to 12	Original language English Norwegian
Doloplus-2 (Wary and Doloplus 1999)	Somatic, psychomotor, psychosocial dimensions of pain Represents changes in pain over time	10	4-point scale Total score range from 0 to 30	Original language French Japanese Italian English Portuguese Spanish Dutch Norwegian Chinese
DS-DAT (Hurley and Volicer 2001)	Noisy breathing; negative vocalizations; content facial expression; sad facial expression; frightened facial expression; frown; relaxed body language; tense body language; fidgeting	9	4-point scale Total score range from 0 to 27	Original language English Italian Dutch
Mobilization-Observation-Behavior-Intensity-Dementia (Husebo et al. 2007)	Pain noises; facial expression; defense Modified version MOBID-2 available includes pain behavior related to head, internal organs/skin, and body diagram	3	11-point NRS	Original language Norwegian Dutch English
Non-Communicative Patient's Pain Assessment Instrument (Snow et al. 2004)	Words; pain faces; noises; bracing; rubbing; restlessness	6	Self-report Pain behaviors on a 6-point Likert scale Pain location VDS proxy pain thermometer	Original language English Italian Portuguese

Table 7.2 (continued)

Scale and developer	Description of the items/ characteristics	Number of items	Scoring method	Languages available
The Pain Assessment Scale for Seniors with Severe Dementia (Fuchs-Lacelle and Hadjistavropoulos 2005)	Facial expression; activity/ body movements; social/ personality/mood; physiological/eating/ sleeping/vocal dimensions of pain Modified shortened version PACSLAC 2 is available (Chan et al. 2013) Modified Dutch version PACSLAC-D is available (Zwakhalen et al. 2007)	60 31 24	Absent or present Total score range from 0 to 60 Total score range from 0 to 31 Total score range from 0 to 24	Original language English French Portuguese Japanese Dutch
The Pain Assessment in Advanced Dementia Scale (Warden et al. 2003)	Breathing; negative vocalizations; facial expression; body language; consolability	5	3-point scale Total score ranges from 0 to 10	Original language English German Chinese Spanish Dutch Italian Portuguese

All available pain observation tools make use of facial expressions of pain. These facial pain cues like frowning and grimacing seem very useful for assessing pain in patients with dementia. Utility and reliability of facial expressions to measure pain in dementia have been frequently debated. However more and more evidence shows that these facial expressions are indeed one of the strongest and key cues to determine pain in dementia (Oosterman et al. 2016; Sheu et al. 2011).

7.4   Management of Pain in Older People

Pain assessment is a must for adequate treatment; however, it does not guarantee successful treatment. Pain management includes both pharmacological and non-pharmacological approaches to reduce the amount of pain and improve functioning and the quality of life. Often a combination of pharmacological and non-pharmacological management is combined and individualized to the patient's needs. A variety of non-pharmacological interventions that may be helpful to reduce pain in older people are available. These are often divided into physical and psychosocial intervention. Physical interventions include massage, exercise, positioning, TENS, etc. Psychosocial interventions include comforting approaches like relaxation, music, and distraction. Many of these non-pharmacological management approaches are easy to use by care workers and family. Non-pharmacological interventions may be effective; however, it must be mentioned that evidence about the effectiveness of non-pharmacological management is often limited. Furthermore the effectiveness may depend on the person's abilities and characteristics (age, health condition, etc.).

Evidence about treatment and side effects of pain in dementia is still limited mainly due to the fact that these patients are often excluded from medical trials (McLachlan et al. 2011). Despite this, pharmacological management of pain is very common in daily practice. However, when people with dementia are prescribed with pain medication, usually the dosage is low, and weak analgesics are often prescribed (Corbett et al. 2012). For a long time, studies consistently reported a lower use of analgesics in patients with cognitive impairment compared to patients without cognitive impairment (Morrison and Siu 2000). However lately the opposite, namely, overuse of analgesics, is also reported in a number of Scandinavian studies on pain in patients with dementia (Haasum et al. 2011; Lovheim et al. 2008). This illustrates the difficulty of tailored and adequate treatment of pain. One could state that either underuse or overuse is inappropriate and undesirable.

Age-related changes are likely to influence how drugs are metabolized and absorbed in older people. When planning pharmacological interventions, the impact of these age-related changes such as comorbidities and use of multiple medications must be considered carefully in order to avoid complications and optimize pain treatment. The overall principle therefore in pain management in older people is "Start low, go slow!" This means that, for example, in the case of opioid use in older adults, an initial dose reduction of up to 50% of the recommended dose is warranted (AGS Panel on Pharmacological Management of Persistent Pain in Older Persons 2009). Most guidelines on pain in older adults provide a clear insight in pharmacological pain treatment options.

7.5   Future Directions

Still many actions need to be taken to optimize the assessment and management of pain in people with dementia. The availability of scales is not sufficient to bridge the gap between assessment and treatment. Even the best-designed tool does not solve the problem. Care workers are challenged with main concerns that cannot be solved solely by using an observational tool. A better understanding of conceptual issues of pain in people with dementia is vital to tailor pain assessment. Better understanding of the factors that affect the mode of pain expression is crucial for improved pain assessment and treatment (Kaasalainen et al. 2013). Furthermore, no information is available on the influence of neuropathology of various subtypes of dementia and its severity on pain cues expressed. For now it remains a guess and daily challenge if the patient's stage of dementia and the type of dementia relate to the pain cues on which the pain tools and users (clinicians and nurses) rely. So far the neuropathology of dementia has not played a major part in pain assessment (Scherder et al. 2003). Only a few empirical studies, which were undertaken in pain in relation to etiology, aimed to identify the impact of

Alzheimer's disease (AD) on central nociceptive processes using MRI investigations. These studies resulted in increasing evidence that patients with AD might experience pain differently. But most of all, current scales available lack usefulness and therefore are only rarely used in daily clinical practice. Improvement of this usefulness is essential and needs to be priority number one in the further development of tools.

References

Abbey J, Piller N, De Bellis A, Esterman A, Parker D, Giles L, Lowcay B (2004) The Abbey pain scale: a 1-minute numerical indicator for people with end-stage dementia. Int J Palliat Nurs 10(1):6–13

Achterberg WP, Gambassi G, Finne-Soveri H, Liperoti R, Noro A, Frijters DH, Cherubini A, Dell'aquila G, Ribbe MW (2010) Pain in European long-term care facilities: cross-national study in Finland, Italy and The Netherlands. Pain 148(1):70–74

Achterberg WP, Pieper MJ, van Dalen-Kok AH, de Waal MW, Husebo BS, Lautenbacher S, Kunz M, Scherder EJ, Corbett A (2013) Pain management in patients with dementia. Clin Interv Aging 8:1471–1482

AGS Panel on Pharmacological Management of Persistent Pain in Older Persons (2009) Pharmacological management of persistent pain in older persons. J Am Geriatr Soc 57(8): 1331–1346

Beiri D, Reeve RA, Champion GD, Addicoat L, Ziegler JB (1990) The faces pain scale for the self-assessment if the severity of pain experienced by children: initial validation and preliminary investigation for ration scale properties. Pain 41:139–150

Chan S, Hadjistavropoulos T, Williams J, Lints-Martindale A (2013) Evidence-based development and initial validation of the pain assessment checklist for seniors with limited ability to communicate-II (Pacslac-II). Clin J Pain 30(9):816–824

Cleeland CS, Ryan KM (1994) Pain assessment: global use of the brief pain inventory. Ann Acad Med Signapore 23:129–138

Closs SJ, Barr B, Briggs M, Cash K, Seers K (2004) A comparison of five pain assessment scales for nursing home residents with varying degrees of cognitive impairment. J Pain Symptom Manage 27(3):196–205

Corbett A, Husebo B, Malcangio M, Staniland A, Cohen-Mansfield J, Aarsland D, Ballard C (2012) Assessment and treatment of pain in people with dementia. Nature reviews. Neurology 8(5):264–274

Elliott AM, Smith BH, Penny KI, Smith WC, Chambers WA (1999) The epidemiology of chronic pain in the community. Lancet 354(9186):1248–1252

Farrar JT, Young JP, LaMoreaux L, Werth JL, Poole RM (2001) Clinical importance of changes in chronic pain intensity measured on an 11-point numerical pain rating scale. Pain 94(2):149–158

Feldt KS (2000) The checklist of nonverbal pain indicators (CNPI). Pain Manag Nurs 1(1):13–21

Fuchs-Lacelle S, Hadjistavropoulos H (2005) Inter-rater reliability and additional psychometric information on the pain assessment checklist for seniors with limited ability to communicate (PACSLAC). IASP Press, Seattle.

Geriatric pain. http://www.geriatricpain.org/. Accessed 31 July 2016

Gordon DB, Dahl JL, Miaskowski C, McCarberg B, Todd KH, Paice JA, Lipman AG, Bookbinder M, Sanders SH, Turk DC, Carr DB (2005) American pain society recommendations for improving the quality of acute and cancer pain management: American pain society quality of care task force. Arch Intern Med 165(14):1574–1580

Grimby C, Fastbom J, Forsell Y, Thorslund M, Claesson CB, Winblad B (1999) Musculoskeletal pain and analgesic therapy in a very old population. Arch Gerontol Geriatr 29:29–43

Haasum Y, Fastbom J, Fratiglioni L, Kåreholt I, Johnell K (2011) Pain treatment in elderly persons with and without dementia: a population-based study of institutionalized and home-dwelling elderly. Drugs Aging 28(4):283–293

Hadjistavropoulos T, Herr K, Turk DC, Fine PG, Dworkin RH, Helme R, Jackson K, Parmelee PA, Rudy TE, Beattie BL, Chibnall JT, Craig KD, Ferrell B, Ferrell B, Fillingim RB, Gagliese L, Gallagher R, Gibson SJ, Harrison EL, Katz B, Keefe FJ, Lieber SJ, Lussier D, Schmader KE, Tait RC, Weiner DK, Williams J (2007) An interdisciplinary expert consensus statement on assessment of pain in older persons. Clin J Pain 23(1 Suppl):S1–43

Herr KA, Garand L (2001) Assessment and measurement of pain in older adults. Clin Geriatr Med 17(3):457–478

Herr K, Bjoro K, Decker S (2006) Tools for assessment of pain in nonverbal older adults with dementia: a state-of-the-science review. J Pain Symptom Manage 31(2):170–192

Herr KA, Mobily PR (1993) Comparison of selected pain assessment tools for use with the elderly. Appl Nurs Res 6(1):39–46

Hurley AC, Volicer L (2001) Evaluation of pain in cognitively impaired individuals. J Am Geriatr Soc 49(10):1397–1398

Husebo BS, Corbett A (2014) Dementia: pain management in dementia-the value of proxy measures. Nat Rev Neurol 10:313–314

Husebo BS, Strand LI, Moe-Nilssen R, Husebo SB, Snow AL, Ljunggren AE (2007) Mobilization-observation-behavior-intensity-dementia pain scale (MOBID): development and validation of a nurse-administered pain assessment tool for use in dementia. J Pain Symptom Manage 34(1):67–80

Huskisson EC (1974) Measurement of pain. Lancet 2(7889):1127–1131

International Association for the Study of Pain, subcommittee on Taxonomy (1986) Classification of Chronic pain. Descriptions of chronic pain syndromes and definitions of pain terms. Pain 3:S1–226

Jensen TS, Karoly P (1992) Self-report scales and procedures for assessing pain in adults. In: Turk DC, Melzack R (eds) The handbook of pain assessment. Guildford Press, New York

Kaasalainen S, Akhtar-Danesh N, Hadjistavropoulos T, Zwakhalen S, Verreault R (2013) A comparison between behavioral and verbal report pain assessment tools for use with residents in long term care. Pain Manag Nurs 14(4):e106–e114

Kalinowski S, Budnick A, Kuhnert R, Konner F, Kissel-Kroll A, Kreutz R, Drager D (2015) Nonpharmacologic pain management interventions in German nursing homes: a cluster randomized trial. Pain Manag Nurs 16(4):464–474

Kolzsch M, Konner F, Kalinowski S, Wulff I, Drager D, Kreutz R (2013) Quality and appropriateness of pain medication Instrument for estimation in nursing home residents. Schmerz 27(5):497–505

Lichtner V, Dowding D, Esterhuizen P, Closs SJ, Long AF, Corbett A, Briggs M (2014) Pain assessment for people with dementia: a systematic review of systematic reviews of pain assessment tools. BMC Geriatr 14:138

Lobbezoo F, Weijenberg RA, Scherder EJ (2011) Topical review: orofacial pain in dementia patients. A diagnostic challenge. J Orofac Pain 25(1):6–14

Lord B (2009) Paramedic assessment of pain in the cognitively impaired adult patient. BMC Emerg Med 9:20

Lovheim H, Karlsson S, Gustafson Y (2008) The use of central nervous system drugs and analgesics among very old people with and without dementia. Pharmacoepidemiol Drug Saf 17(9):912–918

McCaffery M, Beebe A (1989) Pain: clinical manual for nursing practice. Mosby Company, St. Louis

McLachlan AJ, Bath S, Naganathan V, Hilmer SN, Le Couteur DG, Gibson SJ, Blyth (2011) Clinical pharmacology of analgesic medicines in older people: impact of frailty and cognitive impairment. Br J Clin Pharmacol 71(3): 351–364

Melzack R (1987) The short form of the McGill pain questionnaire. Pain 30:191–197

Morrison R, Siu AL (2000) A comparison of pain and its treatment in advanced dementia and cognitively intact patients with hip fracture. J Pain Symptom Manage 19(4):240–248

Oosterman JM, Zwakhalen S, Sampson EL, Kunz M (2016) The use of facial expressions for pain assessment purposes in dementia: a narrative review. Neurodegener Dis Manag 6(2):119–131

Park J, Castellanos-Brown K, Belcher J (2010) A review of observational pain scales in nonverbal elderly with cognitive impairments. Res Soc Work Pract 20(6):651–664

Pasero C, McCaffery M (2002) Pain in the critically ill. Am J Nurs 102(1):59–60

Patel KV, Guralnik JM, Dansie EJ, Turk DC (2013) Prevalence and impact of pain among older adults in the United States: findings from the 2011 national health and aging trends study. Pain 154(12):2649–2657

Pesonen A, KauppilaT TP, Sutela A, Niinisto L, Rosenberg PH (2009) Evaluation of easily applicable pain measurement tools for the assessment of pain in demented patients. Acta Anaesthesiol Scand 53(5):657–664

Royal College of Physicians, British Geriatrics Society, British Pain Society (2007) The assessment of pain in older people: national guidelines 2007, British Pain Society

Scherder EJ, Sergeant JA, Swaab DF (2003) Pain processing in dementia and its relation to neuropathology. Lancet Neurol 2(11):677–686

Sheu E, Versloot J, Nader R, Kerr D, Craig KD (2011) Pain in the elderly: validity of facial expression components of observational measures. Clin J Pain 27(7):593–601

Snow AL, Weber JB, O'Malley KJ, Cody M, Beck C, Bruera E, Ashton C, Kunik ME (2004) NOPPAIN: a nursing assistant-administered pain assessment instrument for use in dementia. Dement Geriatr Cogn Disord 17(3):240–246

Stolee P, Esbaugh J, Aylward S, Cathers T, Harvey DP, Hillier LM, Keat N, Feightner JW (2005) Factors associated with the effectiveness of continuing education in long-term care. Gerontologist 45(3):399–409

Takai Y, Yamamoto-Mitani N, Okamoto Y, Koyama K, Honda A (2010) Literature review of pain prevalence among older residents of nursing homes. Pain Manag Nurs 11(4):209–223

Torrance N, Elliott AM, Lee AJ, Smith BH (2010) Severe chronic pain is associated with increased 10 year mortality. A cohort record linkage study. Eur J Pain 14(4):380–386

van Herk R, van Dijk M, Baar FP, Tibboel D, de Wit R (2007) Observation scales for pain assessment in older adults with cognitive impairments or communication difficulties. Nurs Res 56(1):34–43

Warden V, Hurley AC, Volicer L (2003) Development and psychometric evaluation of the Pain Assessment in Advanced Dementia (PAINAD) scale. J Am Med Dir Assoc 4(1):9–15

Wary B, Doloplus C (1999) Doloplus-2, une echelle pour evaluer la douleur. [Doloplus-2, a scale for pain measurement]. Soins Gerontologie 19:25–27

Wong DL, Baker CM (1988) Pain in children: comparison of assessment scales. Pediatr Nurs 14(1):9–17

Zwakhalen SM, Hamers JP, Abu-Saad HH, Berger MP (2006) Pain in elderly people with severe dementia: a systematic review of behavioural pain assessment tools. BMC Geriatr 6:3

Zwakhalen SM, Hamers JP, Berger MP (2007) Improving the clinical usefulness of a behavioural pain scale for older people with dementia. J Adv Nurs 58(5):493–502

Zwakhalen SM, Koopmans RT, Geels PJ, Berger MP, Hamers JP (2009) The prevalence of pain in nursing home residents with dementia measured using an observational pain scale. Eur J Pain 13(1):89–93

Staff Training and Education

8

Eira I. Klich-Heartt

Abstract

Staff training and development in caring for the client with dementia includes organizational development, evaluation of job descriptions, competencies, programs available, as well as whether to develop training programs in a face-to-face or online learning environment. Utilization of adult learning principles to achieve just-in-time training and daily huddles will assist in offering frequent reminders of principles of the formal educational program.

Keywords

Staff development • Competencies • Online learning

8.1 Introduction

Long-term care facilities, like nursing homes and residential facilities, can vary from a small, quite homelike environment to larger organizations. In such facilities often more than 50% of the clients have dementia (Alzheimer's Association 2013; Hoffmann et al. 2014; Lohrmann et al. 2015; Matthews et al. 2013). Therefore, in-depth knowledge about dementia is essential for health-care staff in order to support high-quality dementia-specific care (Schüssler 2015), but often employees come to long-term care

---

Many thanks to Kiran Sahota, Director of Nursing, Parkview Gardens Post Acute Care.

E.I. Klich-Heartt, DNP, CNS, CNL
Santa Rosa Junior College, Santa Rosa, CA, USA

University of San Francisco, San Francisco, CA, USA
e-mail: eklich-heartt@santarosa.edu

© Springer International Publishing AG 2017
S. Schüssler, C. Lohrmann (eds.), *Dementia in Nursing Homes*,
DOI 10.1007/978-3-319-49832-4_8

facilities with minimal training and education in the care of the client with dementia (Gospel 2015). Staff development begins with the organization's mission and values, policies and procedures, identified learning needs, orientation procedures, and then specific training needs identified. Staff development and training are those activities to promote learning and improve outcomes within an organization (Avillion 2008). Training can be provided as face to face or use computer-based training sessions. Staff development is tied more than ever to positive outcomes for clients, staff, and the organization. Employees need information available to them during their work hours, around the clock, and through a wide variety of caregivers in order to achieve those improved care outcomes. Modern techniques of online or computer-based learning can achieve the goals of educating all staff members at varying levels of caregiving in order to achieve cost-effective and efficient trainings.

8.2   Philosophy, Mission, and Values

Staff training and education should uphold the mission, vision, and philosophy of the organizations which they represent. An organization's mission and values help develop the culture and set the tone for how employees interact with each other, clients, and their families (Avillion 2008). Organizational vision and staff development opportunities were important factors in nurses leaving long-term care (Tummers et al. 2013). Success of staff development depends upon administrative support through commitment and involvement in developing ongoing educational programs and processes that support the quality of life for the dementia client. Werezak and Morgan (2003) emphasize the importance of organizational support, philosophy along with having the facilities and resources in order to implement a successful program (see Fig. 8.1). The organizational values

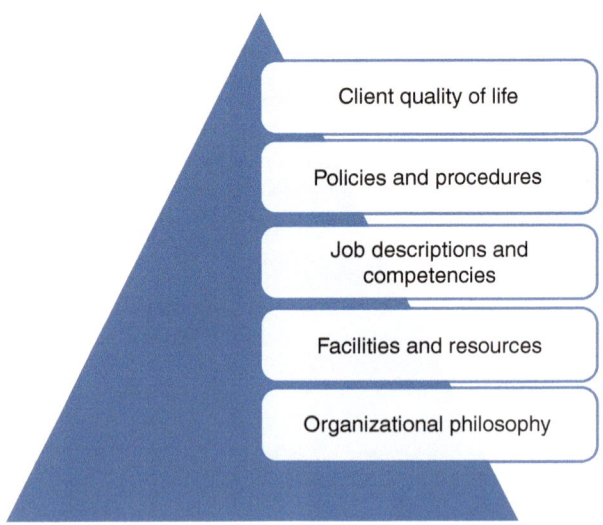

Fig. 8.1 Organizational support for dementia program (Adapted from Werezak and Morgan 2003)

demonstrate the collective beliefs and foundations that a business and their employees are held to. A vision is forward looking as to the future of the organization. It will give the tone of the organization in pulling together to build a united future. A vision statement should be attainable and build trust and support among employees. The mission of a long-term care organization reflects the philosophy, vision, and values of the organization, in particular toward providing care to clients with dementia.

Honoring clients, their values, personality, and preferences are all characteristics that help define how clients will be cared for, with or without dementia. One such philosophy of care, which may be emphasized in the overall organization's mission, is person-centered care (for in-depth knowledge about person-centered care, see Chap. 3 in this book). Person-centered care aims to look specifically at an individual's values and preferences. Therefore it is important for staff members knowing the dementia client's biography and personality. Brooker (2004) describes person-centered care as including valuing patients with dementia, emphasizing a patient's individuality, acknowledging the patient with dementia's individuality, and structuring the environment for optimal well-being. Providing person-centered care for the dementia client involves knowledge of the client as an individual both with the limitation of their dementia and who they were as a patient prior to exhibiting dementia. Such knowledge of the patient's history and past allows for improving communication and connections with the client. Passalaqua and Harwood (2012) describe a series of workshops which demonstrated improved communication techniques among paraprofessionals in caring for dementia clients. Through the organization's mission, values, and philosophy of care, the facility will be able to make decisions to allocate resources for education and training.

8.3   Long-Term Care Facilities and Resources

The majority of the clients living in long-term care facilities, like residential or (skilled) nursing homes, are mainly female and over the age of 80 (Caffrey et al. 2012; Schüssler and Lohrmann 2015; Lohrmann et al. 2015). Over half of the clients had two or more chronic conditions (Caffrey et al. 2012), whereby dementia is one of the most common chronic conditions treated in residential and nursing homes (Caffrey et al. 2012; Fulton 2010). At least four in ten clients needed assistance with three or more activities of daily living (ADL's) (Caffrey et al. 2012).

Long-term care facilities can be either smaller residential care facilities or larger facilities such as a skilled nursing facility or nursing home. The size can be ranging from only four beds (Caffrey et al. 2012; Schüssler et al. 2014) to 400 beds (Schüssler et al. 2014) and more. Taking into consideration the size of a facility may impact the type and kind of training and educational programs which are able to be considered.

In the United States, skilled nursing facilities (size range from 50 to over 200 bed) are licensed by each state and certified by the federal government for receipt of Medicare or Medicaid dollars (Centers for Medicare and Medicaid Services (CMS) 2015).

In 2014 there were around 16,000 skilled nursing homes receiving Medicare/Medicaid dollars, with a slight shift to more for profit agencies and fewer facilities. Three percent of the over-65 population and 9.5% of the over-85 population were listed as permanent residents of skilled nursing facilities, many of these having dementia. In 2015, the CMS developed focused surveys to evaluate, specifically, the provision of dementia care in nursing homes (CMS 2015). These surveys are developed to have metrics to meet in order to provide dementia-specific care. Meeting the survey metrics will help define what is needed to provide optimal care to those residents with dementia as well as provide information to include in the education and training programs. Understanding which type of facility, under which licensure and reimbursement a facility is operating, will help evaluate the type of educational and training programs which can and should be offered to the health-care staff. In addition to understanding the type and licensure under which a facility is operating, evaluating the facility for resources that are available to provide educational and training programs is an ongoing process.

Evaluating facilities for resources available to provide staff development is the responsibility of the administration. An analysis of a facility size, type of licensure, as well as their strengths and weaknesses in providing care for the dementia client is essential in developing education and training programs. Evaluating the facility for time, space for meetings, staff available to free up other staff to attend educational events, and finances available to provide such training becomes a challenge for the leaders of the organization. The size of the organization may determine the size and variety of staffs who are available to both provide the education and attend the training sessions. In smaller residential care facilities, one person may function in the role which in another facility would be covered by several positions. In a smaller facility, the administrator and the human resource staff may be the same individual. Larger organizations have additional concerns with training more staff at varying shifts and through different job descriptions. The organization should evaluate if there is the ability to have a specialist for dementia care available, or if an outside consultant or contract staff resources are available (Warchol 2012; Stein-Parbury et al. 2012).

Education and training of health-care staff can be made available within or outside the long-term care facility, depending on the size and type of organization, and they can be offered face to face or online. A pilot study by Hobday et al. (2010) demonstrated that online education is a cost-efficient and time-saving method for training staff in long-term care facilities. In Sect. 8.11, you can find some resources for online education available for health-care staff working in long-term care.

Whether an education and training program is offered as a face-to-face course or through website technology, organizations would need to review the effectiveness of the educational offerings and ensuring that the educational objectives are being implemented. Having staff available to ensure that the education and training content are applied in the care facility would need to be integrated into the caregiving processes. Evaluating a facility for money, staff, and space to provide education and training programs also entails reviewing and evaluating the facility model of care being implemented to optimize care of the dementia client.

8.4   Models of Care

Several models of care have been developed for clients with dementia. Some models are based upon functional tasks, focusing on supporting activities of daily living, hygiene, and medication management. Kales et al. (2014) utilize a multidisciplinary panel to develop the DICE approach to manage neuropsychiatric behaviors by all caregivers. Newer models of care are focusing more on the individual client and engaging their preferences. Cline (2014) describes in his model that aging is an individual process; however, he makes no reference on how a health-care system, such as a long-term care facility and staff, should interact with an individual. Understanding the individuals' unique aging process, the clients' prior experiences and biography will help collaborating with the client and their family members. In addition to knowing a patient's individual history and biography, other models offer more specific details on how to implement such knowledge of a dementia client.

The capability model of dementia care (CMDC) attempts to provide not only theory of individualized aging but also practical strategies for achieving optimal outcomes (Moyle et al. 2013). Developed by M. Nussbaum, a philosopher and lawyer, the essential ten capabilities are values which are centered on individual human dignity. Moyle et al. (2013) further applied these capability values to enhance the strengths and capabilities of the client with dementia. This focus on the individual is in contrast to the utilitarian care of dementia patient focused on meals and medication administration.

Warchol (2012) describes dementia capable care as facilitating engagement with the client, focusing on abilities the client can achieve, and being able to integrate the client's biography and life story in order to activate the client's long-term memory. Taking a proactive approach to implementing these components has been shown to reduce aggressive behaviors, falls, and weight loss. Konno et al. (2014) also describe implementation of individualized, person-centered care as reducing a client's resistance to care.

A comprehensive model of education for provision of care with the dementia client would include knowing the clients' biography, knowing how to engage the client, focusing on their abilities, and meeting them at their cognitive stages in order to engage them in enjoyable activities. Stinson (2000) offers simple tips for engaging and communicating with the Alzheimer's patient in areas of communication, hygiene, nutrition, elimination, pain control, and comfort. In each of the previous areas, a calm demeanor, gestures and demonstrations, simple language, and limited choices are helpful to engage a client's cooperation. Another person-centered care model is the DementiAbility Method, which focuses on Montessori-based principles to create roles, routines, and activities for the client within a safe and supportive environment (Bourgeois et al. 2015). For this care model, a homelike environment is important, where clients are encouraged to create routines similar to a home environment such as washing dishes, setting tables, or making their bed. The aim is to help people to be as independent as possible and make meaningful contributions to their community. The model includes a strong knowing of the client, creating activities and memory supports to optimize functioning as well as evaluating the clients' preferences and outcomes.

A different model developed by Sheard (2013) uses emotional intelligence to maintain an active engaging environment with dementia clients. His homes are called "Butterfly Care Homes" and allow staff to blend with clients in a way to engage with them in the moment. Staffs eat with clients and are more integrated with the clients. His model focuses on understanding the clients' meanings behind their behaviors and uses positive team relationships in order to deliver personalized care. He emphasizes the lived experience of patients living with dementia and encourages staff to meet clients where they are currently at with their experience and help them develop an emotional connection in order to have a meaningful experience.

All of such models of dementia care emphasize understanding the client with dementia, knowing their prior history, preferences, and values as well as what stage they are currently at. In order to develop education and training materials, an evaluation of staff's current knowledge and performance should be performed.

8.5   Staff Educational Needs Assessment

Staff in a given facility should be assessed as to their knowledge, skills, and attitudes regarding care of the dementia client. Some staff may be hired without any formal training, such as in environmental services. Other challenges include rapid turnover of staff, entailing frequent needs for orientation of new staff with unknown education or training. Evaluating staff upon their hire as to their knowledge, basic training, and experience with dementia-specific clients can help begin the development of an education and training program. All personnel having contact with dementia clients should have a uniform and consistent understanding of their part in providing a therapeutic environment and ensuring positive patient outcomes. Direct patient caregivers may have varying levels of experiences, education, and skills dealing with dementia clients in particular. Evaluating personnel in regard to the existing policies, procedures, and job standards will help develop orientation and ongoing training programs for staff to care for the dementia client.

Job descriptions, policies, and procedures all help develop structure in emphasizing valuing the client with dementia, seeing the client as an individual, and providing person-centered care as well as providing the guidance for the development of the education and training programs. Evaluating such policies, procedures, and job descriptions for evidence of dementia-specific competencies for all staff will ensure that education and training programs meet the needs of the clients. Having clear competencies in place will allow for evaluation of employees to assist in the care of the client with dementia.

In addition to evaluating staff, having knowledge of job descriptions, policies, and procedures regarding care of clients with dementia, having a champion knowledgeable about the best practices in dementia care is essential.

8.6   Coordination of Training for Dementia Care

One person in a leadership position needs to be the coordinator of specific dementia educational learning needs of the employees. This responsibility needs to have the tools and resources to implement learning needs of the organization. This person must be able to understand the needs of the dementia patients as well as best practices for educating staff using adult learning principles. Several programs recommend the use of a care coordinator. The Alzheimer's Society in the United Kingdom has issued a recommendation for developing a dementia champion within facilities to provide support and training and ensure that quality of life is improved for clients (Heath and Sturdy 2009).

In the Healthy Aging Brain Center, the care coordinator is not only in charge of implementing the educational training for caring for clients with dementia but also of ensuring that the plan of care is being implemented. Jeon et al. (2013) mentioned in a study utilizing an educational toolkit that care plans were often not updated, and field notes cited staff mentioning that they did not refer to the care plans when delivering care. A staff specialist in dementia care would be able to ensure that care plans are being implemented and observe teachable moments tying the educational plan to the patients' specific plan of care. Hollister and Chapman 2015 found that in the United States, long-term care facilities receiving government dollars had a wide variety of titles for persons providing such a coordination of care. In some situations the leaders were not nurses but social workers; however, they required a higher level of education or certification specific to providing dementia-specific care.

Another program, the Forget-Me-Not Care Model, uses therapists, either occupational, physical, or speech therapists, as the leaders in providing a cognitive assessment using validated tools in order to develop the care plans for clients with dementia as well as assist with the training of staff in implementing such care. The use of a cognitive assessment and leveling of clients' comprehension and verbal abilities allows for an interdisciplinary model of care which supports the best of staff interaction with clients (Warchol 2004). Activities and programs can be leveled to the clients' ability to maximize their participation in program activities. Direct caregivers are integrated into knowing which level the client is at and may use special approaches during their routine caregiving. Utilizing therapists in such leadership positions allows for a more interdisciplinary approach to understanding the client with dementia as well as allowing clients to function at optimal levels.

Long-term care facilities with dementia clients should have an experienced person in charge of the dementia care program, be knowledgeable regarding dementia-specific competencies, and be able to guide the team into best practices and outcomes.

8.7   Dementia-Specific Competencies

Job descriptions are often the beginning where person-centered care and valuing of the clients' biography are found. Position requirements should define the level of education, licensure, and prerequisites that employees have upon hire. A licensed person has passed a level of examination in the area they are practicing in that demonstrates the necessary knowledge and the ability to work in a defined job role. By itself a license does not assure competence in caring for dementia clients specifically. Certain states are now mandating training for long-term care facilities to ensure initial education and training as well as ongoing trainings to demonstrate competence in caring for dementia clients and their families (CMR 2014). Massachusetts requirements include knowledge about dementia, person-centered care, approaches to caregiving, caregiver strain, working with dementia patients and their families, dietary needs of dementia patients, as well as abuse and neglect of dementia patients. Florida law has also mandated 1 h of dementia training and 3 additional hours of training for direct care staff providing care in long-term care facilities (Florida Administrative Code 58A-4.001). Topics include management of behaviors, activities of daily living assistance, social environment, other activities, environmental issues, family issues, and ethical issues. While each state is mandating required additional training and education regarding dementia care, Williams et al. (2005) describe a process for the development of competencies for nursing staff to accomplish such mandated training. These competencies were directly developed to meet the Florida administrative code, but also leveled for the most common caregivers in all long-term care facilities, that of a licensed practical nurse (LPN) (see Table 8.1). There is the ability to simplify such competencies for certified nursing assistants (CNAs) as well as develop more detailed ones for registered nurses. Competencies are described in terms of knowledge, skills, and attitudes required to care for the dementia patient. In addition, the competencies are addressed as outcomes in relation to a class, as well as being leveled from simple to more complex competencies. Competencies focus on understanding the disease of dementia as well as the ability to facilitate communication and perform in a variety of ways to decrease stress and confrontation for the client with dementia.

Table 8.1 Dementia-specific competency evaluation

Employee name: Evaluator:	M = meets NI = needs improvement DM = does not meet
Competency 1: Understands the characteristics of a dementing illness and the special needs of the person with dementia	

Knowledge, skills, attitudes:
    Defines dementia as decreasing brain function including memory problems, loss of some thinking and communication skills, and changes in personality
    Contrasts dementia with cognitive changes of normal aging and delirium
    Describes the early, middle, and late phases of dementia
    Interprets individual responses, mood, and other feedback as meaningful
    Seeks to create a homelike and comfortable environment
    Seeks a wide range of resources, such as volunteers in daily care
    Uses individual's preferences and social history in daily practice	

Table 8.1 (continued)

Competency 2: Adapts communication to cognitive/emotional needs of the person with dementia	
Knowledge, skills, attitudes: Explains changes in communication skills that occur during progression of dementia Describes the relationship between communication and distress behaviors Demonstrates strategies for effective verbal and nonverbal communication Uses touch to gain person's attention Uses simple sentences Presents one idea at a time Asks one question at a time Avoids negatively worded statements Breaks down tasks Gives simple choices Identifies nonverbal expressions of physical discomfort and pain Demonstrates communication skills and strategies for managing disruptive, aggressive, or other problem behavior Listens and responds to emotional message Uses verbal redirection Uses written and visual cues Allows time to respond Avoids asking "why," arguing, correcting misinformation, confrontation Avoids raising voice Avoids sarcasm with person with dementia Demonstrates desired action Avoids responding to negative language by individual with dementia Uses redirection Reinforces (own) positive (caregiver) self-image using techniques such as positive self-talk Discusses cultural differences in individuals with dementia and how to appropriately adapt communication strategies Includes emotion-focused communication strategies in interactions Gives recognition Expresses positive regard Uses verbal encouragers Explores incomplete expressions of ideas Adopts an attitude of respect for individuality and dignity of the person Uses individual's name in communication Approaches individual in a calm, unhurried manner Avoids confrontation and arguments in communication	

Adapted from Williams et al. (2005)

The Australian state of New South Wales along with the University of Wollongong and the Dementia Collaborative Research Centres has developed online, interdisciplinary competency assessment and training. In addition to direct caregiver training, this online education is for all staff wanting to develop a deeper knowledge and capability in caring for dementia clients using a person-centered approach. Cumming and Traynor (2015) along with associates developed multi-level 40-point levels of competency including the environment, perceptions of dementia, and person-centered care. The main competency areas are *facilitating person-centered and ethical care, working with families/informal carers, understanding living with dementia effectively, communicating, recognizing dementia, assuring diversity and inclusivity, promoting health and well-being, enabling the activities of daily living, implementing therapeutic activities, and promoting a positive environment.* All levels of caregivers should receive orientation and training within each of these levels as they apply to their job descriptions in order to make the best of clients' abilities.

Evaluating the ability to perform such competencies should be done during education and training. As employees evaluate themselves, they would check off their knowledge, skills, and attitudes toward the competencies listed. Such an evaluation would be able to be reviewed with the leader or dementia specialist on an annual basis. Aggregating such staff self-evaluations will assist in further developing a specific continued training program, focused on areas of need or demonstrated need for improvement. The staff educator would be able to then develop educational programs specific to the competencies which are not met.

Using a competency-based approach is helpful for staff during the evaluative process. The validators of the competencies should be staffs who have already demonstrated competency in caring for all elements of the dementia-specific competencies and are trained in how to assess the knowledge, skills, or attitudes of a specific competency. Again, a dementia champion or leader in charge of education and training would be in a position for such evaluation. Competencies should be evaluated with each employee on a yearly basis, with opportunities for further education and development. Certain competencies may be utilized to develop additional training for specific job descriptions or to reinforce particular unit needs.

8.8   Formal Training

Education should follow the competencies which are expected at the completion of a training program. Teri et al. (2005) describe a 2-day modular-based program covering description of dementia, communication, respect, pleasant activities, as well as individualizing care plans. Program training can involve a full-day educational program or be broken up into modules which can be spread out over hour long sessions. Educational programs should focus on changes that can be implemented in the workplace and which are specific to the facility. Kales et al. (2014) describe how an expert panel of multidisciplinary experts developed a four pronged approach for managing and treating neuropsychiatric symptoms. Including all disciplines in educational programs allows for improved evaluation of program effectiveness. Evaluating programs for effectiveness would be done through audits, patient and family satisfaction surveys, employee surveys, as well as investigation of any untoward incidents.

Operationalizing the educational material can be done in a variety of ways. Reminders posted in prominent staff areas help bring home options to remember key

Fig. 8.2 Example of poster for unit – common symptoms of dementia

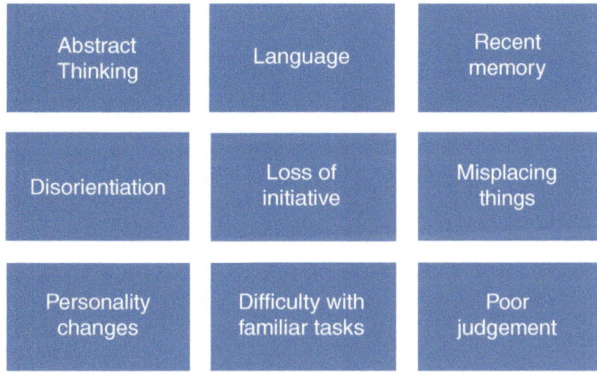

learning activities (see Fig. 8.2). Creating daily huddles can also increase retention of methods which are helpful. A huddle is where staffs come together for a brief 5-minute discussion on topics to remember. The example could be to recall and discuss the common symptoms that certain clients are having which correspond to the module on symptoms of dementia. Gaming activities for use in small bite-sized learning activities can help staff retain concepts. Asking questions in the form of a Jeopardy game can be played quickly and reinforce concepts of communication or barriers to behavior. "Moving a client on to the next activity what is _____ (answer: distraction)?" could be asked of any level caregiver who could identify redirection as appropriate option for a dementia client. Reminders, posters, huddles, and gaming activities are all ways of emphasizing what was taught in formal course content.

8.9 Ongoing Inservice

Continuing education, in addition to the basic education and training, should emphasize and elaborate on development of knowledge, skills, and attitudes related to caring for clients with dementia. Hazelhof et al (2014) describe how ongoing education regarding effective working with challenging behavior can decrease staff stress, improve workplace morale and sustaining improved interventions for patients. Such in-service activities need not be as long as the original course and education. Small inservices could take place during a shift handover, or a shift huddle. Huddles can have flyers or posters developed to remind staff about a specific competency. Posting reminders to staff about specific client abilities is also a helpful way to remind staff how to best engage with clients. Bourgeois et al. (2015) describe knowing a client's cognitive level and matching a caregiver's interaction with the patients' ability. One facility has identified clients by cognitive and developmental levels, as well as integrating the patients' personal interest, history, and tips for care in a color-coded poster for each client's room as reminders to staff on how to engage with clients (see Table 8.2) (Sahota K, 3 June 2016, personal communication).

In addition to huddles and posting specific levels that clients are able to respond to, a unit can use various interactive activities for staff to relate to clients with

Table 8.2 Patient care suggestions

Allen cognitive level	Client strengths	Problems they might have	Tips for care
Red – level 1	Latest stage of dementia Functioning at level of 1–12-month-old infant Look at shiny objects Short attention span Communicate through facial expression Like to be touched, lotion, massage, hair brushed	Usually bedbound May grasp and not let go May bite down and not be able to let go May be incontinent Cannot tell you what they want Will respond if in 12 inches of face	Watch for facial expressions of pain or discomfort; they may not be able to tell you what they need May grasp and not let go, need help releasing their grasp gently May be able to use finger foods – gently help them raise food to their mouth

Adapted from Abilities Care approach, Sahota K, 3 June 2016, personal communication

dementia. Role playing during a staff meeting can be one of those activities. Role playing can be effective in developing empathy and identifying feelings and understanding the clients' reality. In addition to role playing, care workers can be encouraged to attempt to understand behavior from the clients' perspective (Stein-Parbury et al. 2012). Seeing the world through the eyes of a client with dementia can develop empathetic understanding. Role playing activities can also be accomplished by showing small clips of films with patients struggling with memory problems. Asking questions about what is the subject feeling, how are they reacting to a situation, and how would you do this differently are all questions which can allow caregivers, nursing assistants, nurses, or therapists to think out of the box. Other role playing activities could include situations encountered in care. The situation could be replayed at an in-service, with the goal of finding alternate options for responding, asking staff to determine a patient's cognitive level, or level of functioning, and what appropriate responses could be. Another option would be for staff to think of the scenario given to what is behind the scenario, what had the client experienced, and what was their frame of reference or experience which caused certain behaviors. Writing role playing activities should be structured by the education or dementia specialist to achieve certain outcomes, either identifying patients' cognitive level and optional responses or understanding client behaviors.

8.10   Self-Instruction Modules

The decision whether to utilize face-to-face training or online training programs is a decision for every organization to make. Face-to-face classes can develop a positive team spirit; however, getting all staff to one training is expensive and cumbersome. An online program has the advantage of increased flexibility as to when staff can be assigned modules and how long they can have to work on each one. Shift work and replacement of staff for training are overcome with online programs. Barriers to online learning could be the availability of computer terminals available for training purposes or if modules would be expected to be accessed remotely. Hobday et al. (2010) describe an Internet training program for certified nursing assistants caring for dementia clients and found that the online CARES program demonstrated improved knowledge, care competency, and decreased stress regarding caring for dementia clients. Another program from Australia (Traynor 2015) has developed independent training modules which can be purchased and worked on at one's own pace. There are six modules covering the following topics:

1. "What is Dementia"
2. "Recognizing Dementia"
3. "Communication in Dementia Care"
4. "Care Partners and Families across Dementia Care Settings"
5. "Younger Onset Dementia"
6. "Dementia within Culturally and Linguistically Diverse Communities"

Other online learning modules can be accessed either through membership, free, or purchased. The programs available need to have a good fit with the organization's dementia program, job descriptions, and competencies. The overall outcome of online learning would be to improve the care of the clients with dementia, decrease use of psychotropic medications, decrease use of restraints, and improve well-being of dementia clients. The fit of the learning programs available online needs to be matched with the organizational goals.

The development of staff to improve care of clients with dementia includes assessment of the facilities and resources available, evaluation of staff job descriptions and competencies, orientation and ongoing staff training and education, and evaluation of client outcomes. Facilities need to understand what the goals of dementia care would be and develop educational needs to meet those goals. Measurement of such outcome goals would be part of a strong quality improvement and evaluation process.

8.11   Resources

Resources for education and training are available through the Internet. Several resources have been developed by specialty organizations such as the Alzheimer's organizations of various countries, or through government health training centers such as the Oasis Massachusetts Senior Training Program. Below are examples of several sites offering dementia care education. The use of such resources can be utilized in developing staff educational programs.

Internet Resources

Alzheimer's' Association: http://www.hcinteractive.com/ProfessionalCARES?
  GroupID=3
CMS' Hand in Hand Training: http://cms-handinhandtoolkit.info/Downloads.
  aspx
Dementia Care Matters: http://www.dementiacarematters.com/
Dementia Training Study Centers: http://elearning.dtsc.com.au/
Oasis Massachusetts Senior Care Program: http://www.maseniorcarefounda-
  tion.org/OASIS.aspx
NHQCC: http://qio.ipro.org/nursing-homes-hac/qapi/webinar
Nursing Home Toolkit: http://www.nursinghometoolkit.com/
Advancing Excellence in America's Nursing Homes: https://www.nhquality-
  campaign.org/dementiaCare.aspx

Conclusion

Through training and educational programs, long-term care organizations will realize benefits for their facilities and provide further development of all employees. Employees who are able to provide care which demonstrates the organizational mission and values will improve the overall organization's effectiveness. Education and training programs which are aligned with employee job descriptions and competencies which are specific to the client with dementia will improve outcomes for such clients. Developing training programs which emphasize the knowledge of the client will allow all staff to interact with dementia clients in a meaningful way and be able to provide optimal care. Educating staff on best practices, organizations will be able to achieve specialty accreditation and optimal reimbursement. Most importantly active education and training programs allow best practices to be implemented, engage clients in a meaningful way and provide optimal care.

References

Alzheimer's Association (2013) 2013 Alzheimer's disease facts and figures. Alzheimers Dement 9:208–245
Avillion AE (2008) A practical guide to staff development: evidence-based tools and techniques for effective education. HCPro, Marblehead
Bourgeois MS, Brush J, Elliot G, Kelly A (2015) Join the revolution: how montessori for aging and dementia can change long term care culture. Semin Speech Lang 36(3):209–214
Brooker D (2004) What is person-centered care in dementia? Rev Clin Gerontol 13:215–222
Caffrey C, Sengupta M, Park-Lee E et al (2012) Residents living in residential care facilities: United States, 2010, NCHS data brief, no 91. National Center for Health Statistics, Hyattsville
Centers for Medicare and Medicaid Services (CMS) (2015) Nursing home data compendium. https://www.cms.gov/Medicare/Provider-Enrollment-and-Certification/CertificationandComplianc/Downloads/nursinghomedatacompendium_508-2015.pdf. Accessed 10 Apr 2016

Cline DD (2014) A concept analysis of individualized aging. Nurs Educ Perspect 35(3):185–192

Code Mass Regs (2014) Code of Massachusetts Regulations 150–150.029

Cumming A, Traynor V (2015) Dementia care competency framework content: core competencies, domains of practice and levels of practice. http://smah.uow.edu.au/content/groups/public/@web/@smah/@nmih/documents/doc/uow187366.pdf. Accessed 10 Apr 2016.

Florida Administrative Code 58A-4.001.http://www.glrules.org/gateway/reference.asp?no=ref-04001. Accessed 10 Apr 2016

Fulton AT (2010) Nursing home care: an introduction. Med Health RI 93:364

Gospel H (2015) Varieties of qualifications, training, and skills in long-term care: a German, Japanese, and UK comparison. Hum Resour Manage 54(5):833–850. doi:10.1002/hrm.21714

Hazelhof TM, Gerritsen DL, Schoonhoven L, Koopmans RM (2014) "The educating nursing staff effectively (TENSE) study": design of a cluster randomized controlled trial. BMC Nurs 13(1):1–21. doi:10.1186/s12912-014-0046-6

Heath H, Sturdy D (2009) Living well with dementia in a care home: a guide to implementing the national dementia strategy. RCN Publishing Company, Middlesex

Hobday JV, Savik K, Smith S, Gaugler JE (2010) Feasibility of internet training for care staff of residents with dementia. J Gerontol Nurs 36(4):13–21

Hoffmann F, Kaduszkiewicz H, Glaeske G, van den Bussche H, Koller D (2014) Prevalence of dementia in nursing home and community-dwelling older adults in Germany. Aging Clin Exp Res 26(5):555–559

Hollister B, Chapman S (2015) Dementia care coordination workforce and practices in seven duals demonstration states. UCSF Health Workforce Research Center on Long-Term Care, San Francisco

Jeon YH, Govett J, Low LF, Chenoweth L, McNeill G, Hoolahan A, Brodaty H, O'Connor D (2013) Care Planning Practices for behavioural and psychological symptoms of dementia in residential aged care: A pilot of an educational toolkit informed by the Aged Care Funding Instrument. Contemporary Nurse 44(2):156–169

Kales H, Gitlin L, Lyketsos C (2014) Management of neuropsychiatric symptoms of dementia in clinical settings: recommendations from a multidisciplinary expert panel. J Am Geriatr Soc 62(4):762–710. doi:10.1111/jgs.12730

Konno R, Kang HS, Makimoto K (2014) A best evidence review of intervention studies for minimizing resistance-to-care behaviors for older adults with dementia in nursing homes. J Adv Nurs 70(10):2167–2180. doi:10.1111/jan.12432

Lohrmann C, Bauer S, Mandl M (2015) Pflegequalitätserhebung 14. April 2015 (Quality of care survey 14 April 2015). Institute of Nursing Science, Medical University of Graz, Graz

Matthews FE, Arthur A, Barnes LE, Bond J, Jagger C, Robinson L, Brayne C (2013) A twodecade comparison of prevalence of dementia in individuals aged 65 years and older from three geographical areas of England: results of the Cognitive Function and Ageing Study I and II. Lancet 382(9902):1405–1412

Moyle W, Venturato L, Cooke M, Hughes J, van Wyk S, Marshall J (2013) Promoting value in dementia care: staff, resident and family experience of the capabilities model of dementia care. Aging Ment Health 17(5):587–594. doi:10.1080/13607863.2012.758233

Passalaqua SA, Harwood J (2012) VIPS communication skills training for paraprofessional dementia caregivers: an intervention to increase person-centered dementia care. Clin Gerontol 35:425–445. doi:10.1080/07317115.2012.702655

Schüssler S (2015) Care dependency and nursing care problems in nursing home residents with and without dementia. Dissertation, Medical University of Graz, Graz

Schüssler S, Dassen T, Lohrmann C (2014) Care dependency and nursing care problems in nursing home residents with and without dementia: a cross-sectional study. Aging Clin Exp Res. doi:10.1007/s40520-014-0298-8

Schüssler S, Lohrmann C (2015) Change in care dependency and nursing care problems in nursing home residents with and without dementia: a 2-year panel study. PLoS One 10(10):e0141653. doi:10.1371/journal.pone.0141653

Sheard D (2013) Implementing person-centered theories in dementia care: exploring the butterfly approach. Modern Registered Manager 1(3): May/June

Stein-Parbury J, Chenoweth L, Jeon YH, Brodaty H, Haas M, Norman R (2012) Implementing person-centered care in residential dementia care. Clin Gerontol 35:404–424. doi:10.1080/073 17115.2012.702654

Stinson C (2000) Caregiving tips for care of the Alzheimer's patient. Nurs Homes Long Term Care Manag 49(9):64

Teri L, Huda P, Gibbons L, Young H, van Leynseele J (2005) STAR: a dementia-specific training program for staff in assisted living residences. Gerontologist 45:686–693. doi:10.1093/geront/45.5.686

Traynor V (2015) Developing an inter-disciplinary cross-setting dementia care competency framework. Dementia Collaborative Research Center. University of Wollongong, NSW, AU

Tummers LG, Groeneveld SM, Lankhaar M (2013) Why do nurses intend to leave their organization? A large-scale analysis in long-term care. J Adv Nurs 69(12):2826–2838. doi:10.1111/jan.12249

Warchol K (2004) An interdisciplinary dementia program model for long term care. Top Geriatr Rehabil 20(1):59–71

Warchol K (2012) Dementia care model facilitates quality outcomes. Aging Well 5(2):32–34

Werezak LJ, Morgan DG (2003) Creating a therapeutic psychosocial environment in dementia care. J Gerontol Nurs 29(12):18–25

Williams CL, Hyer K, Kelly A, Leger-Krall S, Tappen RN (2005) Development of nurse competencies to improve dementia care. Geriatr Nurs 26:98–105

Communication in Dementia

Paul Watts and Stephen J. O'Connor

Abstract

This chapter will consider principles of communication when caring for someone with dementia. It will start by looking at the role of communication in daily life, the effects of dementia on the individual's ability to communicate and the many barriers that prevent communication in dementia care. The chapter will then cover the moral, professional and ethical issues involved in the common practice of therapeutic deception and that focused on reorientation of the confused or anxious resident. The therapeutic value of person centredness and positive communication will then be discussed, as will the need for effective listening and sensitivity to those with expressive or receptive communication deficits.

Keywords

Dementia • Receptive communication • Expressive communication • Positive communication • Different realities • Therapeutic deception • Reorientation • Legal • Ethical • Principles

P. Watts (✉)
Inchwater Home Care, Dover, Kent, UK
e-mail: paul.watts@inchwater.co.uk

S.J. O'Connor
England Centre for Practice Development, Canterbury Christ Church University, Canterbury, UK
e-mail: stephen.oconnor@canterbury.ac.uk

© Springer International Publishing AG 2017
S. Schüssler, C. Lohrmann (eds.), *Dementia in Nursing Homes*,
DOI 10.1007/978-3-319-49832-4_9

9.1   Communication in Dementia

Communication is vital in every aspect of our lives and relationships. Every day we communicate our needs, wants, feelings and moods in a variety of ways. This innate ability begins from the moment we are born and plays an important part in making us who we are (Veselinova 2014). For the most part, communication is as natural an activity as breathing, a subconscious and forgotten component of our often-busy lives. Consequently, we seldom stop to consider how good or effective we are at communicating, or how others perceive our attempts at communication. If we consciously thought about how good or bad we were at this important life skill, we would quickly become self-conscious of our weaknesses. It is important, however, as professional carers to give the matter deliberate consideration since it is a vital building block in the development of therapeutic relationships and understanding the needs of those we are trying to help (Goode and Booth 2012). In doing so, we must acknowledge that none of us is perfect. Communication is a skill that can always be improved upon, and nowhere is this more appropriate than when communicating with a person affected by dementia. This chapter explores why skilful communication when caring for people with dementia is so important and considers the benefits of taking the time and effort to do so as well as possible.

9.2   Verbal and Non-verbal Communication

The nurse ethicist Verena Tschudin (2003) remarks that 'communication is the vehicle for ethics' and highlights that it should be the basis of all that we do when caring for others in a person-centred, safe and compassionate way. The eighteenth-century American philosopher Henry David Thoreau is also famous for saying that 'It takes two to speak the truth – one to speak and another to hear', and Bramhall (2014) reiterates this when suggesting that communication requires at least two participants, namely, an 'expresser' and a 'receiver' of information. At its most basic, communication is simply the way in which we seek to understand others and make ourselves understood by them verbally or non-verbally, in writing, for instance, or through facial expressions, body language, posture or our tone of voice (Downs and Collins 2015).

At a theoretical level, communication is a relatively simple interaction or transaction between two or more people, and yet we know that it is also much more complex than that. The person we are communicating with needs to be able to interpret not only the content or *meaning* of the information given but also whether there is *congruence* or *material consistency* between the words spoken and the non-verbal signals conveyed by the speaker during the interaction. The *manner* in which information is given is equally important to the *meaning* of the words used, since we use both sets of signals to ascertain how significant or meaningful the information might be. Contrary to popular opinion, the majority of communication in our species, as in most others, is non-verbal, so others' perceptions of *what we say* are greatly influenced by *how we say it*. Individual words or entire conversations are given additional meaning, emphasis or context by the facial expressions, body language or tone of voice used (Downs and Collins 2015), and these are essential in helping full *understanding* to develop. When done badly however, communication is unlikely to achieve its desired effect and may consequently lead to confusion, frustration or agitation, as well as creating social or psychological barriers that prevent further communication being attempted in future (Jootun and McGhee 2011).

Many of us will have been in situations where we feel that others have not really understood what we are trying to say or completely misunderstood the message we were trying to convey. Imagine how much worse it must be for someone affected by dementia in whom the areas of the brain responsible for receiving, processing, understanding, remembering and responding may not be functioning correctly. In addition, areas of the brain connected with feelings and emotion can also be affected in which case communication can be especially challenging. Similarly, communication is made harder when the person being spoken to does not recognise the one who is talking to them, or is suspicious or afraid of their motives. They may not recognise non-verbal cues or reassurances being conveyed alongside our words, or may focus on just one part of the conversation rather than the whole of it, so they do not receive the full message as we intended them to hear it.

Even when the person affected by dementia is the expresser, i.e. the one doing the talking, damage to critical parts of their brain may affect their ability to control facial expression, body posture, tone of voice or gestures as we do. In such cases, much valuable information can be lost as we try to decipher confusing and, at times, opposing verbal or non-verbal cues which have no congruence or are completely dissonant from what is being said (Lindholm 2015). In such circumstances, it is vital that we understand *why this* is the case so that we may understand *how* these problems might be overcome. People communicate for a variety of reasons and not just because there is a 'need'. How and what we communicate are often closely aligned with our personality or identity, so failing to communicate effectively can be damaging emotionally, physically, socially and professionally (Finke et al. 2008). The ability to communicate well is immensely satisfying and promotes self-esteem, good personal relationships and better quality of life. It allows us to connect with others and to establish our needs and wants without confusion or contradiction. Communication can be trivial or important, data laden or merely a social convenience, so an understanding of the nature and purpose of the communication is vital, allowing us to distinguish between what is vital, requiring an immediate response, and that which is not.

9.3 The Consequences of Poor Communication in Dementia

When a person affected by dementia does not understand what is being said to them, or their attempts at communication are ignored or misunderstood, there can be profound and long-lasting effects on the caring relationship. If unable to express their needs or desires adequately, decisions affecting the individual may increasingly be made by others. This may cause of frustration and damage relationships between individuals and family members. It may also have implications for their health, safety, autonomy and wellbeing (Iritura 1999). Poor communication may also place the individual at significant risk of harm in relation to medicine's management or their inability to report incidences of elder abuse or neglect, for example (Dyer et al. 2015). However, whilst concerns for the health and safety of a person affected by dementia must take priority, concerns for their overall wellbeing are equally important which means that we must try to maintain their individual agency and autonomy (King et al. 2013). If an individual feels misunderstood or experiences loss of control over their everyday life, then feelings of frustration, depression, loss, anxiety or agitation may ensue. They may also become increasingly isolated, socially withdrawn or vulnerable as others cease making efforts to communicate with them (Attree 2001).

9.4 Possible Barriers to Communication in Dementia

Recognition of the barriers to good communication is vitally important. These include physical, social and environmental barriers, physiological communication deficits caused by the disease and deficits in our knowledge of the individual's personal background, history, preferences, hopes or aspirations. Careful consideration of these factors can benefit both parties to a discussion or communication encounter and is discussed in more detail below.

9.4.1 Barriers in the Physical and Sociocultural Environment

One of the primary aspects that should be considered is the physical health of the individual. Are they in pain? Can they both see and hear well enough to communicate? Questions such as these allow us to adjust our 'output' and help build a better understanding for future care. Physical problems such as pain, urinary tract infections or hearing loss can all interfere with good communication, but each of these is manageable if we know about them (Veselinova 2014). Mental health difficulties such as depression or anxiety may be harder to identify and more challenging to manage, but it is important to recognise that the person best placed to identify these issues is the person communicating with the individual on a regular basis. Our direct involvement in their daily care can therefore make us the best person to identify and report such issues to others.

The availability of dementia awareness training has increased during the last 30 years and has become a statutory requirement for many health and social care professions. However, the quality of training and receptiveness of learners is often variable, and negative stereotyping of people affected by dementia is still prevalent in some of these courses (NICE 2006; Ward and Dobson 2014). This often leads to a lack of engagement by staff since the person with dementia is considered incapable of effective communication and this potentiates a downward spiral as fewer and fewer attempts are made to communicate with them (Moyle et al. 2010). So-called disabling communication may then occur, in which the person with dementia is increasingly spoken to as a child, and this further limits the degree to which they can make their wishes, needs or preferences known. Eventually, all real attempts at communication cease, reinforcing negative stereotypes and creating a loss of independence and control in the life of the individual (Perry et al. 2005).

Other environmental factors, such as noise, room temperature or strong smells also affect communication (Digby and Bloomer 2014). Noise in particular can distract those who are hard of hearing or already struggling to think of the right words to say. The environments in which we care for dementia patients often have high levels of ambient background noise such as radios or televisions playing, others' conversations being clearly audible or the hustle and bustle of a busy environment. Thus, whilst it is sometimes difficult to ensure a peaceful and quiet environment at all times, we do need to consider finding a quieter space in which to talk alone or undisturbed or at quieter moments in the day. We should also consider whether communication aids such as writing down simple questions or instructions of the use of flash cards might help.

9.4.2 Physiological Impact of the Disease on Understanding and Communication

Damage caused to some areas of the brain can cause receptive dysphasia (Dewitt and Rauschecker 2013). Wernicke's area, for example, located in the left temporal lobe of the brain is responsible for the comprehension of speech. Damage to this part of the brain means that:

- Words may lose their meaning to the person with dementia.
- Words in a sentence may be heard out of sequence or jumbled together.
- Whole sentences may therefore become scrambled and unrecognisable.

However, it is important to recognise that careful attempts to communicate – even with those with receptive dysphasia – can be successful. Common or more frequently used words are likely to be understood better than those used less frequently, and it is useful to think about the vocabulary and words that the individual might use themselves rather than medical jargon or more convoluted speech patterns. Evidence demonstrates that speaking slowly and clearly and using common words and phrases may aid comprehension (Rousseaux et al. 2010). Short words and short sentences should also be used to aid understanding, adding emphasis to keywords in the sentence if necessary so that long sentences and multiple questions are avoided. For example:

'What would you like to drink today, tea or coffee?' (ten words) might become:

'Would you like a drink?' (five words) and then after a moment, 'tea or coffee?' (three words).

Both examples have the same meaning, but the second is much more likely to be understood as the sentences are shorter and the listener is not distracted by more abstract things such as what 'today' might be or what time of the day it is. The delivery of the words needs to be clear and steady, without being exaggeratedly loud or excessively slow (Stanyon et al. 2016). Likewise, infantilising 'baby talk' is neither appropriate nor useful when working with adults and suggests an underlying misunderstanding about the nature of the illness in which the individual is mistakenly considered to have reverted to childhood, which is certainly not the case.

Certain areas of the brain are also involved in encoding language prior to transmission to other parts of the brain (Dewitt and Rauschecker 2013), and damage to these areas can result in abnormal or confusing aspects of speech such as:

- Distorted or 'made-up' words
- Wrong words used in the wrong situations
- Sound substitutions
- Echolalia (repeating what has just been heard)

Sometimes, the person with dementia may use long and complex sentences, which say very little and are largely unintelligible. It is important to recognise, however, that they may not realise that they have expressive communication deficits and that the listener cannot understand what they are saying. Patience, gentleness and kindness as they try to communicate what they are thinking are vital, and seeing the other person's perspective is important, as the following real-life example of a married couple highlights:

Husband (with dementia): *Honestly, I think she ought to go and see someone. She just doesn't seem to understand words any more! I repeat the same thing over and over again, and in the end, I just point.*

Wife: *I can't understand much of what he says any more. His words are often made up and meaningless. It's really just the context that gives clues as to what he means, and I can see him get so frustrated! In the end, he gives up trying and just points to what he wants.*

Similarly, the cues we take from non-verbal communication, such as confirming, regulating or emphasising what is being said verbally, may be confusing or misleading. Care must be taken in interpretation and, as with most communication, context is key (Egan 1990). Focusing on one detail of behaviour over all others may hinder overall understanding, or it may provide a cue upon which further exploration may provide clarification. In expressive communication difficulties, it may be a challenge to differentiate between a 'need' and utterances which are simply meant to be discourse markers or moderators. In circumstances where need is suspected, careful communication to clarify and confirm what they may be asking for is required. In this, context may present further clues to meaning as will a good knowledge of the individual and their normative behaviours, likes, dislikes, etc.

9.4.3 Different Realities: Understanding the Person Affected by Dementia

A person affected by dementia may have a different understanding of the world than we do. Although the causes are an area of academic dispute, it is broadly agreed that cognitive dysfunction associated with dementia can affect visual and auditory interpretation of the world as it is, as well as memory, and executive decision-making functions (Idrizbegovic et al. 2011; Lindholm 2015; Golden et al. 2016). This means that the senses we rely on to inform us about our environment, interactions with others and the basis upon which we understand our world, may be severely impaired. Thus an individual whose lived 'reality' is based on their memories of an earlier life in which they think of themselves as a young man or woman, a son or a daughter and not as an older person may not be easily corrected by means of external stimuli or, indeed, others' attempts to bring them back to 'reality' (Lindholm 2015). As a consequence, strategies intended to relocate the individual in the 'here and now' such as calendars, clocks, daily newspapers, etc. that proclaim today's date may have little or no relevance to the individual and may be ignored or disregarded. Indeed, there is some mileage in considering why it is helpful for us to do so anyway, so long as they are happy, safe and comfortable wherever their mind situates them at the current time.

9.5 The Benefits of Positive Communication

We started this chapter on communication by describing it as the 'vehicle for ethics' and the basis for person-centred, safe effective care, and so indeed it should be. However, issues of morality, ethics and deception in care encounters with those affected by dementia, and especially those living in a different reality, are a deeply contested field of debate. Clinicians, carers, researchers, family carers and others, such as patient advocacy organisations, have all contributed to this debate at some point without coming to agreement. For example, in the UK, one national dementia support charity issued a position statement denouncing a taught ethic of deception in direct conflict with another national (albeit smaller) charitable trust, which advocated that it was perfectly acceptable to collude with an individual's different reality when it might be distressing or harmful to confront this (Alzheimer's Society 2012).

9.5.1 Truth or Lies? The Value of Therapeutic Deception

The debate leading to the difference of opinion evident in the above policy positions of two otherwise similar patient advocacy groups is well documented in the literature and consists primarily of two opposing viewpoints. The first view is that therapeutic deception may alleviate or prevent distress in someone whose reality is not shared by others (Schermer 2007), as, for example, where an individual might believe that their children are still infants who need collecting from school. At such times, the carer may use therapeutic deception or collusion to relieve a potential cause of anxiety or distress by suggesting that the 'children' are safely being collected by someone else. The belief is that in entering into a person's lived reality, we can defuse anxiety or agitation and provide an enhanced sense of psychological health and wellbeing.

There are two difficulties with this approach however. One is an ethical difficulty and the second a practical one. The ethical issue surrounds whether it is ever in a person's best interest to deceive them and there are individuals from academia, practice and those affected by dementia, who agree that there may be circumstances in which therapeutic deception of this kind might be acceptable (Day et al. 2011). Others argue that there are few situations or circumstances in which deception should be employed as a strategy (Culley et al. 2013).

The practical difficulty can be framed by asking what happens if the person realises they are being deceived. Apart from any additional distress this may cause, there are likely to be serious repercussions in terms of future trust relationships with the deceiver, and it is this argument which those critical of therapeutic deception focus upon. As a consequence, a growing consensus suggests that a 'default position' of deception should be avoided if possible (Schermer 2007; Culley et al. 2013) since its use as a first-response strategy fails to empower the individual and removes effective choice and control from their lives. Thus, whilst there may be times in which therapeutic deception may promote a beneficial outcome, and might consequently be considered, this should never be common practice or a primary response to situations which can be managed differently.

9.5.2 The Value of Reorientation Strategies

The second view is one in which the caregiver or professional should attempt to reorient the person affected by dementia to current reality (O'Connell et al. 2007). Using the above example, the caregiver might explain to the individual that their children are now adults and no longer attend school. The belief, particularly found in primary carers such as spouses or immediate family, is that reorientation will allow the individual to recognise their memory deficit and therefore return them to their current reality. However, as with the first position, the difficulties inherent in this approach are ethical as well as practical (Schermer 2007). Reminding an individual that their children are now adults is one example that has limited consequence and may even be welcomed by the individual affected with dementia, but reminding them that they or other family members are dead is arguably of much greater consequence. If, in the individual's reality, this is the first time they have been made aware of it, they are likely to become distressed and need to grieve, and repeating this same piece of information every time the question is raised might be considered cruel or unkind and is unlikely to be in the person's best interest.

Practically speaking, as dementia progresses, it is common for individuals to become repetitive (Hwang et al. 2000). Reorientation, even with minor issues such as the day of the week, can become draining for the primary carer and stressful for the individual; after all, no one enjoys being constantly corrected (Cullen et al. 2005). It is this challenge that can lead to 'compassion fatigue' and place strain on carer relationships (Coetzee and Klopper 2010; Ledoux 2015), especially when the individual concerned makes clear that they see no need for it. Consequently, whilst adhering to the personalisation ethic of control and choice, it can be seen that total honesty and attempts to reorient the individual should be used judiciously with due consideration of the actual circumstances and the reality which they are being reoriented to. As with therapeutic deception, a primary default position of always reorienting the individual may not always be in their best interests and may detrimentally impact upon the resident's quality of life (Barbosa et al. 2015).

9.6   Positive Communication: Seeking to Meet Underlying Need

The opposing views discussed above have one thing in common. Both strategies may be used in the person's best interest in certain circumstances and at certain times, but they may also be equally counterproductive at others. We have argued, however, that adopting either as a simple default position may be ethically unsound and counterproductive in practical terms. In terms of communication, we need to consider how best to engage a person affected by dementia, how best to respond to their communications with us and how these might affect the care we provide. Positive communication aims to address these considerations by seeking an 'alternative path' between the two opposing models based on the individual's underlying need and their known wishes and preferences. It meets the criteria for person-centred communication and establishes a baseline for good care.

Perry et al. (2005) suggest that nurses use several strategies or typologies to promote positive communication with those affected by dementia. These break communication into its component parts and can help us reflect on the interaction and determine how to respond to the messages being received during the discussion.

Clarifying	Ensuring understanding
Exploring	Information gathering
Moderating	Maintaining flow of conversation
Validating	Recognising feelings
Rescuing	Seeking relevance in (isolated/non-connected) statements
Discourse markers	Social conventions (ok, I see, thank-you, uh-huh, etc.)
Connecting	Drawing on personal information to extend links/bonds

Positive communication entails understanding the individual's view of the world without necessarily entering or colluding with it. Note in the above section how validating, for instance, focuses on the patient's emotional and affective state. It does not encompass their view of the world. Similarly, in the above model, moderation is intended to keep the flow of the discussion going rather than shutting it down, which may be the case if we simply try to reorient the individual to 'reality'. Positive communication disregards, to some degree, the words said, and instead, and seeks to find the underlying need behind the words. Returning to our previous example of the married couple, using positive communication as a tool, we would consider the need of the individual as they become anxious about their children. The underlying need, in this example, might be a need for comfort and reassurance. Reassuring the individual their children are safe and well might relieve their anxiety and prevent further agitation. It might require interaction from the caregiver in terms of reassuring words and physical comfort, or it might require distraction first, but once the underlying need is met, the individual is more likely to settle.

The basic communication tools of exploring and clarifying are now coupled with validating and connecting. Validation, or acknowledging the individual's feelings, is an important part of reassuring them that their concerns are being taken seriously. Drawing upon our knowledge of the individual, we can then connect on a very personal level to understand their need. To do this, we neither have to agree with their reality nor disagree. We only have to try to understand it. Once we have recognised the underlying need, we can acknowledge that the individual is anxious and can provide encouragement and support without either reinforcing or challenging their view of the world. For example:

'Peggy Smith' has been living with dementia for 4 years. She is 89 years of age and becoming anxious for her son. She believes him to be in school and that she needs to collect him. It is 10 o'clock at night, and it is cold, raining and dark outside. She is dressed lightly and was preparing for bed before becoming distracted about her son's welfare. For her own safety, she needs to stay indoors.

If we deceive Mrs Smith by suggesting that her son has been collected by someone else, we are not necessarily meeting her underlying need, as she has no evidence for this, or his safety, and may not therefore be reassured. If we attempt reorientation by explaining that her son is now himself retired, we might fail to convince her and still not meet her needs.

By recognising and meeting her needs, we stand a better chance of reducing the risk to Peggy. In this example, acknowledging her concerns would be a good first step. A distraction technique might then be employed, allowing time in which to provide the reassurance and comfort she actually needs.

Therefore, we can ask the following questions:

- What does the individual need?
- What is their reality at the moment?

These questions can be answered by exploring and clarifying the communication. Once we understand these, we can then validate the communication by acknowledging the person's need and connect with them using what we know about them and their needs.

For 'Peggy Smith', the interaction might look something like this:

Individual	Communication	Interpretation
Mrs Smith	I have to pick up my son from school	I am anxious and concerned
Caregiver	Why is that?	Exploring the need
Mrs Smith	It's getting late and he'll be worried!	Clarification of the need
Caregiver	I understand – I have children too	Validating (acknowledging) the concern
Mrs Smith	He needs me, he'll be worried!	Clarification of the need
Caregiver	It is cold and wet outside. Why don't we have a nice cup of tea before we go?	Distraction creating time to connect
Mrs Smith	Maybe just a quick one	Trust in the relationship
Caregiver	<Sits down next to Mrs Smith with cup of tea> Why don't you tell me a bit about your son?	Connecting to meet Mrs Smith's need: finding time to reassure and comfort
Mrs Smith	Well…	

During the course of the conversation, Mrs Smith might recall other events of her and her son's lives, perhaps his graduation or wedding, minimising her natural concern for the safety of her 'school boy' son. Clearly, this is a contrived example. Real-life situations have many more variables and often take place over longer timescales, but it demonstrates the concept that in communication, we should consider not just what is said, but seek a deeper understanding of what needs the words express. This calls for a high degree of patience and attentiveness, or, in other words, effective listening.

9.7 Effective Listening

Effective listening is an essential communication technique that requires skills in listening, empathy and trust. Effective listening includes ideas of 'active' listening, understanding and interpreting the needs of another person correctly, and responding appropriately and effectively to that need (Shipley 2010; Doas 2015). Active listening is therefore a planned and deliberate act which demands the full attention of the listener (Stickley and Freshwater 2006). It requires them to be alert to what is said and how it is said, without necessarily forming judgements. Key to active listening is allowing the individual to speak in their own terms, at their own pace. This may require discourse markers such as 'uh-huh' or 'I see' in order to show attentiveness and enable the speaker to continue, but should avoid potentially judgemental terms such as 'don't worry' or 'it'll be alright' that might appear to discount the value of what is said. To ensure understanding, the communication needs to be reflected back to the individual. The conversation might be paraphrased or summarised; but the basis of the individual's need and their feelings should be included in this summary. By restating the content, both the individual and the carer can be reassured that the communication has been understood clearly (Shipley 2010). It also allows for modification of understanding where required. Clearly, this needs to be done in such a way as to not appear patronising, and part of the skill in effective listening is in achieving a 'natural flow' to the conversation. There are ways in which we can demonstrate active listening, and caregivers should be well rehearsed in both verbal and non-verbal skills:

- *Verbal*
  - Open-ended questions
  - Exploring problems rather than 'leaping' in to solve them
  - Reflecting communication back to the individual
  - Non-judgemental
  - Tone of voice
- *Non-verbal*
  - Eye contact
  - Adopting a mirrored position
  - Open gestures
  - Close proximity

(Stickley and Freshwater 2006)

Non-verbal skills are an essential component in achieving rapport. Good non-verbal skills demonstrate to the individual that they are being listened to (Bryant 2009) and that they have your full attention. As with reflecting, non-verbal communication that is forced may appear patronising, so care needs to be taken to find the 'gentle attentiveness' that signals attention. For example, mirroring the individual's position can seem artificial or pretentious if followed too rigidly resulting in a lack of trust. Performed mindfully, mirroring can reinforce conscientious attentiveness and help build trust.

Similarly, the non-verbal cues that can be picked up from the individual are significant when trying to find the underlying need in their communication (Jootun and McGhee 2011). Facial expressions, body language and the emotional context of the communication may all provide indication of need. The difficulty when communicating with a person affected by dementia, however, is in interpreting non-verbal cues correctly when the verbal content of the conversation may be confusing or misleading. One way to achieve this is to ensure that an overall picture is considered rather than any specific cue. A grimace in itself may not present a need, but may, with other signs, provide a guide to further exploration. In this way, using both verbal and non-verbal indicators, effective listening allows us to respond appropriately to the individual's needs.

9.8   Person-Centred Communication

Person-centred communication is an approach in which the abilities of the individual, rather than their impairment, are considered before and during communication (Downs and Collins 2015). Communication difficulties are likely to increase as the disease progresses, and it is therefore important to understand the context of the communication in order to support the individual. This is achieved by having as full an understanding of the individual as possible in order to respond appropriately, allowing them time in which to respond and enabling them to make choices about their communication.

9.8.1   Know the Person

People communicate using different terms, a variety in language and using a wide range of non-verbal indicators. They may have different understandings of the world based on completely different experiences in life to ours. Of critical importance, in any communication with a person affected by dementia, is to know the individual you are communicating with as fully as possible (Lindholm 2015). Whilst this is not always possible, the better informed you are, the more likely you are to understand their underlying need. In some cases, it may be possible to access detailed information (e.g. a life history album), or it may be the case that the individual is the only source of information and all information is new or incomplete. Gaining insight to their needs will be more likely however, the more you find out about them (Downs and Collins 2015).

9.8.2   Attentive Patience

People who have difficulties communicating often require time and the space in which to understand and be understood. Patience, in its form as a passive act of waiting, is not necessarily useful when we are trying to engage someone in meaningful communication, but it does have a role to play in effective listening. It also indicates that the individual is being heard and listened to, as well as being given the time and space they need (Shipley 2010; Stokes 2013). Non-verbal communications such as eye contact, body positioning and proximity are used to maintain the presence of communication even when verbal communication has paused. Allowing time for the individual to respond, and being mindful of indicators of their under-standing of you, is not a cessation of communication but an aid to successfully understanding the person.

9.8.3   Simplify Choices to Enable Control

Having a degree of control over our lives aids our sense of self-esteem. At a time when control over their life may be felt to be slipping, offering choice to a person affected by dementia is a positive step towards enabling them to retain a sense of control. When the cognitive ability of the individual to make choices diminishes, a reduced range in the choice still allows valid choices to be made (Williams et al. (2005)). For example, offering a person an entire wardrobe of choice may be too great a decision to make. Offering the same person a choice of two shirts may allow a choice to be made successfully as there are just three options available (either shirt or neither). In this way, the individual is able to make a valid choice of a range within their abilities to understand.

9.9   Improving Our Practice: The Importance of Reflection

Reflective practice has become a formal part of many health and social care courses (Payne 2005). Its current theory and models are well documented elsewhere, and we are not going to reproduce them here. What is of importance is the use of reflection to achieve positive communication, i.e. understanding and meeting the underlying need of the individual. In this way, learning from experience by reflecting upon communication interactions can enhance the care experience for the individual and help build confidence in future interactions (Shiau and Chen 2008). Put simply, the act of reflection in communication practice allows the experiences and understand-ings of the communication to be examined and evaluated. In this way positive com-munication might be propagated to others, and, where this hasn't been achieved, future communication might be informed. When reflecting on a communication, we can then ask the following questions:

- What happened?
- What did I do?
- What would I do differently next time?

These questions require a degree of introspection and honesty, but also the time in which to reflect adequately. Of particular importance is the need to inform others of the outcome. In residential care settings where there might be many different staff, the availability of just one or two who are able to communicate effectively with an individual may lead to poor outcomes for that person when they are not on duty. Were the staff able to reflect on why their communications are effective, they may be able to pass on the information to others, allowing more people to commu-nicate well with the individual (Borjesson et al. 2015).

Examining the circumstances of the interaction is important because it might provide clues as to an unmet need. Considering the barriers to communication we outlined earlier, the context of the communication and our knowledge of the individual, we can try to evaluate the interaction afresh. Looking again at the communication without the pressure of direct contact, we can consider aspects such as whether the communication was typical of the individual, whether earlier interactions (or non-interactions) had precipitated this instance and whether our knowledge of the individual is sufficient to enable positive communication. Reflecting on our actions during the communication is also important as we can evaluate our responses in terms of the effectiveness of the outcome. Was the communication a positive one? Were our responses appropriate in terms of the individual's level of comprehension and did they, ultimately, meet the underlying need? Critical consideration of our own performance enables us to determine whether we did everything we were able to, given our understanding of the situation at the time and the circumstances we were working in.

Considering what we might do differently next time is vital in our learning process (Sutton and Dalley 2008). Merely replaying a communication is not enough in terms of adapting our understanding of the individual. Foremost is the question of whether the interaction could be termed positive. Was the need met? Clearly there are different routes to meeting a need, and consideration should be given towards how else the exchange could have been conducted. Once again, whether an interaction has been successful or not, this needs to be communicated to others.

Conclusion

Communication is such an important part of life that we often don't stop to consider how it impacts upon us. Communication, for a person affected by dementia, can present daily difficulties that can be challenging and unsettling. For the family, the inability to communicate effectively can result in feelings of loss and emotional distance. Professionals may have feelings of redundancy or helplessness when faced with these difficulties. In this chapter, we have considered the effects of poor communication and some of the communication barriers a person affected by dementia may experience. Barriers, such as the environment, the physical deterioration of the brain and the resultant changes in understanding, can hinder and challenge us when we attempt to communicate effectively.

Positive communication, in which the individual is placed firmly at the centre of the communication, adopts a different approach to the binary paradigms of reorientation and therapeutic deception. It seeks to enable true person-centred communication by meeting the underlying need. By understanding the concept of positive communication, skills can be developed that assist caregivers on a daily basis and ensure the person affected by dementia enjoys a good quality of life by having their needs met. Communication will become more difficult as the dementia progresses, and it is here that the skill of the caregiver in communicating with the individual will become critical in understanding their needs. In this, there is little substitute for experience, but it is important that it is the right experience of attempting to understand the underlying reason behind the communication. If this has been considered, then a good standard of care will inevitably follow.

References

Alzheimer's Society UK (2012) Position statement – specialised early care for Alzheimer's (SPECAL). Available from: https://www.alzheimers.org.uk/site/scripts/documents_info.php?documentID=1087. Accessed 23 Apr 2016

Attree M (2001) Patients' and relatives' experiences and perspectives of 'Good' and 'Not so Good' quality care. J Adv Nurs 33:456–466

Barbosa A, Sousa L, Nolan M, Figueiredo D (2015) Effects of person-centered care approaches to dementia care on staff: a systematic review. Am J Alzheimer's Disease Other Dementias 30:713–722

Borjesson U, Cedersund E, Bengtsson S (2015) Reflection in action: implications for care work. Reflective Pract 16:285–295

Bramhall E (2014) Effective communication skills in nursing practice. Nurs Stand 29:53–59

Bryant L (2009) The art of active listening. Pract Nurs 37:49–52

Coetzee S, Klopper H (2010) Compassion fatigue within nursing practice: a concept analysis. Nurs Health Studies 12:235–243

Cullen B, Coen R, Lynch C, Cunningham C, Coakley D, Robertson I, Lawlor B (2005) Repetitive behaviour in Alzheimer's disease: description, correlates and functions. Int J Geriatr Psych 20:686–693

Culley H, Barber R, Hope A, James I (2013) Therapeutic lying in dementia care. Nurs Stand 28:35–39

Day A, James I, Meyer T, Lee D (2011) Do people with dementia find lies and deception in dementia care acceptable? Aging Ment Health 15:822–829

Dewitt I, Rauschecker J (2013) Wernicke's area revisited: parallel streams and word processing. Brain Lang 127:181–191

Digby R, Bloomer M (2014) People with dementia and the hospital environment: the view of patients and family carers. Int J Older People Nursing 9:34–43

Doas M (2015) Are we losing the art of actively listening to our patients? Connecting the art of active listening with emotionally competent behaviours. Open J Nurs 5:566–570

Downs M, Collins L (2015) Person-centred communication in dementia care. Nurs Stand 30:37–41

Dyer CB, Pavlik VN, Murphy KP, Hyman DJ (2015) The high prevalence of depression and dementia in elder abuse or neglect. J Am Geriatr Soc 48:205–208

Egan G (1990) The skilled helper: a systematic approach to effective helping. Monterey, Brooks and Cole

Finke E, Light J, Kitko L (2008) A systematic review of the effectiveness of nurse communication with patients with complex communication needs with a focus on the use of augmentative and alternative communication. J Clin Nurs 17:2102–2115

Golden H, Augustus J, Nicholas J, Schott J, Crutch S, Mancini L, Warren J (2016) Functional neuroanatomy of spatial sound processing in Alzheimer's disease. Neurobiol Aging 39:154–164

Goode B, Booth G (2012) Dementia care: a care worker handbook. Abingdon, Hoffer Educational

Hwang J, Tsai S, Yang C, Liu K, Ling J (2000) Repetitive phenomena in dementia. Int J Psychol 30:165–171

Idrizbegovic E, Hedertierna C, Gahlquist M, Kampfe-Nordstrom C, Jelic V, Rosenhall U (2011) Central auditory function in early Alzheimer's disease and in mild cognitive impairment. Age Ageing 40:249–254

Iritura V (1999) Factors affecting the quality of nursing care: the patient's perspective. Int J Nurs Pract 5:86–94

Jootun D, McGhee G (2011) Effective communication with people who have dementia. Nurs Stand 25:40–46

King B, Gilmore-Bykovskyi A, Roiland R, Polnaszek B, Bowers B, Kind A (2013) The consequences of poor communication during transitions from hospital to skilled nursing facility: a qualitative study. J Am Geriatr Soc 61:1095–1102

Ledoux K (2015) Understanding compassion fatigue: understanding compassion. J Adv Nurs 71:2041–2050

Lindholm C (2015) Parallel realities: the interactional management of confabulation in dementia care encounters. Res Lang Soc Interact 48:176–199

Moyle W, Borbasi S, Wallis M, Olorenshaw R, Gracia N (2010) Acute care management of older people with dementia: a qualitative perspective. J Clin Nurs 20:420–428

National Institute for Health and Care Excellence (NICE) (2006) Dementia: supporting people with dementia and their carers in health and social care (section 1.1.9). Available from: https://www.nice.org.uk/guidance/cg42/chapter/1-Guidance. Accessed Online: 1 Apr 2016

O'Connell B, Gardner A, Takase M, Hawkins MT, Ostaszkiewicz J, Ski C, Josipovic P (2007) Clinical usefulness and feasibility of using Reality Orientation with patients who have dementia in acute care settings. Int J Nurs Pract 13:182–192

Payne M (2005) Modern social work theory. Basingstoke, Palgrave Macmillan

Perry J, Galloway S, Bottorff J, Nixon S (2005) Nurse-patient communication in dementia: improving the odds. J Gerontol Nurs 31:43–52

Rousseaux M, Seve A, Vallet M, Pasquier F, Mackowiak-Cordoliani MA (2010) An analysis in conversation in patients with dementia. Neuropsychologia 48:3884–3890

Schermer M (2007) Nothing but the truth? On truth and deception in dementia care. Bioethics 21:13–22

Shiau S, Chen C (2008) Reflection and critical thinking of humanistic care in medical education. Kaohsiung J Med Sci 24:367–372

Shipley S (2010) Listening: a concept review. Nurs Forum 45:125–134

Stanyon M, Griffiths A, Thomas S, Gordon A (2016) The facilitators of communication with people with dementia in a care setting: an interview study with healthcare workers. Age Ageing 45:164–170

Stickley T, Freshwater D (2006) The art of listening in the therapeutic environment. Ment Health Pract 9:12–18

Stokes G (2013) Tackling communication challenges in dementia. Nurs Times 109:14–15

Sutton L, Dalley J (2008) Reflection in an intermediate care team. Physiotherapy 94:63–70

Tschudin V (2003) Ethics in nursing: the caring relationship. Butterworth-Heinemann, Edinburgh

Veselinova C (2014) Influencing communication and interaction in dementia. Nurs Residen Care 16:162–167

Ward A, Dobson M (2014) Lessons learned from a dementia training programme for health professionals: implications for future training provision. J Pract Teaching Learning 12:25–43

Williams C, Hyer K, Kelly A, Leger-Krall S, Tappen R (2005) Development of nurse competencies to improve dementia care. Geriatr Nurs 26:98–105

Polypharmacy in Nursing Home Residents with Dementia

10

Rob J. van Marum

Abstract

Polypharmacy and inappropriate prescribing are common among nursing home residents with dementia. In many cases, medication is not discontinued despite the very limited life expectancy of these individuals, the increased risk of side effects due to drug–drug and drug–disease interactions, and the questionable benefits of medication. A structured approach is essential to managing the medication of nursing home residents with dementia. To facilitate rational prescribing, the WHO six-step method should be used. But it is also important to perform periodical medication reviews in which the appropriateness of the total medication set is evaluated. These medication reviews should be performed in a systematic manner in close collaboration between patient/caregiver, physician, and pharmacist.

At the end of life, it can be expected that pharmacotherapeutic goals gradually chance from largely preventive to more symptomatic therapy. In this chapter, the problems related to polypharmacy are described. Guidelines, based on the WHO six step, are given on how to make rational choices when prescribing for individuals with dementia and on how to perform a medication review. Lastly, attention is given to issues concerning the stopping or withdrawal of medication.

Keywords

Polypharmacy • Inappropriate medication • Medication review

R.J. van Marum, MD, PhD
Professor of Geriatric Pharmacaotherapy, VU University Medical Center Amsterdam,
Department of General Practice and Elderly Care Medicine,
PO Box 7057, 1007 MB, Amsterdam, The Netherlands
e-mail: r.vanmarum@vumc.nl

© Springer International Publishing AG 2017   123
S. Schüssler, C. Lohrmann (eds.), *Dementia in Nursing Homes*,
DOI 10.1007/978-3-319-49832-4_10

10.1   The Problem of Polypharmacy in Nursing Home Residents with Dementia

Old age is often accompanied by multimorbidity. A large general practice database study in the UK showed that patients with a chronic condition, such as diabetes or dementia, generally have 4–5 other chronic conditions (Guthrie et al. 2012). Since most chronic conditions are treated according to guidelines with one or more drugs, it is not surprising that multimorbidity goes hand in hand with polypharmacy (usually defined as the use of 4 or more drugs). Since patients are increasingly treated according to guidelines and life expectancy is steadily increasing, the percentage of people receiving polypharmacy is steadily increasing, even in the oldest old (Melzer et al. 2015).

We can divide the goals of pharmacotherapy roughly into preventive and symptomatic goals. In community-dwelling patients, at least half of the medication used is intended for primary or secondary prevention. It will come as no surprise that a large proportion of this preventive medication consists of medication for cardiovascular risk management (antihypertensive drugs, statins, anticoagulants), although drugs for the prevention of fractures (e.g., vitamin D, calcium, bisphosphonates) or gastric problems (proton pomp inhibitors) are also frequently prescribed to elderly patients. The other half of the medication used is for symptomatic treatment – pain medication, psychiatric medication, treatment of chronic obstructive pulmonary disease, and blood glucose-lowering drugs.

Polypharmacy is very common in long-term care facilities, with worldwide prevalence rates varying between 40% and 90% (Jokanovic et al. 2015). In a study of European long-term care facilities, polypharmacy (5–9 drugs) was observed in half of the residents, and excessive polypharmacy (concurrent use of ≥ 10 drugs) was seen in almost a quarter of the residents (Onder et al. 2012). In addition to chronic drug use, as-needed (pro re nata: PRN) prescriptions are also very common. In a German study, nearly three quarters (74.9%) of all nursing home residents received at least one PRN medication. On average, each resident was prescribed 2.5 ± 2.3 PRN drugs (Dörks et al. 2016). Compared with individuals living in the community, residents of nursing homes tend to use relatively fewer preventive and more symptomatic medications (e.g., psychotropic drugs, pain medication, laxatives).

10.1.1   Polypharmacy and the Risk of Side Effects

Given the high prevalence of chronic diseases in the elderly, polypharmacy often will be indicated. While drugs are undoubtedly started for a specific indication and prescribed according to clinical guidelines, the use of multiple drugs increases the chance of drug-related problems. This is not only due to the increased chance of drug–drug or drug–disease interactions but also as a result of changed pharmacokinetics and pharmacodynamics due to aging (Hajjar et al. 2007; Mangoni and Jackson 2004). Renal function, as estimated by the glomerular filtration rate (eGFR), declines by approximately 1 mL/min/year. This means that in community-dwelling elderly patients, the mean eGFR of a 70-year-old person is about 60 mL/min, whereas it is about 40 mL/min in frail elderly patients. This decreased eGFR leads to a decreased excretion of renally excreted drugs. Moreover, the GFR can be strongly influenced by dehydration and medication that acts on the nephrons (ACE inhibitors, NSAIDs, certain antibiotics). For many drugs, dose adaptation is necessary in case of renal insufficiency in order to prevent toxicity. This is especially the case for drugs with a narrow therapeutic index, such as digoxin, lithium, amino-glycosides, and morphine. But also for many other drugs, such as bisphosphonates, some sulfonylurea derivatives, gout medication, and nitrofurantoin, dose reduction is advised. Given the high risk of ignoring potential renal insufficiency when prescrib-ing medication, physicians should assume that each nursing home resident suffers from renal insufficiency unless proven otherwise. Hepatic blood flow and metabolic capacity may diminish with advancing age, leading to diminished hepatic clearance or activation of drugs by the cytochrome P450 enzymes. Especially in Alzheimer's disease, the blood–brain barrier is less effective, which can lead to higher drug levels in cerebrospinal fluid (which may be relevant for psychotropic drugs) (Zenaro et al. 2016). An altered body composition (less lean body mass, more fat, less water) changes the distribution volume of the body, which may alter the elimination time of drugs (e.g., decreased in lipophilic drugs such as benzodiazepines). But also pharmacody-namics change. For example, cerebral receptors (e.g., dopamine) may become less functional or decrease in number in disease or with advancing age, and cholinergic function in the brain may decrease, increasing the susceptibility to delirium or cogni-tive impairment. Polypharmacy increases the probability of drug–drug interactions (Lindblad et al. 2006). A major pathway of enzymatic degradation (or sometimes activation) of drugs is the cytochrome P450 enzyme system. Many drugs that are known substrates for the CYP450 system also function as inducers or inhibitors of this system, thereby influencing the metabolic processing of other drugs. A good overview of substrates, inducers, and inhibitors can be found at http://medicine. iupui.edu/flockhart/table.htm (Flockhart 2007).

Together, these factors increase a patient's risk of adverse drug events (ADEs) and less efficacious therapy. In frail elderly patients, polypharmacy increases the risk of a loss of function, which can make the difference between independent living and assisted living or between being alert and being sedated. Polypharmacy in the frail elderly in particular increases the likelihood of serious events, such as falls, fractures, stroke, myocardial infarction, or even death. The Dutch Hospital Admission Related to Medicines (HARM) study showed that 6% of all acute hospi-tal admissions are due to adverse drug reactions (Leendertse et al. 2010). In the USA, institutionalized elderly people experience ADEs at a rate as high as 10.8 events per 100 patient–months, often as a result of polypharmacy, multiple comor-bid illnesses, and difficulty with monitoring prescribed medications. This translates into approximately 135 ADEs a year in an average size nursing home (number of beds, 105) or approximately two million events a year among all US nursing home residents (Handler and Hanlon 2010).

Polypharmacy may be especially problematic in patients with dementia. Impaired cognition is a hallmark of dementia, and many drugs (psychotropic drugs, anticholinergic drugs, Parkinson drugs) adversely affect cognitive performance. Being a neurodegenerative disease, dementia also impairs mobility, and many prescribed medicines may further impair mobility by lowering blood pressure (antihypertensive drugs, alpha receptor blocking drugs [e.g., tamsulosin], L-dopa) or by causing dizziness, myopathy (e.g., statins), or Parkinsonism (e.g., antipsychotic drugs). Moreover, some drugs may diminish appetite or the ability to eat and drink, potentially leading to malnutrition and sarcopenia. An additional problem is that demented individuals are often not able to report adverse effects.

10.1.2 Inappropriate Drug Use in Nursing Home Residents with Dementia

As stated earlier, polypharmacy may be indicated when looking at treatment guidelines. Medication that was originally prescribed for a clear indication may become inappropriate in later life, i.e., its potential risks outweigh its potential benefits. This is the case when the risk of side effects is strongly increased (for instance, due to changed pharmacokinetics or pharmacodynamics), but also when the likelihood of potential benefits is very low or when medication is no longer relevant (e.g., the use of cardiovascular preventive medication in end-stage dementia). Whether a drug is inappropriate or not for an individual is not always clear and can only be determined on the basis of all relevant clinical and patient information. There are several lists of potentially inappropriate medications, based on side-effect data from large trials or observational data, numbers needed to treat reported in clinical studies, and expert opinion. Examples of these lists are the Beers criteria and STOPP and START criteria (American Geriatrics Society Beers Criteria Update Expert Panel 2015; O'Mahony et al. 2015). But the underuse of potentially beneficial medication should also be considered inappropriate. Given the problems of polypharmacy in dementia patients, one would expect that medication appropriateness is a key issue in patient management. Yet medication inappropriateness appears to be common among many nursing home residents. In the European Shelter project involving nursing homes in seven European countries and Israel, the appropriateness of drug use was determined using the algorithm of Holmes et al. (Colloca et al. 2012; Holmes et al. 2008). Inappropriate drug use was observed in 44.9% of the residents. Most commonly used inappropriate drugs were lipid-lowering agents (9.9%), antiplatelet agents (9.9%), acetylcholinesterase inhibitors (7.2%), and antispasmodics (6.9%). Inappropriate drug use was directly associated with specific diseases, including diabetes, heart failure, stroke, and recent hospitalization, whereas it was inversely associated with the presence of a geriatrician in the facility.

Roughly the same figures were found in a US study (Tjia et al. 2014). Of 5406 nursing home residents with advanced dementia, 53.9% received at least 1 medication of questionable benefit. Cholinesterase inhibitors (36.4%), memantine hydrochloride (25.2%), and lipid-lowering agents (22.4%) were the most commonly prescribed drugs. In adjusted analyses, having eating problems, a feeding tube, a do-not-resuscitate order, and enrolling in a hospice lowered the likelihood of receiving these medications. The use of feeding tubes increased the likelihood of receiving these medications. The mean (SD) 90-day expenditure for medications of questionable benefit was $816 ($553), accounting for 35.2% of the total average 90-day medication expenditure for residents with advanced dementia who were prescribed these medications.

A systematic review of 43 studies involving nursing home residents also suggested that almost a half of nursing home residents (43%) are exposed to potentially inappropriate medication use, with the estimated prevalence increasing between 1990 and 2014 (Morin et al. 2016). The authors compared this result with that of a systematic review of 12 studies involving community-dwelling elderly (Opondo et al. 2012), in which the average prevalence of inappropriate prescriptions was 20% (i.e., half of our estimate in the nursing home setting). This difference would suggest that institutionalized older adults are at greater risk of receiving potentially inappropriate medications than community-dwelling patients.

A Dutch study focusing on the treatment of heart failure in nursing home residents (mostly with dementia) showed that the recommended medical therapy was often not prescribed, and if it was prescribed, the dosage was usually much lower than the recommended dosage. In most cases, non-pharmacological interventions were not used at all (Daamen et al. 2016). Another, USA-based study of nursing home residents with dementia found that residents were prescribed a mean of 5.9 medications daily and that 37.5% received at least one medication considered "never appropriate" in advanced dementia. Cholinesterase inhibitors (15.8%) and lipid-lowering agents (12.1%) were the most commonly prescribed inappropriate drugs. Twenty-eight percent of the residents took antipsychotics daily. Modest reductions in most daily medications occurred only during the last week of life (Tjia et al. 2010).

The appropriateness of psychotropic drug use in patients with dementia is also subject to much discussion. The use of antipsychotic drugs in the management of the behavioral problems of dementia is common worldwide, even though these drugs are of questionable benefit and have considerable potential to cause harm (Ballard and Waite 2006). Antipsychotic drug use in dementia is associated with an increased incidence of mortality, stroke, pneumonia, falls, and fractures, etc. In 2008, the US Food and Drug Administration issued a warning to all physicians, stating that since both conventional and atypical antipsychotics are associated with an increased risk of mortality in elderly patients treated for dementia-related psychosis, healthcare professionals should consider other management options.

Physicians who prescribe antipsychotics to elderly patients with dementia-related psychosis should discuss this risk of increased mortality with their patients, patients' families, and caregivers. Numbers needed to harm (NNH) for death within 6 months following initiation of antipsychotic drug therapy may be as low as 20–30 (Maust et al. 2015). Despite these warnings, at least a third of all patients with dementia in nursing homes are prescribed an antipsychotic drug (Kamble et al. 2009; Vasudev et al. 2015; Bohlken et al. 2015).

10.2   Prescribing in Dementia Patients: The WHO Six Step

Rational prescribing for patients with dementia is no different from that for non-demented elderly patients. The appropriateness of medication in elderly patients depends upon the remaining life expectancy, the goals of care, and the treatment targets. These factors change in the final years of life and in dementia. Physicians should adopt a systematic approach when prescribing medication for patients in later life, and the WHO six step for rational prescribing is a useful tool for this (de Vries et al. 1994).

Step 1: Define the patient's problem This important first step in daily practice tends to be overlooked, especially in patients with dementia. It is often the caregiver or nurse who comes to the physician with a problem. Physicians should be aware that it is sometimes the caregiver or nurse who has a problem. A patient's behavior may be indicative of illness, pain, or psychiatric suffering. This is especially relevant in the case of behavioral problems associated with dementia – what is the behavior for which medication is requested? When does this behavior occur? What are the triggers for this behavior? Who is actually having a problem with this behavior – the patient or staff and the patient's friends and relatives? If risk factors for disease have been identified (hypertension, cholesterol, vitamin depletion, etc.), the physician should consider whether the presence of a risk factor is really a problem for the patient or just a problem defined by guidelines.

Step 2: Specify the therapeutic objective Defining the goals of therapy is crucial when deciding if and what medication should be described. Therapeutic goals change throughout life and especially in the presence of lifespan-limiting disease (Holmes et al. 2006; Maddison et al. 2011). As the end of life approaches, goals for pharmacotherapy should shift from mostly primary or secondary prevention to symptomatic therapy, to improve the patient's quality of life. Decreasing the 10-year risk of cardiovascular death or morbidity is less relevant in patients with end-stage neurodegeneration. Symptomatic treatment for pain, depression, anxiety, constipation, or dyspnea becomes more important.

Step 3: Verify whether your chosen treatment is suitable for this patient Once the therapeutic goal has been established, the different therapeutic options should be weighed. Since drug therapy is always associated with the risk of harm, the most important question here is: can we attain the formulated goals without prescribing medication. *Primum non nocere* must guide decision-making. When medication is considered, the prescriber must look at the expected number needed to treat (NNT) and expected numbers needed to harm (NNH) of the chosen drug. The effect of age-associated pharmacokinetic and pharmacodynamic changes and the possibility of drug–drug and drug–disease interactions should also be considered. Since this evaluation is often difficult, explicit screening lists, such as the START and STOPP criteria, Beers criteria, or FORTA criteria, may be helpful (American Geriatrics Society Beers Criteria Update Expert Panel 2015; O'Mahony et al. 2015; Pazan et al. 2016). These lists have been developed, mostly based on evaluation of scientific studies and expert opinion, for the elderly population. They clearly indicate which drugs should not be used in elderly patients for reasons of potential to harm or expected low efficacy. The START criteria also indicate which forms of undertreatment occur in elderly patients.

Remaining life expectancy and time until benefit also need to be weighed. The remaining life expectancy for many nursing home patients (at least in the Netherlands, where admission to nursing homes mainly occurs in end-stage dementia) is often less than 1–2 years. This makes the initiation of, for instance, cholesterol-lowering drugs or antihypertensive medication with times until benefit of at least 2 years irrational. But osteoporosis prevention with bisphosphonates may be feasible given that the time until benefit of this therapy is less than 1 year.

The route of drug administration should also be assessed for appropriateness. Inhalation therapy in dementia patients may not always be feasible. Some tablets are hard to swallow, and so another formulation (soluble, liquid, chewable) should be chosen. Medication patches may be better than tablets as route of drug administration.

Step 4: Start the treatment Physicians should use an electronic prescribing system and check the prescription for prescribing errors (correct medication, correct dose, correct dosing interval, etc.). They should pay attention to the formulation (can it be crushed in case of swallowing difficulties, can it be used in a correct way [e.g., inhalation therapy]) and when the medicine should be taken (e.g., statin in evening, bisphosphonate 30 min before breakfast).

Step 5: Give information, instructions, and warnings In the case of nursing home residents with dementia, it is important to inform the nursing staff and the patient's family about possible side effects and correct usage. Since patients with dementia may have difficulties in recognizing and reporting side effects, others must be extra vigilant on their behalf. Incorrect use of drugs may lead to diminished efficacy or harm. For example, the biological availability of bisphosphonates decreases to almost zero when the drug is taken with calcium (milk or tablets) and may cause mucosal irritation. It is therefore important that these drugs are taken at least 20 min before breakfast with a glass of water in an upright position to optimize efficacy and minimize side effects. The uptake of L-dopa drugs used for Parkinson's disease is limited when they are taken together with protein. For drugs that are metabolized by the CYP3A4 enzyme, grapefruit juice is forbidden because it inactivates the intestinal CYP3A4 enzymes, leading to intoxication. The efficacy of inhalation therapy for COPD is strongly dependent on the use of the correct inhalation technique, which must be trained.

Step 6: Monitor the treatment Despite careful consideration of the first five steps, side effects can still occur. Many serious side effects can be prevented by adequate monitoring (Warlé-van Herwaarden et al. 2012). Knowledge of potential major side effects enables physicians or staff to take action to detect these in time. Starting ACE inhibitors means checking renal function and serum potassium within 2 weeks, in order to detect possible renal insufficiency or therapy-induced hyperkalemia. Initiating antihypertensive therapy requires measuring the effects and preventing hypotension. The initiation of cholinesterase inhibitors requires monitoring of intake (and weight). It should be borne in mind that the risk of adverse drug reactions is increased in the first few weeks after medication is changed. It is also important to monitor treatment efficacy. The initiation of psychotropic drugs, being drugs with a low NNH and often questionable benefit, should be carefully monitored and evaluated. If the drug does not have the desired effect, physicians should make a timely decision about whether to increase the dose or to stop the drug.

10.3 Performing a Medication Review

Use of the WHO six step to help prescribe appropriately is one step in achieving rational pharmacotherapy, but it is not enough. In most cases, the medication used by nursing home residents is not initiated by the general practitioner or nursing home physician. Hospital specialists may add medication to the already existing list or stop certain medications. Moreover, as the patient's clinical condition and goals of care change with time, it is not sufficient to focus solely on prescribing. Periodical evaluation of the medications used, a medication review, is necessary to judge whether the current medication regimen is the most appropriate for this patient at a given moment.

Several types of medication review can be distinguished at a hierarchical level. A technical review of the list of the patient's medicines by the physician (*prescription review*) is the lowest and quickest form of medication review. One step higher, in the so-called treatment review, the physician uses the patient's medical record to review treatment. The highest level of medication review is the *clinical medication review*, which is performed with input and consent of the patient and the patient's medical record. If the patient is not considered mentally competent, his or her role can be taken over by a legal representative or the next of kin. This medication review should preferably be performed on admission and thereafter at least once a year or if the patient's health suddenly changes.

In the Netherlands, the broadly accepted guideline *Polypharmacy in the Elderly* states that a true medication review is a review of the complete medical record by physician, pharmacist, and patient together (Dutch General Practitioners et al. 2012). For this purpose, the Dutch guideline proposes a systematic approach, using an implicit screening tool called the *Systematic Tool to Reduce Inappropriate Prescribing (STRIP)* (Keijsers et al. 2014). This tool includes five steps (see Fig.10.1):

Step 1: Pharmacotherapeutic history taking This is a vital element of the medication review. In the case of nursing home residents with dementia, currently used medications are discussed with the legal representative or next of kin. Points for discussion are current experiences, possible side effects, expectations, and usage problems. The input of nursing staff is often necessary in order to get a clear view of current side effects and actual use. The main point of this step is to determine treatment goals.

Fig. 10.1 Systematic tool to reduce inappropriate prescribing

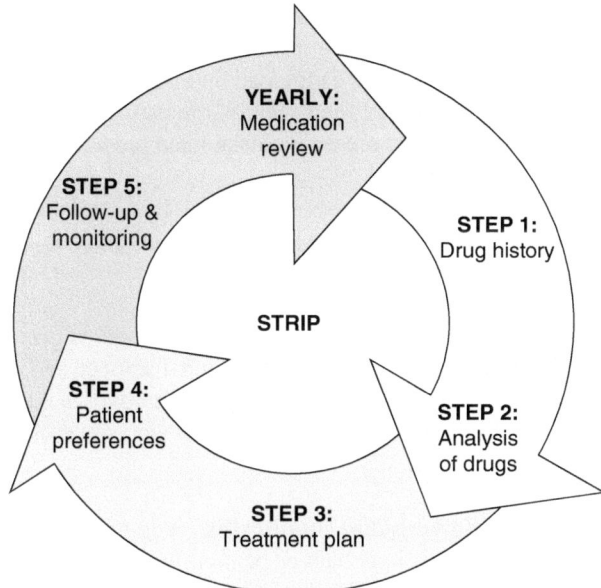

Step 2: Pharmacotherapeutic analysis The purpose of this step is to establish possible drug-related problems. All medicines used should be associated with an underlying medical diagnosis or problem recorded in the patient's medical record (including relevant measurements such as the results of physical examination and laboratory investigations). This helps identify potential therapy-related problems:

(a) *Undertreatment*: Are all medical problems being treated? In nursing home residents, this step is especially important for identifying symptomatic undertreatment (e.g., pain, anxiety, psychosis, obstipation, dyspnea). But it is also useful for detecting guideline deviations. While there may be good reasons to deviate from guidelines, these reasons need to be clearly reported in the patient's medical record.

(b) *Noneffective medication or overtreatment*: Are all medications currently indicated? Are they still beneficial to the patient?

(c) *Potential side effects*: What are the potential side effects of each drug? Are these side effects still acceptable?

(d) *Relevant contraindications and interactions*: Assess drug–drug interactions and drug–disease interactions. Relevant drug–drug interactions may involve the cytochrome P450 (CYP450) family (Flockhart 2007). Also the effect of (especially psychotropic drugs) on cardiac conduction (e.g., prolongation of QTc-time) should be considered (CredibleMeds 2016).

(e) *Incorrect dose*: Is the dose used by the patient safe and adjusted to the indication or renal function?

(f) *Usage problems*: Is all the prescribed medication used in an effective and correct way (e.g., correct use of inhalation therapy, is the bisphosphonate tablet taken in a correct way?)? Is the patient able to swallow all tablets? Can all medicines safely be crushed (and what is the actual current practice if a patient does not accept his pills; are they crushed and hidden in food or liquids?)?

Step 3. Consultation between physician and pharmacist The physician and pharmacist should then draw up a treatment plan based on the pharmacotherapeutic history and analysis.

Step 4. Consultation with the patient's legal representative or next of kin The treatment plan should be presented and discussed and, if necessary, adjusted according to the wishes of the patient's representative. In the case of admitted patients, the nursing staff should be involved in this step since they will administer the medication to the patient.

Step 5. Follow-up and monitoring A monitoring plan is crucial. When will the effects of medication changes be measured? Who will be responsible for doing so?

10.4   Decision-Making Based on Evidence-Based Medicine

Evidence-based medicine is the conscientious, explicit, and judicious use of current best evidence in making decisions about the care of individual patients. The practice of evidence-based medicine means integrating individual clinical expertise with the best available external clinical evidence from systematic research (Sackett et al. 1996). The problem in decision-making is that NNT can only be derived from large published randomized controlled trials (RCTs). These seldom include elderly patients, let alone patients with dementia. The International Conference on Harmonisation (ICH) guideline on geriatrics (E7) states that, for medicines intended for diseases characteristically associated with old age, 50% or more of the participants should be aged 65 and older. For medicines intended to treat diseases present in, but not unique to, older people, 100 or more participants aged 65 and older should be included. Studies show that only 1% of all participants in trials of these medicines are aged 70 years or older (Beers et al. 2014). Thus guidelines are often based on NNT for a selected population that is usually younger and healthier, without multimorbidity or polypharmacy, than the population for which the medicine is destined. For that reason, also the NNH in frail old patients can seldom be derived from these RCTs, which makes it difficult to make choices. Given the frail population in nursing homes, one can assume that the NNH is much lower and that drug efficacy is seldom better, than that reported in RCTs.

Many medicines are used off-label by nursing home residents, and this is especially the case for psychotropic drugs. Moreover, most psychopharmacological interventions for patients with dementia are not evidence based. Bearing this in mind, it is difficult for individual physicians to weigh the benefit and harm of medication in frail elderly patients.

10.5   Screening Tools

Screening tools can help improve rational prescribing in nursing home populations. Implicit screening tools, such as the STRIP or the Medication Appropriateness Index, are judgment based, are patient specific, and consider the patient's entire medication regimen. The use of these tools relies on expert professional judgment, requires good pharmacological knowledge, and is time consuming. Explicit screening tools, on the other hand, are far easier to use. Explicit screening tools contain lists of medicines that are potentially inappropriate for frail elderly patients. Examples of these explicit screening lists are the Beers criteria, the STOPP and START criteria, and the FORTA criteria. Most of these criteria are based on a combination of evaluation of the literature, Delphi panels with experts, and a final evaluation by a small group of experts. For all drugs included in these screening lists, the potential for causing harm outweighs the potential benefit. Drugs can be considered inappropriate based on their potential to cause harm regardless of morbidity (e.g., by causing sedation, anticholinergic properties, causing orthostatic hypotension, etc.) or only in combination with specific morbidity (e.g., decreased renal function, dementia). Some screening lists, such as the STOPP and START criteria and FORTA, also address the risk of underprescribing by listing drugs that can be considered beneficial for elderly patients. These screening lists are easy to use and can be applied with little clinical or pharmacological knowledge. A disadvantage is their rigidity. They should not be used as lists of forbidden drugs but as a warning. It is up to the prescriber to balance potential harms and benefits (using the WHO six step) and to decide whether or not the chosen drug should be prescribed. Multiple studies have shown that the use of screening lists reduces inappropriate prescribing and serious adverse drug reactions, even in nursing home populations. The use of explicit screening lists is not sufficient for a complete clinical medication review, which requires the use of implicit screening lists and patient involvement.

It is difficult to say which explicit screening method is the best for dementia patients in nursing homes. There is a large overlap between most methods, but they may differ with regard to the drugs included. The STOPP and START criteria were developed in Europe and the Beers criteria in the USA. In these regions, but even between countries within Europe, other drugs will be reimbursed or prescribed, so these methods should always be adjusted to the local situation.

10.6   The Problem of Stopping Medication

The high prevalence of potential inappropriate medication use by nursing home residents shows that is not easy to stop medication once it has been started, for several reasons (Reeve et al. 2013a; Schuling et al. 2012; Kalogianis et al. 2016). The first barrier to stopping or withdrawing medication is the attitudes and beliefs of the physician. Some physicians believe there is appropriate evidence for prescribing medication, whereas others may be reluctant to change medication orders made by hospital specialists or feel they lack the education and experience to taper off or stop medications. Physicians may also be concerned that their patients may feel that they are "giving up on them" or "leading them to quicker deaths." In addition, clinicians feel pressured to prescribe according to clinical guidelines, even though they are

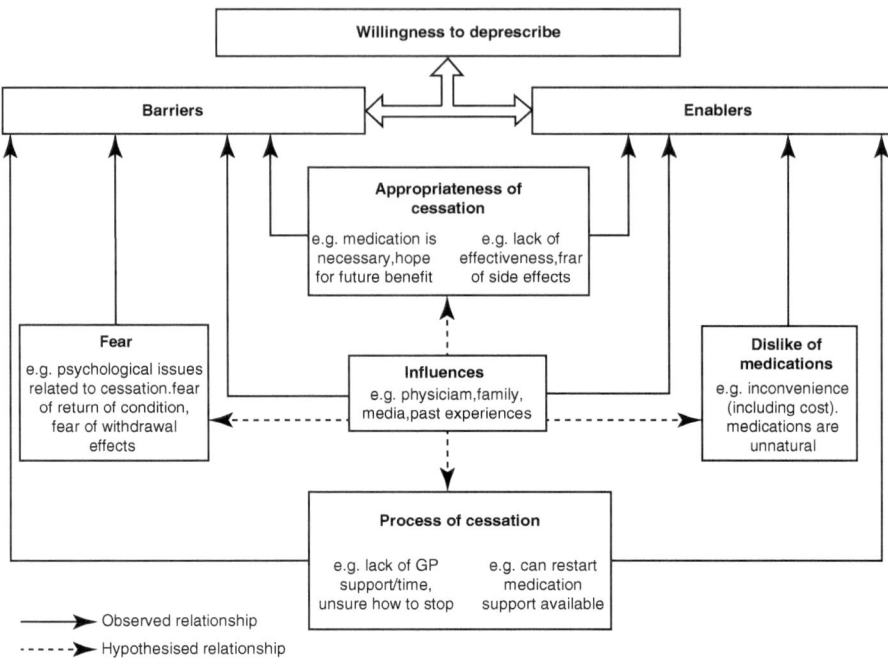

Fig. 10.2 Patient barriers and enablers (From Reeve et al. 2013). Overview of patient barriers and enablers and their observed or hypothesized relationship to medication cessation

aware that such guidelines are rarely based on evidence from studies involving older populations and rarely address the issue of modifying clinical targets with advancing age or care goals. These considerations often lead to "therapeutic inertia" – "recognition of the problem, but failure to act."

Patient's beliefs and attitudes, or those of their caregivers, may also hinder the withdrawal of potentially inappropriate medication (see Fig.10.2). Studies involving community-dwelling elderly patients have shown that most elderly patients have a very limited knowledge of their medications. In majority, they state that they do believe that most medication they use is important since otherwise the doctor would not have prescribed it. On the other hand, studies with the patient's attitude toward deprescribing tool show that the vast majority would reduce their medication use if advised to do so by their physician (Reeve et al. 2013b). Both patients and physicians may be influenced by cognitive bias. Status quo bias means that a preference for continuing with the status quo exists, especially if it has been the default for many years. Omission bias — being more willing to risk harm arising from inaction (continuing medication) than from action (stopping medication) — may also be a problem. For successful cessation of (potential) inappropriate medication, a stepwise approach is best (Best Practice Journal 2010):

Step 1: Create awareness that option of medication cessation is feasible Physicians should talk to patients or their caregivers about possibly stopping or withdrawing medications ("deprescribing") as soon as possible following admission. This does not mean that once a patient is admitted, medication should be stopped as soon as possible. In the context of shared decision-making, the physician should explore with the patient or caregivers how they feel about the current treatment. Since patients and caregivers will have many different barriers and enhancers for deprescribing, it is important to investigate these carefully.

Step 2: Discuss the options and their potential benefits and harms with patient or caregiver Although numbers needed to treat and numbers needed to harm from trials cannot easily be extrapolated to the clinical situation of an individual patient, these numbers can be used as starting point for a discussion. Often, potential benefits will be smaller in frail elderly and harms will be higher.

Step 3: Exploring patient preferences for the different options Preferences from patient or caregiver may differ from those of the physician. Following their opinions may increase the chance of successful deprescribing. Discussing treatment goals as part of advanced care planning is crucial for personalized care.

Step 4: Making a plan A plan for discontinuing medications one at a time should be drawn up, starting with medications with the highest burden and lowest benefit. Discontinuing medicines one at a time makes it easier to know what the likely cause of potential problems is. Although the parties involved (e.g., caregivers, physicians, pharmacists, and nurses) may initially disagree about the order in which medicines should be withdrawn, it is important to reach agreement on this. A lack of agreement might lead to overreporting of assumed side effects or withdrawal symptoms.

Step 5: Discontinue medications and monitor for withdrawal or return of symptoms Stopping medicines may result in withdrawal events/symptoms, including rebound symptoms, such as rebound tachycardia after stopping beta-blocker treatment. Signs or symptoms of the preexisting disease may reappear, such as pain after stopping analgesics and gastric complaints following the cessation of a proton pump inhibitor. Physicians should consider whether tapering is required to prevent rebound effects. They should also check for benefit or harm after each medicine has been stopped.

Conclusion

Despite the fact that the life expectancy of nursing home residents with dementia is limited to a few years, many of them use multiple medications. Studies have shown that most residents use inappropriate medications and that adverse side effects are common in nursing home residents. Pharmacotherapy in nursing homes is essentially different from pharmacotherapy in a community setting. The limited life expectancy, high prevalence of multimorbidity, impaired cognition resulting in a lesser level of shared decision-making, and loss of independence play a role in the decision whether and which medication should be started, continued, or stopped. All physicians working in nursing homes should be trained in the principles of good prescribing and medication review as described in this chapter.

References

American Geriatrics Society Beers Criteria Update Expert Panel (2015) Updated beers criteria for potentially inappropriate medication use in older adults. J Am Geriatr Soc 63(11):2227–2246. doi:10.1111/jgs.13702

Ballard C, Waite J (2006) The effectiveness of atypical antipsychotics for the treatment of aggression and psychosis in Alzheimer's disease. Cochrane Database Syst Rev 25(1):CD003476

Beers E, Moerkerken DC, Leufkens HG et al (2014) Participation of older people in preauthorization trials of recently approved medicines. J Am Geriatr Soc 62(10):1883–1890

Bohlken J, Schulz M, Rapp MA et al (2015) Pharmacotherapy of dementia in Germany: results from a nationwide claims database. Eur Neuropsychopharmacol 25(12):2333–2338

Colloca G, Tosato M, Vetrano DL et al (2012) Inappropriate drugs in elderly patients with severe cognitive impairment: results from the shelter study. PLoS One 7(10):e46669. doi:10.1371/journal.pone.0046669

CredibleMeds (2016) For healthcare providers. https://crediblemeds.org/healthcare-providers/. Accessed 1 July 2016

Daamen MA, Hamers JP, Gorgels AP et al (2016) Treatment of heart failure in nursing home residents. J Geriatr Cardiol 13(1):44–50. doi:10.11909/j.issn.1671-5411.2016.01.001

de Vries TP, Henning RH, Hogerzeil HV, Fresle DA (1994) Guide to good prescribing. WHO, Geneva

Dörks M, Schmiemann G, Hoffmann F (2016) Pro re nata (as needed) medication in nursing homes: the longer you stay, the more you get? Eur J Clin Pharmacol 72(8):995–1001

Dutch General Practitioners, Dutch Geriatric Society, Dutch Order of Medical Specialists (2012) OMS. Multidisciplinary guideline polypharmacy in the elderly. NHG, Utrecht

Flockhart DA (2007) Drug interactions: cytochrome P450 drug interaction table. Indiana University School of Medicine. http://medicine.iupui.edu/clinpharm/ddis/main-table. Accessed 1 July 2016

Guthrie B, Payne K, Alderson P et al (2012) Adapting clinical guidelines to take account of multimorbidity. BMJ 345:e6341. doi:10.1136/bmj.e6341

Hajjar ER, Cafiero AC, Hanlon JT (2007) Polypharmacy in elderly patients. Am J Geriatr Pharmacother 5(4):345–351

Handler SM, Hanlon JT (2010) Detecting adverse drug events using a nursing home specific trigger tool. Ann Longterm Care 18(5):17–22

Holmes HM, Hayley DC, Alexander GC et al (2006) Reconsidering medication appropriateness for patients late in life. Arch Intern Med 166(6):605–609

Holmes HM, Sachs GA, Shega JW et al (2008) Integrating palliative medicine into the care of persons with advanced dementia: identifying appropriate medication use. J Am Geriatr Soc 56(7):1306–1311. doi:10.1111/j.1532-5415.2008.01741.x

Jokanovic N, Tan EC, Dooley MJ et al (2015) Prevalence and factors associated with polypharmacy in long-term care facilities: a systematic review. J Am Med Dir Assoc 16(6):535.e1–535.12

Best Practice Journal (2010) A practical guide to stopping medicines in older people. http://www.bpac.org.nz/BPJ/2010/April/stopguide.aspx. Accessed 1 July 2016

Kalogianis MJ, Wimmer BC, Turner JP et al (2016) Are residents of aged care facilities willing to have their medications deprescribed? Res Social Adm Pharm 12(5):784–788

Kamble P, Chen H, Sherer JT et al (2009) Use of antipsychotics among elderly nursing home residents with dementia in the US: an analysis of National Survey Data. Drugs Aging 26(6):483–492

Keijsers CJ, van Doorn AB, van Kalles A et al (2014) Structured pharmaceutical analysis of the systematic tool to reduce inappropriate prescribing is an effective method for final-year medical students to improve polypharmacy skills: a randomized controlled trial. J Am Geriatr Soc 62(7):1353–1359

Leendertse AJ, Egberts AC, Stoker LJ et al (2010) Frequency of and risk factors for preventable medication-related hospital admissions in the Netherlands. Arch Intern Med 168(17):1890–1896

Lindblad CI, Hanlon JT, Gross CR et al (2006) Clinically important drug-disease interactions and their prevalence in older adults. Clin Ther 28(8):1133–1143

Maddison AR, Fisher J, Johnston G (2011) Preventive medication use among persons with limited life expectancy. Prog Palliat Care 19(1):15–21

Mangoni AA, Jackson SH (2004) Age-related changes in pharmacokinetics and pharmacodynamics: basic principles and practical applications. Br J Clin Pharmacol 57(1):6–14

Maust DT, Kim HM, Seyfried LS et al (2015) Antipsychotics, other psychotropics, and the risk of death in patients with dementia: number needed to harm. JAMA Psychiatry 72(5):438–445. doi:10.1001/jamapsychiatry.2014.3018

Melzer D, Tavakoly B, Winder RE et al (2015) Much more medicine for the oldest old: trends in UK electronic clinical records. Age Ageing 44(1):46–53

Morin L, Laroche ML, Texier G et al (2016) Prevalence of potentially inappropriate medication use in older adults living in nursing homes: a systematic review. J Am Med Dir Assoc 17(9):862. e1–862.e9. doi:10.1016/j.jamda.2016.06.011

O'Mahony D, O'Sullivan D, Byrne S et al (2015) STOPP/START criteria for potentially inappropriate prescribing in older people: version 2. Age Ageing 44(2):213–218. doi:10.1093/ageing/afu145

Onder G, Liperoti R, Fialova D et al (2012) Polypharmacy in nursing home in Europe: results from the SHELTER study. J Gerontol A Biol Sci Med Sci 67(6):698–704

Opondo D, Eslami S, Visscher S et al (2012) Inappropriateness of medication prescriptions to elderly patients in the primary care setting: a systematic review. PLoS One 7(8):e43617. doi:10.1371/journal.pone.0043617

Pazan F, Weiss C, Wehling M, FORTA (2016) The FORTA (Fit fOR The Aged) List 2015: update of a validated clinical tool for improved pharmacotherapy in the elderly. Drugs Aging 33(6):447–449

Reeve E, To J, Hendrix I, Shakib S et al (2013a) Patient barriers to and enablers of deprescribing: a systematic review. Drugs Aging 30(10):793–807

Reeve E, Wiese MD, Hendrix I et al (2013b) People's attitudes, beliefs, and experiences regarding polypharmacy and willingness to Deprescribe. J Am Geriatr Soc 61(9):1508–1514

Sackett DL, Rosenberg WM, Gray JA et al (1996) Evidence based medicine: what it is and what it isn't. BMJ 312(7023):71–72

Schuling J, Gebben H, Veehof LJ et al (2012) Deprescribing medication in very elderly patients with multimorbidity: the view of Dutch GPs. A qualitative study. BMC Fam Pract 13:56

Tjia J, Rothman MR, Kiely DK et al (2010) Daily medication use in nursing home residents with advanced dementia. J Am Geriatr Soc 58(5):880–888. doi:10.1111/j.1532-5415.2010.02819.x

Tjia J, Briesacher BA, Peterson D et al (2014) Use of medications of questionable benefit in advanced dementia. JAMA Intern Med 174(11):1763–1771. doi:10.1001/jamainternmed.2014.4103

Vasudev A, Shariff SZ, Liu K et al (2015) Trends in psychotropic dispensing among older adults with dementia living in long-term care facilities: 2004-2013. Am J Geriatr Psychiatry 23(12):1259–1269

Warlé-van Herwaarden MF, Kramers C, Sturkenboom MC et al (2012) Targeting outpatient drug safety: recommendations of the Dutch HARM-Wrestling Task Force. Drug Saf 35(3): 245–259

Zenaro E, Piacentino G, Constantin G (2016) The blood-brain barrier in Alzheimer's disease. Neurobiol Dis pii S0969-9961(16):30165–30166. doi:10.1016/j.nbd.2016.07.007

Quality of Life of People with Dementia in Nursing Homes

Martin N. Dichter and Gabriele Meyer

Abstract

This chapter summarizes the theoretical knowledge on quality of life (QoL) and health-related quality of life (HRQoL) of people with dementia and its development. Based on this information, the principles of the measurement of dementia-specific QoL will be explained. The chapter will describe the following measurements which can be applied for the assessment of QoL or HRQoL of people with dementia in nursing homes: Activity and Affect Indicator Quality of Life (AAIQOL), Cornell-Brown Scale for Quality of Life in Dementia (CBS-QoL), Dementia Quality of Life questionnaire (DEMQOL & DEMQOL-proxy), Heidelberg instrument for the assessment of quality of life in dementia (H.I.L.DE), Quality of Life in Alzheimer's Disease (QoL-AD), Quality of Life in Alzheimer's Disease Nursing Home version (QoL-AD-NH), Quality of Life Assessment Schedule (QOLAS), Alzheimer Disease-Related Quality of Life (ADRQL), Dementia Care Mapping (DCM), Observing Quality of Life in Dementia (OQOLD), Observed Quality of Life in Dementia Advanced (OQOLDA), Quality of Life for Dementia (QoL-D), Quality of Life in Late-Stage Dementia Scale (QUALID), QUALIDEM, and Vienna List. Moreover,

M.N. Dichter, MScN, RN (✉)
German Center for Neurodegenerative Diseases (DZNE),
Stockumer Straße 12, 58453 Witten, Germany

School of Nursing Science, Witten/Herdecke University,
Stockumer Straße 12, 58453 Witten, Germany
e-mail: Martin.Dichter@dzne.de

G. Meyer
School of Nursing Science, Witten/Herdecke University,
Stockumer Straße 12, 58453 Witten, Germany

Institute for Health and Nursing Science, Medical Faculty, Martin Luther University,
Halle-Wittenberg, Germany
e-mail: gabriele.meyer@medizin.uni-halle.de

© Springer International Publishing AG 2017
S. Schüssler, C. Lohrmann (eds.), *Dementia in Nursing Homes*,
DOI 10.1007/978-3-319-49832-4_11

questions for the selection of the appropriate measurement will be recommended and associated factors with QoL of people with dementia are described. Finally, we summarize the effectiveness of non-pharmacological interventions targeting the maintenance or promotion of dementia-specific QoL.

Keywords
Dementia • Nursing homes • Quality of life • Measurements • Psychometrics • Models • Definition

11.1 Introduction

Healthcare and healthcare research that focus on person-centered outcomes (e.g., quality of life) are an international priority (Federal Ministry of Education and Research 2011; Institute P-COR – Patient-Centered Outcomes Research Institute 2015). This applies particularly for care (Gibson et al. 2010; Haberstroh et al. 2010) and research (Moniz-Cook et al. 2008) for people with dementia because this is a chronic and currently incurable syndrome. During recent years, science in this field has been increasingly productive (Fig. 11.1).

There is no general accepted definition about what is meant by quality of life (QoL). This applies for the most part for QoL and also for dementia-specific QoL. A recently published article addresses the indiscriminate use of the terms quality of

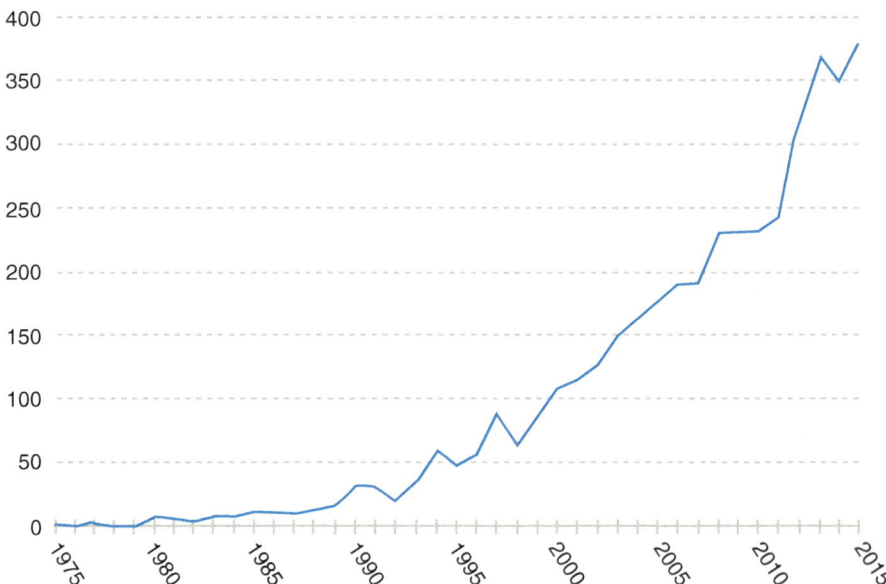

Fig. 11.1 Number of publications indexed in Medline [PubMed] using quality of life and dementia as search terms, search date: 28.09.2016

life, health-related quality of life (HRQoL), and health status (Karimi and Brazier 2016). In contrast to the indiscriminate use were the different definitions available for the concepts QoL and HRQoL.

An influential definition of QoL is the definition by the World Health Organization, which defines QoL as "individuals' perceptions of their position in life in the context of the culture and value systems in which they live and in relation to their goals, expectations, standards and concerns" (WHO 1995). This definition highlights the individuality, the culture-specific influence, and the breadth of the concept of QoL.

In contrast, HRQoL is defined, for example, as "how well a person functions in their life and his or her perceived well-being in physical, mental, and social domains of health" (Hays and Reeve 2010). In this definition, functioning refers to the individual ability to realize predefined activities, and well-being refers to individual subjective feelings (Karimi and Brazier 2016; Wilson and Cleary 1995). Based on this and similar definitions of HRQoL, Karimi and Brazier (2016) conclude that HRQoL is a particular type of health description, hence the World Health Organization defines health as "a state of complete physical, mental and social well-being, and not merely the absence of disease and infirmity" (WHO 2014). This means that HRQoL measurements reflect health in a wider sense (well-being and functioning) than clinical outcomes. However, this wide description targets health and not QoL. Therefore, HRQoL assesses a self-perceived health status and not QoL (Karimi and Brazier 2016). Based on this differentiation of both terms, this chapter focuses on the concept of quality of life for people with dementia. In cases where only research results were available for HRQoL of people with dementia, these will be highlighted in the text.

11.2   Models of Quality of Life for People with Dementia in Nursing Homes

Due to the indiscriminate use of the terms QoL and HRQoL and a lack of theoretical work targeting dementia-specific QoL, no consensus exists for the definition of QoL of people with dementia. One early and influential theoretical model describes dementia-specific QoL as consisting of objective (e.g., behavioral competence and environment) and subjective (e.g., perceived QoL and psychological well-being) components (called "sectors") (Lawton 1991, 1994). Based on this theoretical approach, Jonker et al. developed a hierarchical model called "Lawton's next step." This model defines psychological well-being as the starting point and central indicator for dementia-specific QoL (Jonker et al. 2004), and the authors argue for the consideration of non-dementia-related domains of QoL, such as personal factors (e.g., religion, income, age), next to environmental characteristics and dementia-related domain. The development from Lawton's first model to the model by Jonker and colleagues reflects the increasing importance of subjectivity for the concept of dementia-specific QoL. For both models it must be noted that they are based on the interpretation of selected evidence and experience of the authors and not on direct empirical data, a systematic review, or a concept analysis.

In contrast, a current key publication (O'Rourke et al. 2015) about factors which influence the QoL is based on self-expression of people with dementia in qualitative studies. The objective of this meta-synthesis was the identification of factors that affect QoL and not the concept of QoL in particular. Nevertheless, the results provide interesting information for the interpretation of QoL of people with dementia. In summary, the meta-synthesis identified four overlapping factors which affect QoL: relationships, sense of place, wellness perspective, and agency in life today. Connectedness is the link between all four factors. The results demonstrate the experience of connectedness (being purposeful or together) within one factor affecting QoL in a positive way. In addition, connectedness is associated with happiness. The feeling of disconnectedness within a factor (e.g., loneliness, worthlessness) negatively influences QoL. Moreover, it is associated with sadness (O'Rourke et al. 2015). In summary, this model underlines the relevance of the individual experience of people with dementia with their QoL. With connectedness as the central factor, the model focuses on how people with dementia and their individual environment (e.g., direct care, living arrangement) adapt to the consequences of dementia and general life changes, and not on their abilities (e.g., functional, cognitive). The results of this meta-synthesis were confirmed by the preliminary results of an ongoing meta-synthesis on factors influencing QoL of people with dementia (Dichter et al. 2016b).

A literature-based definition specifies dementia-specific QoL as "the multidimensional evaluation of the person-environment system of the individual, in terms of adaption to the perceived consequences of the dementia" (Ettema et al. 2005b). Based on this definition, the seven adaptive tasks of the adaption coping model (Dröes 1991) were interpreted as dementia-specific QoL dimensions: "(1) *dealing with own disability*, (2) *developing an adequate care relationship with the staff*, (3) *preserving an emotional balance*, (4) *preserving a positive self-image*, (5) *preparing for an uncertain future*, (6) *developing and maintaining social relationships, and* (7) *dealing with the nursing home environment*" (Ettema et al. 2007b). In addition, this model highlights the importance of psychosocial dimensions, which is supported by a review that showed ten psychosocial (e.g., attachment, social contact, spirituality) as well as three physical and practical domains (e.g., physical health, financial situation) of QoL judged by people with dementia (Scholzel-Dorenbos et al. 2010).

The focus on psychosocial domains and adaptation in contrast to abilities and functional domains allow the theoretical assumption that a high quality of life is also possible in the advanced stages of the dementia syndrome. This is an important perspective for affected persons and caregivers as well as researchers providing interventions to have the possibility of being effective with regard to QoL and other psychosocial outcomes. In addition, this perspective does not stigmatize the situation for people with dementia by an inevitable, continued decrease of quality of life during the course of their disease.

11.3 Measuring of Dementia-Specific Quality of Life in Nursing Homes

During the course of the theoretical developments, several dementia-specific QoL instruments have been developed, using self-ratings, proxy-ratings, or direct observations as the data sources (Ettema et al. 2005a; Scholzel-Dorenbos et al. 2007).

Dementia-specific QoL measurements are preferable to generic measures, because they focus on domains which are important for people with dementia (Gräske et al. 2012). Their items are helpful to reflect the special situation of people with dementia and the components of interventions for the care of people with dementia. These advantages of dementia-specific measurements suggest a higher potential for the responsiveness to change that these measurements have.

11.3.1 Different Measurement Perspectives

QoL is a subjective, multidimensional, and independent construct (Rabins and Black 2007). Therefore, self-reports from people with dementia are acknowledged as the gold standard for measuring QoL in this population (Brod et al. 1999; Kane et al. 2003). Although one study indicates the reliable self-rating of people with dementia in advanced stages (Hoe et al. 2005), people with severe or very severe dementia are usually not able to rate their QoL when based on standardized questions (Fuh and Wang 2006; Huang et al. 2009). The cognitive decline among people with dementia is characterized by memory and concentration deficits and results in a decrease in decision-making and communicative abilities. For people with dementia, it will be problematic to understand questions in the right way and to recall relevant situations as a basis for their ratings (Streiner et al. 2015). Therefore, the reliability and validity of QoL self-reports has been questioned in the later stages of the disease (Ettema et al. 2005a), and the use of proxy measures is preferred in advanced dementia and for longitudinal QoL evaluation (Ettema et al. 2005b).

The proxy-assessment is typically applied by family members or caregivers in a close relationship to the person with dementia. However, proxy-rated QoL measurements are associated with numerous methodological difficulties. Scores are systematically lower than self-rated QoL values (Gräske et al. 2012; Huang et al. 2009). In the last years, numerous studies investigated the difference between self and proxy-ratings and possible influencing factors (Gräske et al. 2014). Proxy-ratings by family caregivers are influenced by the burden, depression, and noncognitive symptoms (Sands et al. 2004; Fuh and Wang 2006), whereas proxy-ratings by professional caregivers are influenced by attitudes (Winzelberg et al. 2005), life satisfaction, the assessment circumstances, and the challenging behavior of people with dementia living in nursing homes (Gräske et al. 2014).

The key problem is that with regard to the proxy perspective, the subjectivity of the QoL assessment is partly lost (Thorgrimsen et al. 2003). Following Pickard and Knight (2005), two different perspectives, the proxy-patient and the proxy-proxy perspective, have to be differentiated. Based on a proxy-proxy perspective, the family or professional caregiver assesses the QoL of a person with dementia from the proxy perspective (e.g., "How do you rate her/his QoL?"). This perspective differs more from a QoL self-rating than it does from a patient-proxy perspective. In the latter perspective, a proxy assesses the QoL of a person with dementia just as he/she thinks that the person with dementia would rate him or herself (e.g., "How do you think the resident would judge her/his QoL"). Ratings of QoL from a proxy

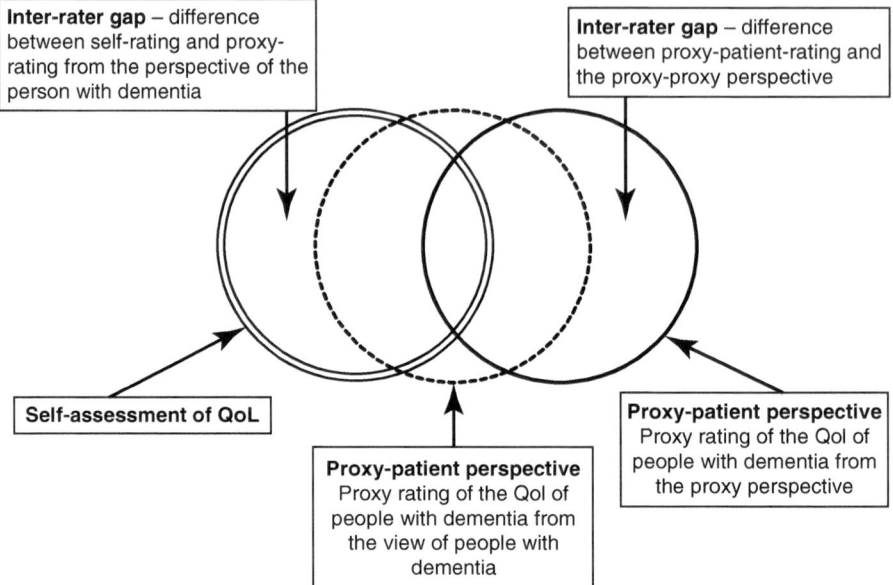

Fig. 11.2 Differentiation of proxy perspectives in the assessment of QoL based on Pickard and Knight (2005)

perspective differ more from a self-rating than ratings of a proxy taken from the patient's perspective (Pickard and Knight 2005). Figure 11.2 illustrates the different rating perspectives.

Next to self- and proxy-based measurements, a third category of measurements is based on direct observations. This means that a rater repeatedly assesses the behavior of a person with dementia for a defined period of time. Observed behavior includes, for example, interaction between people with dementia, interaction with the environment, activities and affect (Bowling et al. 2015). Observer ratings are preferred for people with late stage dementia. The major challenge is the often weak inter-rater reliability of observation-based QoL ratings (Dichter et al. 2016d).

11.3.2 Quality of Life Measurements for People with Dementia in Nursing Homes

Existing dementia-specific QoL measurements can be distinguished on the base of the mentioned perspectives. In addition, the measurements can be differentiated according to their feasibility, psychometric properties, stage of dementia, and the care setting in which the application of the measurement is possible, as well as the underlying QoL definition and domains (Ettema et al. 2005a; Ready and Ott 2003).

Hereinafter dementia-specific QoL and HRQoL measurements that can be applied in nursing homes are described. This list of measurements is based on a systematic review (Dichter et al. 2016d). Depending on the country, these measurements are applied often in research or care. We describe these QoL measurements, because in the literature all of them were reported under the term QoL measurements. Based on the definitions distinguished between QoL and HRQoL, we assign the measurements to one of these concepts.

The measurements will be described without a detailed description of their psychometric properties. For the respective psychometric properties of each measurement, several systematic reviews exist (Dichter et al. 2016d; Bowling et al. 2015).

11.3.2.1 AAIQOL (Activity and Affect Indicator Quality of Life)

The AAIQOL, which is also sometimes called "QoL-D", consists of two subscales for the assessment of activity and affect as dimensions of HRQoL. The activity scale is derived from the Pleasant Events Schedule (Teri and Logsdon 1991) and the component scale is derived from the Affect Rating scale (Lawton et al. 1996). The activity subscale covers 15 activity items inside and outside the home, and the affect subscale contains six affect items (three reflecting positive affect and three negative affect). The frequency of activities and affect is rated over 1 or 2 weeks, respectively. The AAIQOL allows a proxy-rating using both subscales and a self-rating where only the activity subscale is applied. The application of the measurement is possible for mild to severe dementia (Albert et al. 1996). Only the original US version exists; there is no linguistically validated version for other countries available (Dichter et al. 2016d).

11.3.2.2 CBS-QoL (Cornell-Brown Scale for Quality of Life in Dementia)

The CBS-QoL consists of 19 bipolar items covering four dimensions of HRQoL: positive affect, negative affect, satisfaction, and physical complaints. All 19 items are summarized in a total score. The HRQoL rating is applied by a clinician after semi-structured interviews with the respective person with dementia and a caregiver. The time frame for the HRQoL rating is the previous month (Ready et al. 2002). The clinical rating is based on joint interviews between a clinician, the person with dementia, and a caregiver and results in a questionable feasibility for the application of the CBS scale in the nursing home practice. The CBS-QoL was developed for people with mild to moderate dementia. It is available in its original US version (Ready et al. 2002) and a Spanish version (Lucas-Carrasco et al. 2013).

11.3.2.3 DEMQOL and DEMQOL-Proxy (Dementia Quality of Life Questionnaire)

The DEMQOL consists of 28 items for the self-rating version and 31 for the proxy version (Smith et al. 2005). Both measurements can be applied for the measurement of HRQoL for people with mild to moderate dementia (proxy version: mild to severe dementia). The self-rating version allows the assessment of the HRQoL domains daily activities, memory positive emotion, and negative emotion. With the proxy version, the domains functioning and emotion can be assessed. Both versions are applied during an interview. The proxy version was developed for the assessment by caregivers. Both DEMQOL versions were originally developed in England (Smith et al. 2005). Both versions were translated to German (Berwig et al. 2009) and Spanish (Lucas-Carrasco et al. 2010).

11.3.2.4 H.I.L.DE (Heidelberg Instrument for the Assessment of Quality of Life in Dementia)

H.I.L.DE. is a QoL measurement for people with mild to severe dementia in nursing homes. It is mainly based on proxy-rating; however, for some items, self-rating or observations are required (Becker et al. 2005, 2011). H.I.L.DE. contains 48 QoL indicators which allow the assessment of the following domains: medical care and perceived pain, living environment, activities, social relations, emotions, and life satisfaction. An advantage of H.I.L.DE. is the presence of competence groups (mild dementia, moderate dementia, severe dementia with somatic disabilities, severe dementia with Behavioral and Psychological Symptoms of Dementia (BPSD)), which facilitate the interpretation of H.I.L.DE. results. Unfortunately, QoL rating based on H.I.L.DE. is very time-consuming, thus the application is not recommended in research. For the application in clinical practice, shorter measurement versions are under development. Apart from the original German version, no further version exists for any other country.

11.3.2.5 QoL-AD (Quality of Life in Alzheimer's Disease)

The QoL-AD is a 13-item scale for the assessment of HRQoL in people with Alzheimer's disease (Hylla et al. 2016). The QoL-AD has two versions; one is completed by self-rating and one by the caregiver (proxy-rated). When both self and proxy versions are used, a weighted composite score is calculated by giving greater weight (2:1) to the self-rating in relation to the proxy-rating. The QoL-AD results in a score that ranges from 13 to 52, with higher scores indicating a higher QoL (Logsdon et al. 1999, 2002). The QoL-AD items cover the following HRQoL domains: physical health, mental health, social and functional abilities, social contacts, financial situation, and overall QoL. The scale was primarily developed for the HRQoL ratings of people living in their own home with mild to severe dementia. In addition, a QoL-AD nursing home version is available (see below). But the original 13-item version is also applied in nursing homes.

The QoL-AD is the most often used dementia-specific HRQoL measurement in research (Bowling et al. 2015), and the self-rating version demonstrated almost satisfactory psychometric properties (Dichter et al. 2016d; Bowling et al. 2015). In contrast, the proxy version is also applied in a number of studies, but we have only insufficient information on its psychometric properties (Dichter et al. 2016d). In addition, it is unclear whether the items have to be rated from a proxy-proxy or patient-proxy perspective.

There are translated versions of the QoL-AD available for Great Britain (Selai et al. 2001b), Brazil (Novelli et al. 2005), Taiwan (Fuh and Wang 2006), Japan (Matsui et al. 2006), Mandarin (Lin Kiat Yap et al. 2008) and Cantonese China (Chan et al. 2011), France (Wolak et al. 2009), Spain (Gomez-Gallego et al. 2014), Turkey (Akpinar and Kücükgüclü 2012), and Portugal (Barrios et al. 2013).

11.3.2.6 QoL-AD NH (Quality of Life in Alzheimer's Disease Nursing Home Version)

The Qol-AD nursing home version is based on the original 13-item version, which is also used for people with mild to severe dementia (Logsdon et al. 1999). For the adaption to the nursing home setting, two of the original 13 items were deleted, four items were added, and the wording of three items was changed (Edelman et al. 2005). As in the case of the original version, there is a self and a proxy version available for the QoL-AD NH. Based on the 15 items, the scale' total score ranges between 15 and 60, with higher scores indicating a higher QoL. In addition to the US version, a German translation of the measurement is obtainable (Dichter et al. 2016e).

11.3.2.7 QOLAS (Quality of Life Assessment Schedule)

The QOLAS is a dementia-specific measurement for the individualized QoL rating of people with mild to moderate dementia (Selai et al. 2001a). The QOLAS has five domains: physical, psychological, social relationships/family, activities, and cognitive-related QoL. The QOLAS is applied during a semi-structured interview where people with dementia have to rate their current score and their target score on a scale from 0 to 5. Apart from the original British version, no other version is available. Currently, a linguistically validated German version is under development (Dichter et al. 2013).

11.3.2.8 ADRQL (Alzheimer Disease-Related Quality of Life)

The ADRQL is a proxy-rated HRQoL measurement for people with mild to severe dementia (Rabins et al. 1999). It is available in several versions with 40 to 48 items. These items cover the HRQoL dimensions social interaction, awareness of self, feelings and mood, enjoyment of activities, and response to surroundings. The proxy-ratings are applied by family caregivers or professional caregivers. These ratings are based on observations during the previous 2 weeks. In addition to the original US version, translated and adapted versions are available for Switzerland (Menzi-Kuhn 2006) and Japan (Yamamoto et al. 2000). The Japanese version is called AD-HRQL-J or QLDJ. This Japanese version consists of 20 translated ADRQL and four new developed items.

11.3.2.9 DCM (Dementia Care Mapping)

DCM is a dementia-specific QoL measurement that is based on structured proxy observations (Kitwood and Bredin 1992). By means of observing different behaviors, the dimensions activity, well-being, and quality of care were assessed. The observation procedure differs depending on the research questions or the reasoning in clinical practice. In general, observations take place at 5 min intervals over 4 or 5 h. The domain's activity and quality of care result in frequency and percentage scores. For the domain well-being, a six response option scale results in a range between +5 (well-being) and −5 (ill-being). In addition to the English language version, several translations, e.g., to German, Dutch, and Norwegian, exist.

11.3.2.10 OQOLD (Observing Quality of Life in Dementia) and OQOLDA (Observed Quality of Life in Dementia Advanced)

The OQOLD version for mild to moderate and the OQOLDA version for severe dementia are observation-based proxy QoL measurements that were developed in the USA (Edelman et al. 2007). With both measurements, six items on verbal cues and indicators of engagement as well as affect (OQOLD) or subtle signs of positive and negative affect and engagement (OQOLDA) were observed. To facilitate the most accurate observation, a professional caregiver with a close relationship to the person with dementia is most appropriate. The observation ratings were based on a seven-point scale ranging from −3 (extremely pleasant experience) to +3 (extremely unpleasant experience). No version in a language other than the US version exists.

11.3.2.11 QoL-D (Quality of Life for Dementia)

The proxy-based QoL-D was developed in Japan (Terada et al. 2002). It consists of 31 items which cover the six QoL domains positive affect, negative affect and actions, ability of communication, restlessness, attachment with others, and spontaneity and activity. All items are to be answered on a four-point scale based on the present judgment of the proxy-rater. No version in a language other than Japanese is available (Dichter et al. 2016d).

11.3.2.12 QUALID (Quality of Life in Late-Stage Dementia Scale)

The QUALID allows QoL in particular for the assessments of institutionalized people with severe or very severe dementia (Weiner et al. 2000). The measurement is based on Lawton's model (Lawton 1991) and covers positive and negative emotions, discomfort and satisfaction. The 11 items were based on proxy observations during the previous week. The five-point response scale for each item results in a total score from 11 to 55, lower scores indicate a higher QoL. In addition to the original US version (Weiner et al. 2000), translated versions are available for Sweden (Falk et al. 2007), Spain (Garre-Olmo et al. 2010), Norway (Mjorud et al. 2014), and Germany (Brandenburg 2013).

11.3.2.13 QUALIDEM

QUALIDEM is a proxy-based measurement that consists of two consecutive versions (Ettema et al. 2007a, 2007b). The 37-item version for people with mild to severe dementia covers nine QoL domains: care relationship, positive affect, negative affect, restless tense behavior, positive self-image, social relations, social isolation, feeling at home, and having something to do. Thus, the QUALIDEM is the only dementia-specific instrument that enables assessment of the QoL domains of "care relationship" and "feeling at home." Both domains are important for people with dementia who live in nursing homes. The 18-item version for people with very severe dementia covers the same QoL domains with the expectations of positive self-image, feeling at home, and having something to do. All items are rated based on the observations of the previous 2 weeks by one or more professional caregivers with a close relationship to the person with dementia. Since 2016, a definition and complementary items are available for each QUALIDEM item. Based on this, the QoL rating by one professional caregiver is possible (Dichter et al. 2016a, 2016c). Without the application of the item definitions and examples, the collaborative QoL rating by two or more caregivers is recommended (Ettema et al. 2007b).

The developers of the measurement advise the calculation of subscale scores and not a measurement total score. This will result in a QoL-profile which shows more information than only one total score. Nevertheless, it can sometimes be necessary to calculate an overall score for statistical or methodological reasons. In such cases, the authors recommend calculating an overall QUALIDEM score with additional computations for each subscale. This approach is demonstrated in several studies (Dichter et al. 2015; Verbeek et al. 2010).

In addition to the original Dutch version, translations to English and German are available. In a recent study, the German version was applied with a seven-response scale demonstrating a sufficient item distribution and inter-rater reliability (Dichter et al. 2016c).

11.3.2.14 Vienna List
The Vienna List allows HRQoL proxy-ratings for people with severe dementia (Porzsolt et al. 2004). The measurement consists of 40 items which reflect the dimensions communication, negative affect, bodily contact, aggression, and mobility. These items were answered with a five-point response scale based on the present situation. As a result, a score for each HRQoL is calculated. The original version was developed in Austria, and no other version is available.

11.3.2.15 Selection of the Appropriate Measurement
The illustrated measurements demonstrate the heterogeneity of the available dementia-specific measurements. Therefore, the question of how to select the most appropriate measurement for the right purpose is of great interest. Currently, no general recommendation exists for this question. We recommend a stepwise process according to the following questions. These questions are based on a recommendation by Schölzel-Dorenbos and colleagues (2007) and supplemented by our own experience:

- Which concept should be measured, i.e. overall QoL or HRQoL?
- Which measurement perspective is preferred and possible, i.e. self, proxy, observation?
- At what stage of dementia are the people who are to be assessed?
- In which setting should the instrument be applied?
- Does the measurement assess the QoL domains that the research question or intervention focus on? Does the measurement assess the QoL domains that the professional caregiver focuses on in clinical practice?
- How are the psychometric properties of the measurements in question? In particular, how are the feasibility and the reliability of these measurements?
- Should the QoL values of people with dementia be comparable to those of significant others (family caregivers, professional caregivers)?

After answering these questions, an appropriate measurement selection is possible. However, it has to be noted that despite the large number of measurements, the ideal scale is often missing. In such cases we believe that the questions 5 and 6 are the most important ones. This applies in particular in cases where the QoL of people with dementia and without dementia has to be assessed (e.g., studies evaluating the effectiveness of a psychosocial intervention on the whole nursing home population). The usage of a dementia-specific measurement is also appropriate in such cases, because of the advantages of these measurements regarding the feasibility and the validity for people with dementia. The validity of these measurements for people without dementia has to be assessed by the user in advance (question 5).

11.4 Factors Associated with Quality of Life of People with Dementia in Nursing Homes

QoL is seen as a major outcome in dementia research and practice since it is important to know which factors are associated with the QoL of people with dementia. The knowledge of factors which affect QoL in a positive way will be helpful for the development of interventions in research and also for the creation of daily care and the care environment in nursing homes.

Unfortunately, little is known about this issue. Moreover, the indiscriminate use of the terms QoL and HRQoL has led to the fact that factors associated with QoL or HRQoL or both are discussed together without distinction. In the literature, both concepts are discussed under the name QoL, irrespective of which specific measurement was applied. In the following summary, we have omitted such a separation/distinction. Nevertheless, we recommend a separation and clear definition of QoL and HRQoL in future studies and reviews.

11.4.1 Personal Characteristics Not Related to Dementia

The first systematic review (Beerens et al. 2013) demonstrated that only two individual studies identified an association between objective sociodemographic characteristics (e.g., age, gender, marital status) of people with dementia and their QoL. In one study, female gender was negatively associated with QoL (Barca et al. 2011), and one other study showed a negative association between QoL and being widowed (Samus et al. 2005). The majority of studies included in the mentioned review identified no association. This seems to be logical based on the theoretical approaches mentioned earlier in this chapter. The investigation of associations between nonobjective individual characteristics like self-image and QoL would seem to be of interest for future studies.

11.4.2 Personal Factors Related to Dementia

Cognition of people with dementia is only related to QoL if this QoL is proxy-based. No association was found between self-rated QoL and cognition (Beerens et al. 2013). Similar results are obtained for severity of dementia. Only statistically weak results indicate a negative association between severity of dementia and proxy-assessed QoL. Knowledge about a possible association between self-rated QoL and severity of dementia is missing. Only ambiguous evidence exists also for a relationship between dependencies in activities of daily living and QoL. Thus, a number of studies demonstrated a negative association and others did not (Beerens et al. 2013). In summary, these results highlight that QoL does not necessarily depend on the direct effects of dementia-related personal factors. As mentioned above, this is an important conclusion as it provides options for action for caregivers and researcher. Based on theoretical assumptions, it might be possible to maintain or promote QoL of people with dementia in all stages of the disease.

11.4.3 Challenging Behavior and Mood

Challenging behavior like agitation or apathy was negatively related to proxy-rated QoL (Beerens et al. 2013). This seems to be logical if we interpret challenging behavior as an indication of stress, unmet needs, or a low QoL. This view is also in the line with several studies which apply the frequency or severity of challenging behavior as an outcome in intervention studies and as an indicator for a good or bad QoL (Chenoweth et al. 2009; Dichter et al. 2015). However, all available studies were based on a proxy perspective and not on a self-perspective. It would be helpful to investigate the relationship on challenging behavior and self-rated QoL in future studies to confirm this interpretation.

Several studies investigated a possible association between depressive symptoms and anxiety as indicators of mood (Beerens et al. 2013). These studies demonstrated a clear negative relationship between depressive symptoms and self-rated QoL. The identified association between depressive symptoms and proxy-rated QoL was not linear. Wetzels et al. (2010) and González-Salvador et al. (2000) showed a stronger association between depressive symptoms and proxy-rated QoL for people with mild to moderate dementia than for people with advanced dementia. The presence of anxiety demonstrated in one study a negative association with self-reported QoL of people with dementia (Hoe et al. 2006). Two other studies showed no association (Samus et al. 2005; Nakanishi et al. 2011). The results on the two indicators of mood (depressive symptoms and anxiety) suggest the possibility to improve or maintain the QoL of people with dementia by interventions which target the reduction of depressive symptoms or anxiety.

11.4.4 Pain

Only a few studies have investigated the association between pain and QoL of people with dementia. Here, observed pain (Beer et al. 2010) and also self-rated pain (Torvik et al. 2010) were related to a lower self-rated QoL. Based on these results and the evidence on insufficient pain medication in nursing homes, further research on interventions dealing with that topic is needed.

11.5 Effectiveness of Non-pharmacological Interventions Targeting Quality of Life of People with Dementia in Nursing Homes

Although QoL is widely applied as outcome, only a few studies demonstrate a positive effect on the QoL of people with dementia. A meta-analysis demonstrated ambiguous results on quality of life (Cooper et al. 2012). The authors categorized the interventions in nursing homes, based on the study availability, in three groups: cognitive simulation therapy in groups, staff training, and individualized care planning as well as other interventions. In summary, only one study investigating a group-based cognitive stimulation in comparison to usual care demonstrated in a reanalysis an effect on self-reported QoL of people with dementia (Spector et al. 2003). All other studies identified no effect or a tendency toward a negative effect on QoL (Chenoweth et al. 2009; Dichter et al. 2015).

This unsatisfactory evidence has to be explained with the need for the further improvement of interventions. However, most importantly, it is necessary to increase the theoretical knowledge on QoL of people with dementia and to improve the available dementia-specific QoL measurements. This is an important task which is also described in the UK MRC framework for the development and evaluation of complex interventions (Craig et al. 2013). All currently available measurements need further scientific work. Two findings which underline this fact are the lack of studies on the sensitivity to change of dementia-specific QoL measurements and the lack of well-designed cross-cultural adaptations and reliability studies (Dichter et al. 2016d).

11.6 Summary

QoL is a person-centered outcome for people with dementia, and it is widely applied in dementia research and care. However, it is also an outcome which raises several questions. The currently available theoretical approaches have changed their interpretation and definition of QoL of people with dementia. The stronger focus on psychosocial QoL domains in contrast to abilities and functional domains describes the view of people with dementia more. This shift has only partly influenced the available dementia-specific QoL measurements and their evaluation (Missotten et al. 2016). This fact makes it difficult to select the most appropriate measurement, although several measurements are available. Therefore, we recommend further research on the psychometric properties of the available measurements. This means particularly a methodologically strong linguistic validation and evaluation of reliability, a validity evaluation based on theoretical models and predefined hypotheses, and studies for the determination of the sensitivity to change and interpretability.

There is also a need for more longitudinal studies investigating associations between dementia-specific self-rated QoL and possible influencing factors (e.g., personal dementia-related factors, pain, mood and depression, care models). More evidence about factors which influence the QoL of people with dementia and methodological stronger measurements will help to improve the quality and possibility to identify effective non-pharmacological interventions which maintain or promote the QoL of people with dementia.

References

Akpinar B, Kücükgüclü Ö (2012) The Validity and Reliability of the Turkish version of the Quality of life scale for patients with Alzheimer's Disease (Qol-AD). J Neurol Sci 29(3):554–565

Albert SM, Del Castillo-Castaneda C, Sano M, Jacobs DM, Marder K, Bell K, Bylsma F, Lafleche G, Brandt J, Albert M, Stern Y (1996) Quality of life in patients with Alzheimer's disease as reported by patient proxies. J Am Geriatr Soc 44(11):1342–1347

Barca ML, Engedal K, Laks J, Selbaek G (2011) Quality of life among elderly patients with dementia in institutions. Dement Geriatr Cogn Disord 31(6):435–442

Barrios H, Verdelho A, Narciso S, Goncalves-Pereira M, Logsdon R, de Mendonca A (2013) Quality of life in patients with cognitive impairment: validation of the Quality of Life-Alzheimer's Disease scale in Portugal. Int Psychogeriatr 25(7):1085–1096

Becker S, Kruse A, Schroder J, Seidl U (2005) The Heidelberg instrument for the assessment of quality of life in dementia (H. I. L. DE.) – dimensions of quality of life and methods of organization. Z Gerontol Geriatr 38(2):108–121

Becker S, Kaspar R, Kruse A (2011) The Heidelberg instrument for the assessment of quality of life in dementia (H. I. L. DE.). Hans Huber, Bern

Beer C, Flicker L, Horner B, Bretland N, Scherer S, Lautenschlager NT, Schaper F, Almeida OP (2010) Factors associated with self and informant ratings of the quality of life of people with dementia living in care facilities: a cross sectional study. PLoS One 5(12):e15621

Beerens HC, Zwakhalen SM, Verbeek H, Ruwaard D, Hamers JP (2013) Factors associated with quality of life of people with dementia in long-term care facilities: a systematic review. Int J Nurs Stud 50:1259–1270

Berwig M, Leicht H, Gertz HJ (2009) Critical evaluation of self-rated quality of life in mild cognitive impairment and Alzheimer's disease – further evidence for the impact of anosognosia and global cognitive impairment. J Nutr Health Aging 13(3):226–230

Bowling A, Rowe G, Adams S, Sands P, Samsi K, Crane M, Joly L, Manthorpe J (2015) Quality of life in dementia: a systematically conducted narrative review of dementia-specific measurement scales. Aging Ment Health 19(1):13–31

Brandenburg H (2013) Quality of life of people with severe dementia in nursing oases: empirical results and methodological implications. Z Gerontol Geriatr 46(5):417–424

Brod M, Stewart AL, Sands L, Walton P (1999) Conceptualization and Measurement of Quality of Life in Dementia: The Dementia Quality of Life Instrument (DQoL). Gerontologist 39(1):25–35

Chan I, Chu L, Lee P, Li S, Yu K (2011) Effects of cognitive function and depressive mood on the quality of life in Chinese Alzheimer's disease patients in Hong Kong. Geriatr Gerontol Int 11:69–76

Chenoweth L, King MT, Jeon YH, Brodaty H, Stein-Parbury J, Norman R, Haas M, Luscombe G (2009) Caring for Aged Dementia Care Resident Study (CADRES) of person-centred care, dementia-care mapping, and usual care in dementia: a cluster-randomised trial. Lancet Neurol 8(4):317–325

Cooper C, Mukadam N, Katona C, Lyketsos CG, Ames D, Rabins P, Engedal K, de Mendonca Lima C, Blazer D, Teri L, Brodaty H, Livingston G, World Federation of Biological Psychiatry – Old Age T (2012) Systematic review of the effectiveness of non-pharmacological interventions to improve quality of life of people with dementia. Int Psychogeriatr 24(6):856–870

Craig P, Dieppe P, Macintyre S, Michie S, Nazareth I, Petticrew M (2013) Developing and evaluating complex interventions: the new Medical Research Council guidance. Int J Nurs Stud 50(5):587–592

Dichter MN, Halek M, Dortman O, Meyer G, Bartholomeyczik S (2013) Measuring the quality of life of people with dementia in nursing homes in Germany – the Study Protocol for the Qol-Dem Project [Die Erfassung der Lebensqualität von Menschen mit Demenz in stationären Altenpflegeeinrichtungen in Deutschland – Studienprotokoll des Qol-Dem Projektes]. GMS Psychosoc Med 10:Doc07. doi:10.3205/psm000097

Dichter MN, Quasdorf T, Schwab CG, Trutschel D, Haastert B, Riesner C, Bartholomeyczik S, Halek M (2015) Dementia care mapping: effects on residents' quality of life and challenging behavior in German nursing homes. A quasi-experimental trial. Int Psychogeriatr:1–18

Dichter MN, Schwab CG, Meyer G, Bartholomeyczik S, Halek M (2016a) Item distribution, internal consistency and inter-rater reliability of the German version of the QUALIDEM for people with mild to severe and very severe dementia. BMC Geriatr 16:126

Dichter MN, Ettema TP, Schwab CGG, Meyer G, Bartholomeyczik S, Halek M, Dröes RM (2016b) QUALIDEM – user guide. DZNE/VUmc, Witten/Amsterdam

Dichter MN, Schwab CG, Meyer G, Bartholomeyczik S, Halek M (2016c) Linguistic validation and reliability properties are weak investigated of most dementia-specific quality of life measurements-a systematic review. J Clin Epidemiol 70:233–245

Dichter MN, Palm R, Halek M, Bartholomeyczik S, Meyer G (2016d) Die Lebensqualität von Menschen mit Demenz. Eine Metasynthese basierend auf den Selbstäußerungen von Menschen mit Demenz. In: Kovács L, Kipke R, Lutz R (eds) Lebensqualität in der Medizin. Konzept, Praxis, Ethik. Springer VS, Wiesbaden, pp 287–302

Dichter MN, Wolschon EM, Meyer G, Kopke S (2016e) Cross-cultural adaptation of the German version of the quality of life in Alzheimer's disease scale – nursing home version (QoL-AD NH). Int Psychogeriatr 28:1–2

Dröes RM (1991) In movement; on psychosocial care for elderly people with dementia [In beweging: over psychosociale hulpverlening an demente ouderen]. PhD Thesis. Vrije Universiteit

Edelman P, Fulton BR, Kuhn D, Chang CH (2005) A comparison of three methods of measuring dementia-specific quality of life: perspectives of residents, staff, and observers. Gerontologist 45 Spec No 1(1):27–36

Edelman P, Fulton BR, Kuhn D, Gallager M, Dougherty J, Long C (2007) Assessing quality of life across the dementia continuum. Two new observational tools for researchers and practitioners. Azheimer's Care Today 8(4):332–343

Ettema TP, Dröes RM, de Lange J, Mellenbergh GJ, Ribbe MW (2005a) A review of quality of life instruments used in dementia. Qual Life Res 14(3):675–686

Ettema TP, Dröes RM, de Lange J, Ooms ME, Mellenbergh GJ, Ribbe MW (2005b) The concept of quality of life in dementia in the different stages of the disease. Int Psychogeriatr 17(3):353–370

Ettema TP, Dröes RM, de Lange J, Mellenbergh GJ, Ribbe MW (2007a) QUALIDEM: development and evaluation of a dementia specific quality of life instrument – validation. Int J Geriatr Psychiatry 22(5):424–430

Ettema TP, Dröes RM, de Lange J, Mellenbergh GJ, Ribbe MW (2007b) QUALIDEM: development and evaluation of a dementia specific quality of life instrument. Scalability, reliability and internal structure. Int J Geriatr Psychiatry 22(6):549–556

Falk H, Persson LO, Wijk H (2007) A psychometric evaluation of a Swedish version of the Quality of Life in Late-Stage Dementia (QUALID) scale. Int Psychogeriatr 19(6):1040–1050

Federal Ministry of Education and Research (2011) Age has future. Research agenda of the federal goverment for demographic change [Das Alter hat Zukunft. Forschungsagenda der Bundesregierung für den demographischen Wandel]. Federal Ministry of Education and Research, Bonn

Fuh JL, Wang SJ (2006) Assessing quality of life in Taiwanese patients with Alzheimer's disease. Int J Geriatr Psychiatry 21(2):103–107

Garre-Olmo J, Planas-Pujol X, Lopez-Pousa S, Weiner MF, Turon-Estrada A, Juvinya D, Ballester D, Vilalta-Franch J (2010) Cross-cultural adaptation and psychometric validation of a Spanish version of the Quality of Life in Late-Stage Dementia Scale. Qual Life Res 19(3):445–453

Gibson MC, Carter MW, Helmes E, Edberg AK (2010) Principles of good care for long-term care facilities. Int Psychogeriatr 22(7):1072–1083

Gomez-Gallego M, Gomez-Garcia J, Ato-Garcia M (2014) Confirmatory factor analysis of the quality of life in Alzheimer's disease scale in patients with Alzheimer's disease. Exp Aging Res 40(3):266–279

Gonzalez-Salvador T, Lyketsos CG, Baker A, Hovanec L, Roques C, Brandt J, Steele C (2000) Quality of life in dementia patients in long-term care. Int J Geriatr Psychiatry 15(2):181–189

Gräske J, Fischer T, Kuhlmey A, Wolf-Ostermann K (2012) Quality of life in dementia care – differences in quality of life measurements performed by residents with dementia and by nursing staff. Aging Ment Health 16(7):819–827

Gräske J, Meyer S, Wolf-Ostermann K (2014) Quality of life ratings in dementia care – a cross-sectional study to identify factors associated with proxy-ratings. Health Qual Life Outcomes 12(1):177

Haberstroh J, Hampel H, Pantel J (2010) Optimal management of Alzheimer's disease patients: Clinical guidelines and family advice. Neuropsychiatr Dis Treat 6:243–253

Hays RD, Reeve BB (2010) Measurement and modeling of health-related quality of life. In: Killewo J, Heggenhougen HK, Quah SR (eds) Epidemiology and demography in public health. Academic Press, San Diego, pp 195–102

Hoe J, Katona C, Roch B, Livingston G (2005) Use of the QOL-AD for measuring quality of life in people with severe dementia – the LASER-AD study. Age Ageing 34(2):130–135

Hoe J, Hancock G, Livingston G, Orrell M (2006) Quality of life of people with dementia in residential care homes. Br J Psychiatry 188:460–464

Huang HL, Chang MY, Tang JS, Chiu YC, Weng LC (2009) Determinants of the discrepancy in patient- and caregiver-rated quality of life for persons with dementia. J Clin Nurs 18(22):3107–3118

Hylla J, Schwab CGG, Isfort M, Halek M, Dichter MN (2016) Internal consistency and construct validity of the quality of life in Alzheimer's disease (QoL-AD) proxy – a secondary data analysis. Pflege. doi:10.1024/1012-5302/a000xxx

Institute P-COR – Patient-Centered Outcomes Research Institute (2015) National priorities for research and research agenda. Patient-Centered Outcomes Research Institute, Washington

Jonker C, Gerritsen DL, Bosboom PR, Van der Steen JT (2004) A model for quality of life measures in patients with dementia: Lawton's next step. Dement Geriatr Cogn Disord 18(2):159–164

Kane RA, Kling KC, Bershadsky B, Kane RL, Giles K, Degenholtz HB, Liu J, Cutler LJ (2003) Quality of life measures for nursing home residents. J Gerontol A Biol Sci Med Sci 58:M240–M248

Karimi M, Brazier J (2016) Health, health-related quality of life, and quality of life: what is the difference? PharmacoEconomics 34:645–649

Kitwood T, Bredin K (1992) A new approach to the evaluation of dementia care. J Adv Health Nurs Care 1(5):41–60

Lawton MP (1991) A multidimensional view of quality of life in frail elders. In: Birren EJ, Lubben EJ, Rowe CJ, Deutchman ED (eds) The concept and measurement of quality of life in the frail elderly. Academic Press, San Diego, pp 3–23

Lawton MP (1994) Quality of life in Alzheimer disease. Alzheimer Dis Assoc Disord 8(Suppl 3):138–150

Lawton MP, Van Haitsma K, Klapper J (1996) Observed affect in nursing home residents with Alzheimer's disease. J Gerontol B Psychol Sci Soc Sci 51(1):P3–14

Lin Kiat Yap P, Yen Ni Goh J, Henderson LM, Min Han P, Shin Ong K, Si Ling Kwek S, Yi Hui Ong E, Pui Kwan Loh D (2008) How do Chinese patients with dementia rate their own quality of life? Int Psychogeriatr 20(3):482–493

Logsdon RG, Gibbons LE, McCurry SM, Teri L (1999) Quality of life in Alzheimer's disease: patient and caregiver reports. J Ment Health Aging 5(1):21–32

Logsdon RG, Gibbons LE, McCurry SM, Teri L (2002) Assessing quality of life in older adults with cognitive impairment. Psychosom Med 64(3):510–519

Lucas-Carrasco R, Lamping DL, Banerjee S, Rejas J, Smith SC, Gomez-Benito J (2010) Validation of the Spanish version of the DEMQOL system. Int Psychogeriatr 22(4):589–597

Lucas-Carrasco R, Gomez-Benito J, Rejas J, Ott BR (2013) The Cornell-Brown scale for quality of life in dementia: Spanish adaptation and validation. Alzheimer Dis Assoc Disord 27(1):44–50

Matsui T, Nakaaki S, Murata Y, Sato J, Shinagawa Y, Tatsumi H, Furukawa TA (2006) Determinants of the quality of life in Alzheimer's disease patients as assessed by the Japanese version of the Quality of Life-Alzheimer's disease scale. Dement Geriatr Cogn Disord 21(3):182–191

Menzi-Kuhn C (2006) [Quality of life of people with dementia in institutional care] Lebensqualität von Menschen mit Demenz in stationären Langzeitpflegeeinrichtungen. Master in Nursing Science Unpublished Masterthesis, Maastricht University

Missotten P, Dupuis G, Adam S (2016) Dementia-specific quality of life instruments: a conceptual analysis. Int Psychogeriatr 28:1245–1262

Mjorud M, Kirkevold M, Rosvik J, Engedal K (2014) Principal component analysis of the Norwegian version of the quality of life in late-stage dementia scale. Dement Geriatr Cogn Disord 37(5–6):265–275

Moniz-Cook E, Vernooij-Dassen M, Woods R, Verhey F, Chattat R, De Vugt M, Mountain G, O'Connell M, Harrison J, Vasse E, Droes RM, Interdem MO (2008) A European consensus on outcome measures for psychosocial intervention research in dementia care. Aging Ment Health 12(1):14–29

Nakanishi K, Hanihara T, Mutai H, Nakaaki S (2011) Evaluating the quality of life of people with dementia in residential care facilities. Dement Geriatr Cogn Disord 32:39–44

Novelli MM, Dal Rovere HH, Nitrini R, Caramelli P (2005) Cross-cultural adaptation of the quality of life assessment scale on Alzheimer disease. Arq Neuropsiquiatr 63(2A):201–206

O'Rourke HM, Duggleby W, Fraser KD, Jerke L (2015) Factors that affect quality of life from the perspective of people with dementia: a metasynthesis. J Am Geriatr Soc 63(1):24–38

Pickard AS, Knight SJ (2005) Proxy evaluation of health-related quality of life: a conceptual framework for understanding multiple proxy perspectives. Med Care 43(5):493–499

Porzsolt F, Kojer M, Schmidl M, Greimel ER, Sigle J, Richter J, Eisemann M (2004) A new instrument to describe indicators of well-being in old-old patients with severe dementia – the Vienna List. Health Qual Life Outcomes 2:10

Rabins PV, Black BS (2007) Measuring quality of life in dementia: purposes, goals, challenges and progress. Int Psychogeriatr 19(3):401–407

Rabins PV, Kasper JD, Kleinman L, Black BS, Patrick DL (1999) Concepts and methods in the development of the ADRQL: an instrument for assessing health-related quality of life in persons with Alzheimer's disease. J Ment Health Aging 5:33–48

Ready RE, Ott BR (2003) Quality of Life measures for dementia. Health Qual Life Outcomes 1:11

Ready RE, Ott BR, Grace J, Fernandez I (2002) The Cornell-Brown scale for quality of life in dementia. Alzheimer Dis Assoc Disord 16(2):109–115

Samus QM, Rosenblatt A, Steele C, Baker A, Harper M, Brandt J, Mayer L, Rabins PV, Lyketsos CG (2005) The association of neuropsychiatric symptoms and environment with quality of life in assisted living residents with dementia. Gerontologist 45:19–26

Sands LP, Ferreira P, Stewart AL, Brod M, Yaffe K (2004) What explains differences between dementia patients' and their caregivers' ratings of patients' quality of life? Am J Geriatr Psychiatry 12(3):272–280

Scholzel-Dorenbos CJ, Ettema TP, Bos J, Boelens-van der Knoop E, Gerritsen DL, Hoogeveen F, de Lange J, Meihuizen L, Droes RM (2007) Evaluating the outcome of interventions on quality of life in dementia: selection of the appropriate scale. Int J Geriatr Psychiatry 22(6):511–519

Scholzel-Dorenbos CJ, Meeuwsen EJ, Olde Rikkert MG (2010) Integrating unmet needs into dementia health-related quality of life research and care: introduction of the Hierarchy Model of Needs in Dementia. Aging Ment Health 14(1):113–119

Selai C, Trimble MR, Rossor MN, Harvey RJ (2001a) Assessing quality of life in dementia: preliminary psychometric testing of the quality of life assessment schedule (QOLAS). Neuropsych Rehabil 11:219–243

Selai C, Vaughan A, Harvey RJ, Logsdon R (2001b) Using the QOL-AD in the UK. Int J Geriatr Psychiatry 16(5):537–538

Smith SC, Lamping DL, Banerjee S, Harwood RH, Foley B, Smith P, Cook JC, Murray J, Prince M, Levin E, Mann A, Knapp M (2005) Measurement of health-related quality of life for people with dementia: development of a new instrument (DEMQOL) and an evaluation of current methodology. Health Tech Assess NHS R&D HTA Program 9(10):1–110

Spector A, Thorgrimsen L, Woods B, Royan L, Davies S, Butterworth M, Orrell M (2003) Efficacy of an evidence-based cognitive stimulation therapy programme for people with dementia: randomised controlled trial. Br J Psychiatry 183:248–254

Streiner DL, Norman GR, Cariney J (2015) Health measurement scales: a practical guide to their development and use. Oxford University Press, Oxford

Terada S, Ishizu H, Fujisawa Y, Fujita D, Yokota O, Nakashima H, Haraguchi T, Ishihara T, Yamamoto S, Sasaki K, Nakashima Y, Kuroda S (2002) Development and evaluation of a health-related quality of life questionnaire for the elderly with dementia in Japan. Int J Geriatr Psychiatry 17(9):851–858

Teri L, Logsdon RG (1991) Identifying pleasant activities for Alzheimer's disease patients: the pleasant events schedule-AD. Gerontologist 31(1):124–127

Thorgrimsen L, Selwood A, Spector A, Royan L, de Madariaga LM, Woods RT, Orrell M (2003) Whose quality of life is it anyway? The validity and reliability of the Quality of Life-Alzheimer's Disease (QoL-AD) scale. Alzheimer Dis Assoc Disord 17(4):201–208

Torvik K, Kaasa S, Kirkevold O, Rustoen T (2010) Pain and quality of life among residents of Norwegian nursing homes. Pain Manag Nurs 11:35–44

Verbeek H, Zwakhalen SM, van Rossum E, Ambergen T, Kempen GI, Hamers JP (2010) Dementia care redesigned: effects of small-scale living facilities on residents, their family caregivers, and staff. J Am Med Dir Assoc 11(9):662–670

Weiner MF, Martin-Cook K, Svetlik DA, Saine K, Foster B, Fontaine CS (2000) The quality of life in late-stage dementia (QUALID) scale. J Am Med Dir Assoc 1(3):114–116

Wetzels RB, Zuidema SU, de Jonghe JF, Verhey FR, Koopmans RT (2010) Determinants of quality of life in nursing home residents with dementia. Dement Geriatr Cogn Disord 29(3):189–197

WHO (1995) The world health organization quality of life assessment (WHOQOL): position paper from the World Health Organization. Soc Sci Med 41(10):1403–1409

WHO (2014) Constitution of the World Health Organization. Basic documents of the Word Helath Organization, Geneva

Wilson IB, Cleary PD (1995) Linking clinical variables with health-related quality of life. A conceptual model of patient outcomes. JAMA 273(1):59–65

Winzelberg GS, Williams CS, Preisser JS, Zimmerman S, Sloane PD (2005) Factors associated with nursing assistant quality-of-life ratings for residents with dementia in long-term care facilities. Gerontologist 45 Spec No 1(1):106–114

Wolak A, Novella JL, Drame M, Guillemin F, Di Pollina L, Ankri J, Aquino JP, Morrone I, Blanchard F, Jolly D (2009) Transcultural adaptation and psychometric validation of a French-language version of the QoL-AD. Aging Ment Health 13(4):593–600

Yamamoto N, Abe T, Yamada Y, Yamazato C, Amemiya H, Sugishita C, Kamata K (2000) Reliability and validity of a Japanese quality of life scale for the elderly with dementia. Nurs Health Sci 2:69–78

End-of-Life Care and Advance Care Planning in Dementia

12

Stephen J. O'Connor

Abstract

This chapter will describe the principles of end-of-life care in relation to the care and management of people with dementia and highlight why end-of-life care is such an important aspect of care in many nursing homes. It will explain why accurate end-of-life prognostication is difficult in so many cases and look at residents', family members' and healthcare professionals' perspectives on the delivery of end-of-life care to those with dementia in nursing homes. The chapter will also address some of the challenges commonly affecting people with dementia at the end of life, the importance of timely assessment and symptom management and some of the tools which can be used to assist carers in the assessment, planning, delivery and evaluation of the care provided in such circumstances. The contribution of specialist palliative and end-of-life care input from the local hospital, hospice or family physician will also be discussed. Finally, the importance of identifying resident's concerns, anxieties and wishes as early as possible will be considered so that care at the end of life can be delivered as far as possible in line with their wishes, and their physical, psychological, emotional, social and spiritual needs are addressed in a timely and appropriate manner as life draws to an end.

Keywords

Dementia • End-of-life care • Palliative care • Terminal care • Dying • Nursing home • Care home • Residential home • Principles • Symptoms • Advance care planning • Advance directives • Family and resident perspectives • Healthcare professional perspectives

S.J. O'Connor
England Centre for Practice Development, Canterbury Christ Church University, Canterbury, UK
e-mail: stephen.oconnor@canterbury.ac.uk

© Springer International Publishing AG 2017
S. Schüssler, C. Lohrmann (eds.), *Dementia in Nursing Homes*,
DOI 10.1007/978-3-319-49832-4_12

12.1   Introduction

It has been estimated that more than 35 million people are living with dementia across the world at the present time. This figure is expected to rise to 65 million people by the year 2030 and more than 115 million by the year 2050 (Ryan et al. 2012). No wonder, then, that dementia has been described as one of the greatest palliative and public health challenges facing our generation at the present time (Hospice UK 2015). Unlike many other illnesses or long-term medical conditions, it is likely that a person diagnosed with dementia will die much sooner than antici- pated in many cases and often more quickly than people with other life-threatening or long-term conditions including most cancers. Guhne et al.'s (2006) study of 1692 elderly people over 75 years of age in Leipzig, Germany, showed that people with dementia were more likely to die sooner than those who did not have dementia with a mean survival time of 3.1 years compared to 4.0 years ($p < 0.001$) when other disease, demographic and lifestyle factors were taken into account.

   Even more worryingly, another study of people with Alzheimer's disease by Monroe et al. (2012) showed that advanced dementia was negatively associated with opioid use and other symptom control measures, meaning that those who are less able to speak for themselves receive less analgesia and have pain and other disturbing symptoms assessed less frequently or comprehensively during the last weeks or months of life than those with other conditions. As a consequence of these and many other scientific studies, the European Association for Palliative Care (EAPC) has called for greater collaboration between policy makers and health and social care professionals working in the fields of primary care, gerontology, long- term residential care, hospice and specialist palliative or end-of-life care services, so that end-of-life care for people with dementia can be better coordinated and the quality, safety and person-centredness of care improved both in Europe and else- where (EAPC 2013; Van-de-Steen 2014). They initially identified the need for improvements in eight domains of care as a result of the initial rounds of their Delphi study of 64 international experts from 23 different countries though later adding three more, namely, prognostication and timely recognition of dying, educa- tion of the healthcare team; and societal and ethical issues. The last of these is beyond the scope of this chapter, but we shall discuss the other two in addition to those directly concerned with care delivery in residential or care home settings as illustrated in Fig. 12.1. First, however, it is necessary to define what is meant by end-of-life care and how this term differs from other terms such as palliative or terminal care.

12.2   What Is End-of-Life Care?

End-of-life care is a separate and distinctive entity from palliative or terminal care and has its origins in the work of Lorenz et al. (2006, 2008) although use of the term is somewhat ambiguous (O'Connor 2016; Froggatt and Payne 2006; Frogatt et al. 2009). It has been variously used to describe the care given to patients in the last

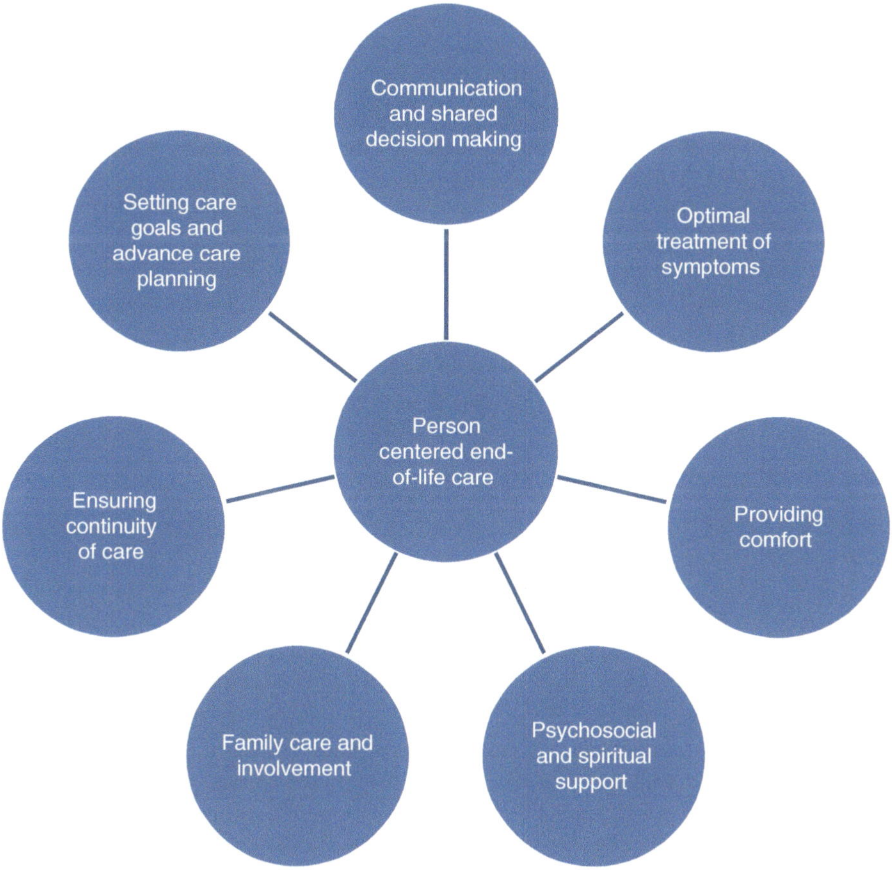

Fig. 12.1 The clinical domains for end-of-life care when caring for people with dementia (Adapted from the EAPC 20014, van der Steen et al. (2014))

year, months, weeks or days of life, with the UK's Gold Standards Framework describing it as care for those 'nearing' the end of life, although they go on to suggest that it includes care given in the 'final year' of life to people with an end-stage illness, though acknowledging that it is not always easy to ascertain when this is the case (http://www.goldstandardsframework.org.uk/ accessed 14th October 2016). The UK's National Council for Palliative Care (2006) describes it as a general rather than a medical term which may be easily understood by the general public to mean that stage where death can no longer be prevented by treatment and when death is likely to occur sooner rather than later.

Physical indicators in addition to worsening cognitive function include increasing weight loss, frailty, poor appetite, breathlessness or recurring respiratory problems, poor performance status, increasing dependence on others for assistance with activities of daily living, and potentially, increased pain or other terminal symptoms (Porock and Oliver 2007; Porock et al. 2005). The UK's National Council for

Palliative Care (2006) suggests, therefore, that it is 'the provision of supportive and palliative care in response to the assessed needs of patient and family during the last phase of life', adding that 'in most cases, end-of-life care does not begin earlier than 1 year before death' (p3), though no evidence is provided to support this somewhat arbitrary timescale. Generally speaking, however, this does provide a good indicator as to when end-of-life care should begin for most people, although the cognitive problems associated with dementia mean that end-of-life (or advance care) planning should be started even earlier whilst the individual is still able to make their end-of-life preferences known and be involved in discussions about what these should include to ensure that the individual's wishes are respected and optimal end-of-life care provided. Hence, knowing when a person is likely to die and recognizing that this is actually happening are crucial in determining the quality of death experienced by a person with dementia as we shall now discuss.

12.3   Prognostication and Timely Recognition of Dying

One of the reasons why care is often suboptimal for those dying of or with dementia is related to the lack of a clear terminal trajectory such as those commonly observed in cancer or other life-limiting conditions including heart failure, chronic obstructive pulmonary disease and renal failure. It is important to note however, that people affected by dementia may also have one or more of these conditions in addition to dementia, so comorbidity is an important 'confounding variable' when trying to ascertain whether a resident is approaching the end of their life and how soon this may happen. As a consequence, attempts to predict the remaining lifespan for people with dementia over periods longer than a few weeks or months have met with varying degrees of success since it can be extremely difficult to predict a person's remaining lifespan with certainty, even though there may be indicators like those listed above, that the individual has entered the final stage of their life. Mitchell et al. (2010), for instance, tried to estimate life expectancy in advanced dementia using the ADEPT score so that nursing home residents could be transferred to hospice to die in a timelier and more appropriate manner; but even when completed at the bedside on a regular basis, the tool only marginally improved nurses' ability to identify which residents with advanced dementia were likely to die within 6 months and plan their management and care accordingly. This is not surprising for dementia masks many of the signs and symptoms which might otherwise indicate terminal malaise, and residents are usually unable to voice their thoughts or feelings at this time, even though they may have some months left to live.

Conversely, another study by Casarett et al. (2012) of 21074 patients admitted to hospice over a two-and-a-half-year period found that 5562 or 26.4% of those transferred to hospice died within 7 days of admission though this means that nurses and other staff overestimated the individual's remaining lifespan in three out of every four cases since the prognostic model used in the study, which included the Palliative Performance Scale (PPS) score, proved to be less reliable for people with advanced dementia and those with cancer than conditions such as end-stage pulmonary disease. This clearly demonstrates that end-of-life prognostication for people with dementia is extremely difficult in comparison to other client groups, whether in the long or short term, and another study by Powers and Watson (2008) highlights this difficulty, given that long-term residential care in a nursing home needs to balance the need to help residents live active 'normal' lives for as long as possible whilst recognising that at some point in the future, they will need to prepare the individual, though more usually his or her family members, for the imminent likelihood of death. It is a very imprecise science however, and even though dementia is a leading cause of death in American nursing homes, its terminal nature is often forgotten, in spite of the fact that 54.8% of the 323 nursing home residents admitted with advanced dementia in one study died within 18 months of their admission, often within 6 months of that date, though the reasons leading to death may have been multifactorial (Mitchell et al. 2009). This does mean however, that a palliative approach to the management of nursing home residents may be justified from the point of admission to the care home, and there is some evidence that this can actually improve outcomes for such patients no matter how soon they might die once there.

12.4   Optimal Treatment of Symptoms in People with Dementia

In spite of the EAPC's recommendations, and indications that dementia is at last becoming a policy priority in many countries, the palliative and end-of-life needs of those affected by dementia in all its forms are only now beginning to be fully understood. Studies show that end-of-life care has often been suboptimal, even in those countries with established policies, guidelines or national frameworks for people with the condition. Often, this is because policies or guidelines focus on long-term care needs to the detriment of end-of-life care planning or, as the EAPC suggests, there is too little emphasis on staff education, training or the competencies needed to deliver better end-of-life care and more comprehensive services to those dying with dementia (van der Steen et al. 2014). This is regrettable since everyone affected by dementia is likely to benefit from palliative approaches to care which emphasize comfort, dignity, autonomy, meticulous symptom assessment and timely intervention at every stage of their illness, and not just in their final weeks or months of life. In spite of this, many still fail to receive adequate support from palliative or end-of-life care specialists whilst living in long-term care institutions, and still fewer during the crucial, early stages of the illness when meaningful conversations may still be had about the individual's anxieties, fears and preferences regarding the end of life before they become unable to express these for themselves more fully (Karikari-Martin et al. 2012).

12.4.1 The Consequences of Poor Prognostication in Dementia Care

The consequences of poor prognostication are clear. Sampson et al. (2011), for instance, demonstrated that people with advanced dementia often receive inadequate end-of-life care, and although small in scope ($n = 32$), this longitudinal study showed that patients with dementia tended to be frailer than others, with over half (62%) having decubitus ulcers and almost half dying during the 6-month follow-up period, indicating that they should have had an advance care plan in place and been in receipt of intensive end-of-life interventions to promote quality of life in the time which remained to them (O'Connor 2016). Sampson et al.'s study showed that 95% (or 30 of the 32 patients) had unalleviated pain on those occasions when it was assessed by the research team, and only seven had an advance care plan in place at the time of their death, all of which had been written by a carer or close family member rather than the individual themselves. This suggests that the individual's wishes, needs and preferences with regard to end-of-life care planning had not been considered whilst they were still capable of playing a central role in those decisions or leading the discussion themselves.

Mitchell et al.'s (2009) longitudinal study of 323 nursing home residents identified weight loss and malnutrition as the commonest problems identified in residents with advanced dementia with 85.8% of their sample being unable to maintain an adequate dietary intake to preserve their health or functional status effectively. It is generally understood that parenteral feeding is unlikely to improve on this situation, yet many in the advanced stages of dementia are subjected to futile interventions which have little hope of benefit. Infections too are also common, with 52.6% of residents experiencing a severe febrile event requiring medical intervention during Mitchell et al.'s study, and 41.1% developing pneumonia at some point during this time. After adjusting for age, sex and disease duration, the 6-month mortality rate for residents who developed pneumonia after admission in this study was 46.7%; 44.5% for those developing another form of infection, and 38.6% for those suffering from malnourishment or weight loss, indicating that the commonest symptoms are not necessarily the most life threatening, though all of them offer significant challenges to the care of residents and none should be ignored. Other distressing symptoms include dyspnea (46.0%) and pain severe enough to warrant hospitalization (39.1%), a visit to the emergency room, or other 'burdensome' interventions such as tube feeding or invasive medical tests in 40.7% of residents. Interestingly, the likelihood of these interventions occurring was reduced when family members or other proxies, such as nursing home staff or attending physicians, had a good understanding of the individual's likely prognosis and recognized these problems as indicators that death was imminent, allowing symptomatic management to take place without subjecting the individual to futile measures which were not warranted.

12.4.2 Polypharmacy and Inappropriate Interventions at the End of Life

Parsons et al. (2011, 2012) reviewed the medication administration records of 115 care home residents and followed this up with a review of 112 and 105 records on two subsequent occasions. They found that approximately two-thirds of residents (66.9%) were regularly given one or more psychotropic medications with more than 10% of these having a high sedative load score at baseline (12.2%) increasing to

14.3% at time points 2 and 3. Multiple drugs, particularly serotonin reuptake inhibitors, were most often used, but these drugs are not without side effects, including sedation. The study confirmed the findings of others such as Blass et al. (2008) and Tjia et al. (2010) which question the overuse of non-beneficial medications in advanced dementia as death approaches which may be compounded by the lack of monitoring for adverse effects. Thus, whilst medication undoubtedly does have a role to play in advanced dementia, it should always be tailored to the primary goals of care, namely the provision of supportive and palliative care in response to the assessed needs of both the patient and family members during the last phase of life. This encompasses continuous assessment, goal setting, the promotion of comfort and dignity, psychosocial and spiritual care, good symptom management, excellent communication and family involvement in the delivery of coordinated care which is person centred and based on shared decision making (EAPC 2013).

Notwithstanding this, Teno et al.'s (2011a) survey of 486 family members asked to provide information on the circumstances surrounding the death of a loved one from dementia showed that 10.8% died with a feeding tube in place, 17.6% made a decision not to use a feeding tube and 71.6% reported playing no part in any decision about the use of feeding tubes. Of those respondents whose family member died with a feeding tube in place, 13.7% stated that there was no discussion with them about its insertion, and 41.6% of those who did reported that the discussion lasted less than 15 minutes. The risks associated with the use of feeding tubes were not discussed with them in one-third of cases, and 12.6% felt pressured into agreeing to a feeding tube by the attending physician. Residents were physically restrained in order to insert the feeding tube in 25.9% of cases and pharmacologically restrained in 29.2%. It is perhaps not surprising therefore, that family members of individuals who died with a feeding tube in place were less likely to rate the care of their loved one as being 'excellent' at the end of life than those treated more palliatively without a feeding tube in place.

Pressure to insert a feeding tube in patients with advanced dementia is by no means unusual, with Sharp and Shega (2009) demonstrating that 56% of the healthcare professionals questioned in their survey ($n = 326$) had recommended the insertion of a percutaneous endoscopic gastrostomy (PEG) tube to feed patients with advanced dementia and dysphagia in spite of there being little evidence that they improve nutritional status or increase the survival of the individual concerned, and the fact that they did not consider them useful in improving functional status or the individual's quality of life! Interestingly, whilst almost 40% believed, in spite of their own negative experiences, that tube insertion was the recommended standard of care which should be offered routinely, only 15% believed it should be, and only 11% said that they would want such an intervention themselves if they had advanced dementia. Another study in Italy by Toscani et al. (2013) looking at the incidence and intensity of prevailing signs and symptoms, treatment options and the use of measures such as parenteral hydration and nutrition, cardiopulmonary resuscitation and life-sustaining drugs in the last 48 hours of life showed that 71.6% were inappropriately prescribed antibiotics, i.e. with curative rather than palliative (symptomatic) intent, and 29 patients (20.5%) were receiving nasogastric or percutaneous endoscopic feeding. Two-thirds (66.6%) were receiving parenteral fluids which may worsen pulmonary symptoms at the time of death, and 58.2% were immobilized by bed rails or other immobilizers which in the view of most experts, including many in the EAPC, should not be used at all. Not surprisingly, therefore, almost half the residents in the study were suffering from decubitus ulcers at the time of data collection, and many had still not formally been classified as dying during the final 48 hours of their life, meaning that palliative or end-of-life measures which may have been needed were not being considered, including those of a psychosocial or spiritual nature within hours of death.

Apart from the human cost of such failures, futile interventions on dying residents are unlikely to be cost effective, though relatively few economic analyses of the cost of these interventions have been conducted (Goldfeld et al. 2012). In contrast, when a palliative approach to end-of-life care is taken, a relatively limited pharmacopeia of palliative drugs can elicit better patient outcomes when titrated to individual symptoms and assessment of need which, together with the provision of information and advice about the dying process, can improve care outcomes for those who are dying and, equally importantly, those who remain behind after the death. The range of drugs needed for the effective management of terminal symptoms is even more limited, and can usually be managed quite effectively in the care home with the support of the resident's GP or community nursing team, especially when given via the preferred routes, namely, oral, transdermal, sublingual, buccal or subcutaneous (via a 'butterfly cannula' or syringe driver) as follows (see Table 12.1):

12.4.3 The Benefits of Hospice or Specialist Palliative Care Interventions at the End of Life in Dementia

A study by Miller et al. (2012) of 4344 nursing home residents with advanced dementia demonstrated that residents referred for hospice or specialist palliative care support as part of their management plan were prescribed fewer inappropriate medications, invasive intravenous or intramuscular injections, feeding tubes or intravenous fluids, and received better management of agitation and restlessness in the last 90 days of their life in comparison to those not referred to palliative care services. They also had a lower incidence of dyspnea, meaning that respiratory symptoms were better controlled; and they were also less likely to die in an unfamiliar hospital environment as opposed to the care environment they were most familiar with and felt safest in.

A controlled study of 538 family members of people officially certified as dying of dementia by Teno et al. (2011b) found that those being treated with palliative intent by hospice service services (260 or 48.3% of their sample) reported fewer unmet needs or concerns regarding the quality of the care received, and felt that the process of dying had been more peaceful for their loved one, accentuating the importance of recognizing when a resident with dementia is actively dying in order to determine the most appropriate management plan for the final weeks or months

Table 12.1 Drugs commonly used at the end of life in dementia

Opioid drugs for pain	Alfentanil Rapifen® Buprenorphine for non-malignant pain unresponsive to non-opioid analgesics, e.g. BuTrans® Transtec® Diamorphine hydrochloride Fentanyl – as transdermal patches for severe chronic pain, e.g. Fencino® Fentalis® Matrifen® Mezolar® Opiodur® Osmanil® Tilofyl® Victanyl® Fentanyl – as sublingual tablets for breakthrough pain in adults where other short-acting opioids are unsuitable, e.g. Abstral® Recivit® Fentanyl – as buccal tablets/lozenges for breakthrough pain in adults where other short-acting opioids are unsuitable, e.g. Effentora® Actiq® Morphine sulphate MST® MXL® Oramorph® Sevredol® Zomorph® Oxycodone hydrochloride OxyNorm® OxyContin®
Anti-emetics (to control nausea and vomiting)	Metoclopramide Haloperidol Cyclizine Levomepromazine
Anxiolytics (to control anxiety)	Diazepam Lorazepam Midazolam
Anti-muscarinic/antispasmodic drugs (to control terminal secretions or muscle spasms)	Hyoscine hydrobromide Hyoscine butylbromide Glycopyrronium bromide

of their life. Parsons et al. (2012) found that older people in general, and specifically care home residents, are at greater risk of suboptimal or inappropriate prescribing behaviors by physicians in comparison to other client groups. The researchers found that over two-fifths of older people with dementia residing in six residential care homes in England were prescribed at least one potentially inappropriate medication at each point in their data collection which might normally be discontinued as life draws to a close had a more palliative approach been taken.

12.5 Continuity of Care

End-stage dementia patients commonly have a relatively long terminal trajectory which invariably makes it difficult for families to sustain adequate levels of care in the home, even with intensive home care support. They are also often older than those with other conditions and are more likely to experience problems or symptoms which remain unalleviated or difficult to manage. As a consequence, about 70% of people with dementia in the USA die in a nursing home or similar long-term care facility (Fulton et al. 2011), highlighting the importance of transitions in care for those diagnosed with any form of dementia as the therapeutic intent of their management plan changes. For the most part, admission to a long-term facility should indicate a change in focus towards palliative or end-of-life priorities including the prevention and management of infection, appropriate treatment of comorbidities, evidence-based decisions around tube feeding or artificial hydration and excellent pain and symptom assessment (Ryan et al. 2012). However, this focus group study of healthcare professionals' opinions about the end-of-life care needs of patients with dementia only elicited the opinions of staff working in acute hospitals, hospices and primary care, rather than those nursing homes or long-term care facilities where the majority of people affected with dementia die. This is by no means unique to the USA however, since another international study conducted in five European countries (the Netherlands, Belgium, England, Scotland and Wales) by Houttekier et al. (2010) found that the commonest place of death for someone with dementia was a nursing home or similar long-term care facility, although there was considerable variation across different countries. As in the USA, home deaths were comparatively rare, with the highest proportion occurring in Belgium (11% of dementia-related deaths), whilst hospital death was commonest in Wales where 46% of people affected by dementia died.

It is worth noting however, that new approaches to the management of advanced dementia in the community are being posited, and within the UK, advocated as an effective and cost efficient way of managing projected increases in the number of people living with dementia by the middle of the century. Treloar et al. (2009) have described a novel service predicated around the provision of the necessary equipment, medicines management expertise, nutritional and social care needs, as well as improved funding support to commission necessary informal care in the home. The study showed that the needs of people with advanced dementia can be improved and sustained until the time of death where good palliative care can be provided in the community, and posit that enabling the individual to die at home may lead to few bereavement issues and more satisfactory outcomes than transferring the individual to other settings, though the provision of comprehensive domiciliary care for people affected by dementia is still quite scarce.

12.5.1 Hospice Versus Residential Home Deaths

Great efforts are being made in the UK and many other countries to improve access to hospices for people with dementia, but whilst people with dementia undoubtedly benefit from hospice or specialist palliative care at the end of their life, it is questionable whether transferring patients to a hospice in the days or weeks before death is useful or appropriate. The transfer of individuals who may be confused, distressed or frightened to an unfamiliar care setting with a new set of carers prior to death may increase their anxiety and accentuate behavioral or psychological problems in the individual concerned. There is little evidence to date which indicates that the benefits residents derive from admission to a hospice in the last weeks or days of life outweigh these drawbacks, partly because hospices have been slow to embrace those with dementia or study the impact and effectiveness of these admissions. Many of the studies conducted to date, especially within the USA and countries with similar health insurance systems, have been developed with a view to minimizing the cost of sending residents to a hospice who may not actually die within the very narrow timeframe (usually 5–10 days) for which reimbursement for end-of-life care is made; whereas in other countries such as the UK, it has been difficult to find hospices willing to accept people with dementia until relatively recently.

12.5.2 Education and Training for Care Home Staff

Mitchell et al. (2010) concluded from their study that end-of-life care should be provided on the basis of the individual's presenting symptoms, known preferences and identified care goals rather than on the basis of estimated life expectancy alone. This is also why specific educational programs have been developed to equip nursing home staff with the confidence and skills to deliver good palliative and end-of-life care in the place which residents most recognize under the care of staff who know them best. Such programmes have proven effective in enabling nursing homes to deliver end-of-life care without transferring residents to hospital or a hospice at the end of their lives with support instead, from specialist palliative care practitioners from the local hospice, generic community nursing services; or the resident's family physician who are all vital in achieving this goal (Hart and O'Connor 2013), particularly when comorbidities are present (Bartlett and Clarke 2012). Appropriate training prevents inappropriate admissions to hospital or the need to transfer residents to a hospice at the end of their life, increases the resident's visibility to palliative care services locally, and ensures that pain and other symptoms are successfully managed by home care staff whilst reducing futile or unnecessarily invasive interventions. It also increases the confidence, competence and job satisfaction of residential or care home staff (Hart and O'Connor 2013). These authors delivered a series of educational workshops based on a national training framework, 'The Six Steps Programme' to staff in 12 residential or long-term care settings. The program succeeded in reducing the number of inappropriate referrals to emergency rooms or acute hospitals, reducing the number of hospital deaths and increasing the number of residents dying in the place of their choosing, usually their nursing home; increasing the prescription of anticipatory drugs necessary to manage common symptoms at the end of life, and increasing the number and proportion of care home residents having an advance care plan and 'do not attempt cardiopulmonary resuscitation' (DNACPR) order in place in those care homes completing the program. It also increased the number of care homes maintaining an end-of-life care register so that residents could benefit from better integrated health and social care services. The contents, which were delivered to senior care home staff as well as a 1-day workshop for other carers consisted of the following:

- Step 1 – Necessary discussions as the end-of-life approaches
- Step 2 – How to assess, plan and review end-of-life care
- Step 3 – How to coordinate end of-life-care for residents with other service providers
- Step 4 – How to deliver high-quality end-of-life care
- Step 5 – How to provide care in the last days of life (terminal care)
- Step 6 – Care for the individual, family members and home staff after death

The program also included the services of a facilitator to assist care home managers in implementing policies and procedures to improve end-of-life care in the care home, carry out a self-assessment of the quality of care provided, and audit the impact of the program in respect of the outcomes already discussed above. Interestingly however, an 18-month follow-up telephone interview study of care home staff carried out in the same homes found that the most beneficial skills acquired from the program was the ability to conduct those very necessary end-of-life discussions either on admission to the home, or when it became apparent that residents were entering the final year of life, and it is to this important domain that we now turn.

12.6   Communication, Shared Decision Making and Advance Care Planning

Until relatively recently, patients and families were rarely informed of the terminal nature of dementia, and advance care planning discussions were therefore comparatively rare. However, even in the current day, patients' and family members' understanding and perceptions about dementia and its likely prognosis are not as well informed as they should be (Thuné-Boyle et al. 2010). Their in-depth interview study of the end-of-life care needs of 20 family carers and 21 professional carers of people with advanced dementia was conducted in an acute hospital in London, but it outlines the situation which many of those being admitted to a nursing or residential home face. Hence, admission to the home provides opportunity to discuss at greater depth, information concerning the likely progress of the condition and the need to prepare for the eventuality of death, particularly when so many are known to die within a year of their arrival. Interestingly, their study also showed that those told about the long-term impact of their dementia early in its progress were more likely to discuss or initiate discussions about their wishes and preferences than those who were not, suggesting that it is sometimes care professionals' anxieties about such discussions which hold them back from initiating them, with proxy decision making by family carers or professional carers being much more common where residents are not given adequate information about the likely course of their illness. Poor communication can also limit the quality of care, with negative attitudes and an unwillingness to share information acting as a barrier to the provision of person-centered, safe and effective care at the end of life, effective symptom control, adequate need assessments and the mis-attribution of behavior in those unable to express what they are feeling and experiencing so that signs which might otherwise indicate pain, distress, discomfort or other symptoms are attributed to a decline in cognitive function or challenging behaviour if this has been a feature of their condition hitherto (Chang et al. 2009).

12.6.1 Engaging in Advance Care Planning Discussions

Advance care planning is a process by which people can plan ahead to make decisions and express preferences about what they would wish to happen with their care and treatment if they lost the capacity to make decisions for themselves and other people had to make decisions for them. It usually takes place in the context of an anticipated deterioration in an individual's physical or cognitive state, but may be made by anyone at any time. In some countries, they have the force of law, and professionals are obliged to adhere to them in so far as it is reasonably possible to do so. The fact that they are a process is important, as many people may find them too emotionally draining to complete in one long interview. It is perfectly acceptable for them to be drawn up over a period of time, as the individual feels more able to talk about the implications that advance care planning brings to mind, but they also have a right not to be forced into making a plan or feeling coerced into doing so by healthcare professionals or family members. The UK Alzheimer's Society website points out that 'it should not be assumed that people with dementia are unable to make their own decisions' and argue that 'individuals should be supported in making their own advance care plans where possible'. On the same page, they also point out that 'the rate at which a person's condition deteriorates varies from individual to individual' whilst reminding us that 'with earlier diagnosis and new treatments, people are retaining capacity for longer', a fact often forgotten in the overwhelmingly negative policy and media coverage given to Alzheimer's and other forms dementia (https://www.alzheimers.org.uk/site/scripts/documents_info.php?documentID=1036 accessed 14th October 2016). Knowing how and when to initiate discussions about the end of life is fraught with difficulty however, and the skill and preparation of the individual concerned in doing so is paramount. On the whole, it is better to allow the resident to settle into the home or come to terms with their worsening condition before broaching the subject, and the following are also important considerations to be borne in mind when engaging in such a discussion or ascertaining whether the individual would like to:

- Choose the right time – be guided by the resident, family member or their changing condition but start as early as possible whilst the resident has as much capacity to think and respond for themselves as possible.
- Choose the right place – this should be quiet, relaxed and unthreatening without risk of being disturbed or being overheard, though conversely, some residents may prefer to talk about such issues more generally within a group setting, perhaps as a facilitated discussion in the first instance which may be less intense or threatening.
- Consider whether or not a family member or members should be present – this depends on the health and legal competence of the resident, but also known responsibilities and dynamics within the family support system. Include the partner, spouse or those family members who the resident has indicated are most important to them only.
- Consider whether there is a need for one or more family members to have lasting power of attorney in the event that the resident's cognitive state/legal capacity deteriorates quickly.
- Make sure that the results of the process and your rationale for including others in the discussion(s) are noted prominently in the resident's care record where they can be found easily in the event of the resident's deterioration.

Having discussed the advance care plan with the resident and/or family members, it is also important to review this regularly to ascertain whether the resident's wishes have changed, whether other medical conditions have been diagnosed in the interim period, and whether the advance care plan remains appropriate in that situation. It should also take account of changes in the resident's social and physical environment, such as the loss of a spouse or other significant person and any other changes that may impact on the relevance of the advance care plan. Any new decisions will be shaped by the resident's current capacity to make their own decisions and whether or not, in the absence of family or friends to help, a 'best interest' decision needs to be made on their behalf by the GP, other physicians or care home staff caring for the resident as they deteriorate.

12.6.2 When Is It Best to Initiate Advance Care Planning Discussions?

No matter what the resident's condition when admitted to the home, or the day to day fluctuations in their physical, emotional or cognitive state, it should be remembered that dementia is progressive and ultimately fatal, so early discussions about the resident's wishes and preferences, together with those of family members, can be useful if the individual wishes to talk about them. Dementia is often associated with other conditions in its advanced stages, which make effective communication and discussion of these priorities even harder. Infection, dehydration, physical malaise, hypercalcemia and the required use of opiate analgesics may all cloud the individual's legal capacity and decision making ability (Burton et al. 2012).

Likewise, verbal communication skills including verbal learning, verbal memory and verbal fluency may vary considerably with these conditions with or without the effect of the underlying dementia, so it is important that individuals are at least given an opportunity to have such a discussion if they feel able to and want to.

Many situations and circumstances may avail themselves in a residential or care home to initiate discussions with a resident or residents about what they would wish for at the end of their life or lives. These may include admission to the care home as stated above but may also be relevant on the resident's return from an inpatient admission to hospital for treatment of a comorbid condition or 'routine' surgery such as a knee or hip replacement. It may also be pertinent if a resident's condition worsens or deteriorates, as their care needs and functional status change, or following the death of a family member or other resident. It is also, of course, opportune to do so when a resident prompts the question themselves; but in the event that they do not, the following questions may prove helpful depending on the capacity of the individual to answer them:

- Tell me how you feel about your illness?
- Tell me what the most important things are to you at the moment?
- Who is/are the most important person/people in your life at the moment?
- Do they know you feel that way about them?
- Who would you like to care for you as your health gets worse?
- How would you like to be cared for as your health gets worse?
- Are your worried about your future?
- What worries you about your future?
- What things give you hope for the future?
- What things would give you most comfort as your life draws to a close?
- Where would you like to be cared for as your life draws to a close?
- Who would you like to care for you as your life draws to a close?
- What worries you most about dying?
- What might make the process of dying more bearable for you?
- Who would you like to be with you when you die?
- Where would you prefer to die?
- What would you like to happen to you in the immediate aftermath of your death?
- What preferences do you have about your funeral arrangements?
- What would you like to happen to your property when you die?
- Who would you like to implement your last wishes after your death?
- Have you discussed these issues with them?
- Would you like to discuss these issues with them?
- Would you like help discussing these issues with them?

The individual's readiness and ability to answer these questions will vary enormously depending on the extent to which their dementia and other comorbidities are affecting them. If residents are palpably unable or unwilling to discuss anything beyond the here and now as represented in the first of these questions, then it is perfectly alright to end the conversation there for days, weeks or months, until such a time as their situation changes and it is advisable to start the process again or they clearly indicate they are ready to do so. The main thing is not to become discouraged by residents' or family members' seeming reluctance, and not to persist when this becomes apparent. A semi-structured interview study by Stewart et al. (2011) showed that both care home staff and family members held positive opinions towards advance care planning in general, but contemplating the death of a resident or family member is understandably more difficult. Other barriers include the dementia itself, and the residents' ability to communicate their wishes, as well as fear or reluctance among less senior members of the care home staff. On the whole, such discussions seemed to go better the earlier and more natural or 'matter of fact' they seemed, stressing that the purpose of the discussion(s) is to identify the residents' and families' wishes only, and reassuring both that the care plan could be reviewed or changed at any time in the light of new circumstances. The involvement of staff known to residents and family members was also key to their success, as was the degree of training staff received, and the confidence they felt in undertaking this important aspect of end-of-life care. It is perfectly okay, however, for staff to opt out of this task permanently or on a temporary basis if they feel the need to do so, or as their personal experience of death and dying dictate.

If the resident's condition is such that the questions are too long or complicated, these can be broken down into shorter, closed questions as demonstrated in Chap. 9: 'Communication in Dementia', and simpler words such as 'scared' used instead of 'worried'. It may also be necessary to phrase questions in the present tense and only deal with how the individual is feeling in the 'here and now' where appropriate, bearing in mind that only the first of the questions listed above may be relevant to someone who has lost all sense of time in the advanced stages of the illness. More details about advance care planning, including an online open learning program which includes units on legal and ethical issues, advance care planning in dementia and advance care planning in residential homes developed by the author in collaboration with local GPs, hospice, care home and community nurses, can be found in: https://www.canterbury.ac.uk/health-and-wellbeing/advance-care-planning/home. aspx (O'Connor et al. 2016).

Conclusion

This chapter has outlined the principles of end-of-life care in so far as they relate to the care and management of people with dementia with particular reference to the dementia-specific 'domains of care' developed by an international panel of experts on behalf of the European Association of Palliative Care. It has considered why end-of-life care is an important issue for everyone working in residential, nursing or long-term care homes in relation to the irreversible and progressive nature of the illness, and the fact that residents with dementia will almost certainly die with, if not from the condition. Research findings have been used to highlight the difficulties associated with end-of-life prognostication in dementia and the propensity for people with dementia to die more suddenly and unexpectedly than other care home residents. These demonstrate the need to consider end-of-life care planning as soon as possible where indicated, and the commonest physical signs that death is likely to occur soon have been highlighted. The benefits derived from taking a palliative approach to the care of such residents have been discussed, and the importance of open awareness contexts, improved communication, and better education for professional carers has been described with examples drawn from the author's own experience. The contribution which specialist palliative and end-of-life professionals can make to the assessment, delivery and evaluation of high-quality dementia care in long-term care settings has been evaluated in the light of research findings and the importance of identifying residents' concerns, anxieties and wishes in the form of an advance care plan explained. Practical advice about the ways in which these can be discussed has been provided, but the importance of not forcing individuals – whether residents or family members – to discuss such issues until they are ready to do so has also been highlighted. The nature of dementia is such that it may never be possible to elicit the fears, concerns and preferences of all those likely to die of dementia in residential or care homes; but the importance of aspiring to this as a means of delivering safe, effective, person-centered dementia care of the very highest quality to residents at the end of their lives has clearly been demonstrated.

References

Alzheimer's Society (2016) Decision-making and advanced planning. https://www.alzheimers. org.uk/site/scripts/documents_info.php?documentID=1036. Accessed 14 Oct 2016

Bartlett A, Clarke B (2012) An exploration of healthcare professionals' beliefs about caring for older people dying from cancer with a coincidental dementia. Dementia 11:559–565

Blass DM, Black BS, Phillips H et al (2008) Medication use in nursing home residents with advanced dementia. Int J Geriatr Psychiatry 23:490–496

Burton CZ, Twamley EW, Lee LC et al (2012) Undetected cognitive impairment and decision-making capacity in patients receiving hospice care. Am J Geriatr Psychiatry 4:306–316

Casarett DJ, Farrington S, Craig T et al (2012) The art versus science of predicting prognosis: can a prognostic index predict short-term mortality better than experienced nurses do? J Palliat Med 15:703–708

Chang E, Daly J, Johnson A et al (2009) Challenges for professional care of advanced dementia. Int J Nurse Pract 15:41–47

European Association for Palliative Care (EAPC) (2013) EAPC white paper: recommendations on palliative care and treatment of older people with Alzheimer's disease and other progressive dementias. EAPC, Brussels

Frogatt K, Vaughan S, Bernard C et al (2009) Advance care planning in care homes for older people: an English perspective. Palliat Med 23:332–338

Froggatt K, Payne S (2006) A survey of end-of-life care in care homes: issues of definition and practice. Health Social Care Community 14:341–348

Fulton AT, Rhodes-Kropf J, Corcoran AM et al (2011) Palliative care for patients with dementia in long-term care. Clin Geriatr Med 27:153–170

Goldfeld KS, Hamel MB, Mitchell SL (2012) Mapping health status measures to a utility measure in a study of nursing home residents with advanced dementia. Med Care 50:446–451

Guhne U et al (2006) Incident dementia cases and mortality. Results of the leipzig Longitudinal Study of the Aged (LEILA75+). Dement Geriatr Cogn Disord 22:185–193

Hart M, O'Connor SJ (2013) Final report of the Maidstone area 'Six Steps End of Life Care Programme' prepared for the West Kent Clinical Commissioning Group. Canterbury Christ Church University, Canterbury. ISBN 978-1-909067-22-6

Hospice UK (2015) Hospice enabled dementia care: the first steps. Hospice, London. ISBN: 978-1-871978-90-2

Houttekier D, Cohen J, Bilsen J et al (2010) Place of death of older persons with dementia. A study in five European countries. J Am Geriatr Soc 58:751–756

Karikari-Martin P, McCann JJ, Hebert LE et al (2012) Do community and caregiver factors influence hospice use at the end of life among older adults with Alzheimer disease? J Hosp Palliat Nurs 14:225–237

Lorenz KA, Shugarman LR, Lynn J et al (2006) Health care policy issues in end-of-life care. J Palliat Med 9:731–748

Lorenz KA, Lynn J, Dy SM et al (2008) Evidence for improving palliative care at the end of life: a systematic review. Ann Intern Med 148:147–W28

Miller SC, Lima JC, Mitchell SL (2012) Influence of hospice on nursing home residents with advanced dementia who received Medicare-skilled nursing facility care near the end of life. J Am Geriatr Soc 60:2035–2041

Mitchell SL, Teno JM, Kiely DK et al (2009) The clinical course of advanced dementia. N Engl J Med 361:1529–1538

Mitchell SL, Miller SC, Teno JM et al (2010) Prediction of 6-month survival of nursing home residents with advanced dementia using ADEPT vs hospice eligibility guidelines. JAMA 304:1929–1935

Monroe T, Carter M, Feldt K et al (2012) Assessing advanced cancer pain in older adults with dementia at the end-of-life. J Adv Nurs 68:2070–2078

National Council for Palliative Care (2006) End of life care strategy: the National Council for Palliative Care submission. NCPC, London

O'Connor SJ (2016) End of life care definitions and triggers for assessment: a summary and discussion of the literature. Canterbury Christ Church University, Canterbury. ISBN 978-1-909067-59-2

O'Connor SJ, Hart M, Kirk M et al (2016) Advance care planning programme. https://www.can-terbury.ac.uk/health-and-wellbeing/advance-care-planning/home.aspx. Accessed 14 Oct 2016

Parsons C, Haydock J, Mathie E et al (2011) Sedative load of medications prescribed for older people with dementia in care homes. BMC Geriatr 11:56

Parsons C, Johnston S, Mathie E et al (2012) Potentially inappropriate prescribing in older people with dementia in care homes: a retrospective analysis. Drugs Aging 29:143–155

Porock D, Parker-Oliver D (2007) Recognizing dying in nursing home residents. J Hosp Palliat Nurs 9:270–278

Porock D, Oliver DP, Zweig S et al (2005) Predicting death in the nursing home: development and validation of the 6-month Minimum Data Set Mortality Risk Index. J Gerontol A Biol Sci Med Sci 60:491–498

Powers BA, Watson NM (2008) Meaning and practice of palliative care for nursing home residents with dementia at end of life. Am J Alzheimers Dis Other Demen 28:723–733

Ryan T, Gardiner C, Bellamy G et al (2012) Barriers and facilitators to the receipt of palliative care for people with dementia: the views of medical and nursing staff. Palliat Med 26:879–886

Sampson EL, Jones L, Thune-Boyle IC et al (2011) Palliative assessment and advance care planning in severe dementia: an exploratory randomized controlled trial of a complex intervention. Palliat Med 25:197–209

Sharp HM, Shega JW (2009) Feeding tube placement in patients with advanced dementia: the beliefs and practice patterns of speech-language pathologists. Am J Speech Lang Pathol 18:222–230

Stewart F, Goddard C, Schiff R et al (2011) Advanced care planning in care homes for older people: a qualitative study of the views of care staff and families. Age Ageing 40:330–335

Teno JM, Mitchell SL, Kuo SK et al (2011a) Decision-making and outcomes of feeding tube insertion: a five-state study. J Am Geriatr Soc 59:881–886

Teno JM, Gozalo PL, Lee IC et al (2011b) Does hospice improve quality of care for persons dying from dementia? J Am Geriatr Soc 59:1531–1536

The Gold Standards Framework (2016) Introduction to the GSF. http://www.goldstandardsframe-work.org.uk/. Accessed 14 Oct 2016

Thuné-Boyle ICV, Sampson EL, Jones L et al (2010) Challenges to improving end of life care of people with advanced dementia in the UK. Dementia 9:285–298

Tjia J, Rothman MR, Kiely DK et al (2010) Daily medication use in nursing home residents with advanced dementia. J Am Geriatr Soc 58:880–888

Toscani F, Di Giulio P, Villani D et al (2013) Treatments and prescriptions in advanced dementia patients residing in long-term care institutions and at home. J Palliat Med 16:31–37

Treloar A, Crugel M, Adamis D (2009) Palliative and end of life care of dementia at home is feasible and rewarding: results from the 'Hope for Home' study. Dementia 8:335–347

Van de Steen J, Radbruch L, Hertogh C et al (2014) White paper defining optimal palliative care in older people with dementia: a Delphi study and recommendations from the European Association for Palliative Care. Palliat Med 28:197–209

Depression in Nursing Home Residents with Dementia

13

Debby L. Gerritsen, Roeslan Leontjevas, Sandra A. Zwijsen, Raymond T.C.M. Koopmans, and Martin Smalbrugge

Abstract

Depression is highly prevalent in nursing home residents with dementia. It is negatively associated with a resident's well-being and daily functioning and can increase mortality and use of healthcare services. However, depression is under-recognized and undertreated in nursing homes. To improve depression management in residents with dementia, procedures are necessary for detecting and diagnosing depression and for psychosocial and pharmacological treatment strategies. Furthermore, monitoring the effects of any given treatment is highly important for improving depression management. This chapter describes a care program that encompasses procedures for a multidisciplinary approach to depression recognition and treatment in residents with dementia and that has been developed and shown to be effective in the nursing home setting. Additionally, the chapter goes into requirements for adequate depression management and implementing care programs in daily practice.

D.L. Gerritsen, PhD (✉)
Department of Primary and Community Care, Centre for Family Medicine,
Geriatric Care and Public Health, Radboud University Medical Centre,
Huispost 117 ELG, P.O. Box 9101, 6500 HB Nijmegen, The Netherlands
e-mail: Debby.Gerritsen@radboudumc.nl

R. Leontjevas
Faculty of Psychology and Educational Sciences, Open University of the Netherlands,
Heerlen, The Netherlands

S.A. Zwijsen • M. Smalbrugge
Department of General Practice and Elderly Care Medicine, Amsterdam Public Health
Research Institute, VU University Medical Center, Amsterdam, The Netherlands

R.T.C.M. Koopmans
Department of Primary and Community Care, Centre for Family Medicine,
Geriatric Care and Public Health, Radboud University Medical Centre,
Huispost 117 ELG, P.O. Box 9101, 6500 HB Nijmegen, The Netherlands

Joachim en Anna, Center for Specialized Geriatric Care, Nijmegen, The Netherlands

© Springer International Publishing AG 2017
S. Schüssler, C. Lohrmann (eds.), *Dementia in Nursing Homes*,
DOI 10.1007/978-3-319-49832-4_13

Keywords
Depression • Assessment • Treatment • Monitoring • Implementation

13.1   Introduction

Depression is a major problem in nursing homes (NHs); on average, about 29% of NH residents have a depression diagnosis (Mitchell and Kakkadasam 2011). Important risk factors for depression in nursing home residents are pain, functional limitations, visual impairment, stroke, loneliness, lack of social support, and negative life events (Jongenelis et al. 2004). It is negatively associated with a resident's well-being and daily functioning and can increase mortality and use of healthcare services. Depression also causes distress for relatives and care personnel (Smalbrugge et al. 2006; Gutzmann and Qazi 2015). Nevertheless, depressive symptoms often go unnoticed, for instance, because depressive symptoms can also be attributed to medical illness, functional impairments, and dementia (AGS/AAGP 2003) (Thakur and Blazer 2008). For NH residents with dementia, it is even more complicated to detect depression, because many have language and memory impairments that impede reliable communication about their feelings. Therefore, involving nursing staff in recognizing depression is the first step for improvement of depression care in NH residents with dementia. Thereto, it is important that nursing staff is trained in recognizing depressive symptoms and that screening instruments validated in nursing home residents with dementia are available. To improve depression recognition, it is also important to involve (gero)psychologists and (elderly care) physicians, who are skilled in screening and diagnosing depression. The use of a validated depression instrument may help a psychologist to further evaluate the observations of the nursing staff, his or her own observations, and information from the resident. Accordingly, a diagnostic procedure should also account for possible cognitive problems. Depressive symptoms in persons with dementia can be considered different from the symptoms of depression in persons without dementia (Barca et al. 2008; Olin et al. 2002). Since the often used criteria of the *Diagnostic and Statistical Manual of Mental Disorders* (APA 2000) do not account for that, it may be advisable to use diagnostic criteria that do, such as the Provisional Diagnostic Criteria for Depression of Alzheimer's Disease for residents with dementia (Olin et al. 2002). Given the under-recognition of depression in NHs, care programs for depression management should certainly include structural depression screening and diagnosing (assessment) procedures (AGS/AAGP 2003).

Treatment of depression in NH residents with dementia also requires improvement. Up till now, depression has merely been treated with antidepressants despite scarce evidence and indications that pharmacological treatment of depression in dementia may not be beneficial compared with placebo (Nelson and Devanand 2011; Banerjee et al. 2011). Alternatively, evidence for psychosocial interventions is available: many studies have reported significant benefits on depression and various psychological well-being outcomes (Bharucha et al. 2006; Konnert et al. 2009; Hyer et al. 2008; Buettner and Fitzsimmons 2002; Verkaik et al. 2011). Considering that adverse outcomes of drug treatment of depression can be serious (Coupland et al. 2011), behavioral and psychosocial interventions should be considered as first-line treatment in NH residents. Recent literature also shows that collaborative care of depression is more effective than a monotherapy (Oestergaard and Moldrup 2011; Brodaty et al. 2003). For instance, a study on behavioral management in nursing and residential homes, training of caregivers by an old-age psychiatric hospital outreach team, and ongoing support to individual workers has shown positive effects on depression outcomes (Proctor et al. 1999).

This chapter describes a multidisciplinary approach to depression recognition and treatment in residents with dementia that has been developed and investigated in the nursing home setting: Act in case of Depression (AiD) (Leontjevas et al. 2013a, b). AiD prescribes procedures for detecting depression, psychosocial and pharmacological treatment strategies, and a procedure for monitoring the effects of the given treatment. The program was developed by a working group of geropsychologists within the context of the University Network of Nursing Homes, Nijmegen. It is based on national (Dutch) and international guidelines (AGS/AAGP 2003: www. ggzrichtlijnen.nl) and scientific evidence, combined with the clinical expertise of the developers. AiD was shown to have an effect on the motivational aspects of mood: in a large randomized controlled trial, it appeared effective in decreasing depression on units for somatically frail residents and in decreasing apathy on dementia special care units. On both types of units, residents' self-reported quality of life scores improved. Furthermore, the effects of AiD were far stronger in units on which the implementation process had been successful; especially improved recognition of depression led to larger effects (Leontjevas et al. 2013a, b).

13.2   How to Act in Case of Depression in Dementia?

AiD aims to reduce depression prevalence and to increase the quality of life of NH residents by educating NH personnel and providing procedures for multidisciplinary collaboration regarding the assessment and treatment of depression, which are tailored to individual residents regarding their cognitive abilities and personal needs. Thus, the core aim of AiD is to provide a structure toward depression management that is broadly applicable. All assessment and treatment procedures are evidence based and leave room for decisions based on clinical expertise of professionals. The program suggests assessment instruments and treatments, but these may be replaced by other valid tools. AiD has three core elements: assessment, treatment, and monitoring and evaluation (Fig. 13.1).

13.2.1 Element 1: Stepwise Depression Assessment

For depression assessment, a stepped care approach involving three steps is advised. In the first step, "detection," a nursing staff member uses a screening instrument to recognize residents who may have depressive symptoms. An observer-rated instrument focusing on nonverbal symptoms is advised for this step, since this is not dependent on communication abilities which can be impaired in residents with dementia. To this end, the five-item Nijmegen Observer-Rated Depression (NORD) scale (see gray box) was developed and validated, which can be used for screening for depression on a regular basis in NH residents with and without dementia. It appeared sensitive, short, and easy to score (Leontjevas et al. 2012b).

The Nijmegen Observer-Rated Depression (NORD) Scale
Instruction: Answer "yes" when the behavior was present in the last 2 weeks and "no" when the behavior was not present or not applicable to your client. "Often" means that the behavior was present for several hours during at least 8 days of the last 2 weeks.

1. Does the client often look sad, gloomy, or cheerless?
2. Does the client often cry or is he/she often emotionally distressed?
3. Does the client often lack a positive response to social contacts or pleasant events?
4. Does the client often need to be encouraged to do something or participate in joint activities?
5. Does the client often have problems with sleep (falling asleep, maintaining sleep, waking up) or appetite (no appetite, unusually hungry)?

If more than one question is answered with "yes," further screening is indicated.

Updated from Leontjevas et al. (2012b). Permission conveyed through Copyright Clearance Center, Inc.

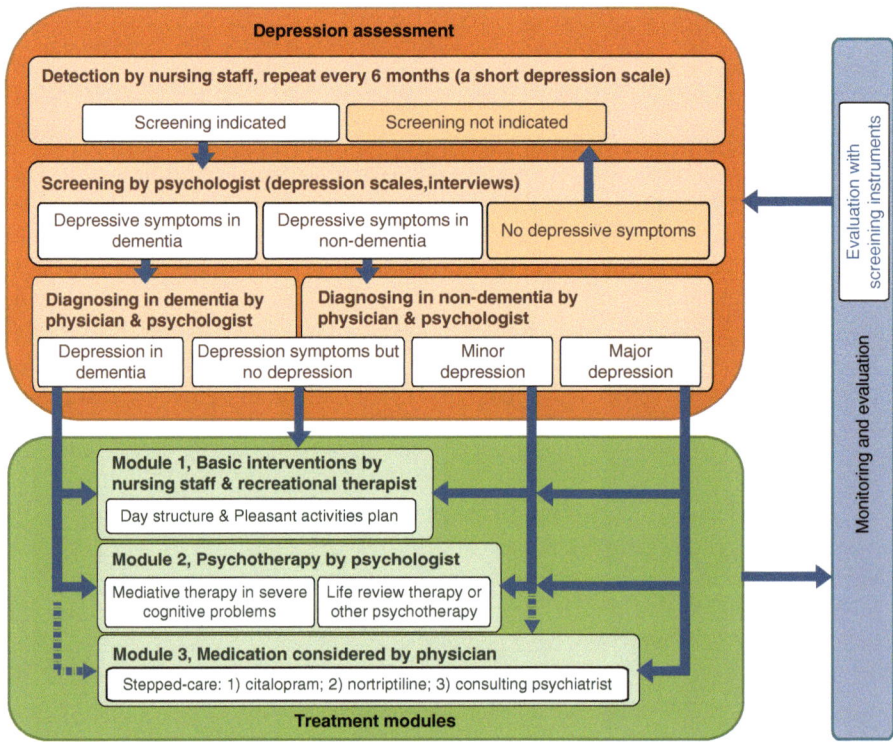

Fig. 13.1 The care program act in case of depression (Updated from Leontjevas et al. (2013a). Permission conveyed through Copyright Clearance Center, Inc.)

In the Netherlands, where psychologists are staff members in most care organizations, the second assessment step, "extensive screening," is to be conducted by a psychologist when this is indicated by the detection instrument used in the first step. For residents who cannot be interviewed because of the severity or type of their (cognitive) impairments, the use of a proxy-based depression screening instrument is advised. For residents who can self-report, the Geriatric Depression Scale 8-item version is suggested ((Jongenelis et al. 2007) GDS8, cutoff score > 2). When observation is more appropriate, the Cornell Scale for Depression in Dementia ((Alexopoulos et al. 1988) CSDD, cutoff score > 7) has acceptable accuracy when professional caregivers are the only source of information, both in residents with and without dementia (Leontjevas et al. 2012a).

When indicated by the second step, in the third step of depression assessment, a psychologist and/or a physician undertake a diagnostic procedure. AiD advises the use of the Provisional Diagnostic Criteria for Depression of Alzheimer's Disease for residents with dementia (Olin et al. 2002), instead of the *Diagnostic and Statistical Manual of Mental Disorders* (APA 2000).

Usually, the second and third assessment steps are combined in one session with the residents and/or nursing staff member. In countries where psychologists and/or physicians are not affiliated to the NH, this is even more advisable.

13.2.2 Element 2: Treatment Strategies

As described, there is limited evidence for the effects of antidepressants in NHs, especially in residents with dementia. Therefore, the focus should be on psychosocial treatment of depression. AiD emphasizes psychosocial treatment, and the revealed effects of the care program underpin that a multidisciplinary approach is advisable (Leontjevas et al. 2013a, b). AiD has three treatment modules that also reflect a stepped care approach.

Module 1 is to be performed for NH residents with depressive symptoms or depression and comprises environmental and behavioral strategies by nursing or care staff and/or an activity therapist. They develop and execute a day structure program (DSP) and a pleasant activities plan (PAP) (Teri et al. 1997; Verkaik et al. 2011). A DSP structures the way days are spent, thereby preventing disruptions of the circadian rhythm and realizing meaningful ways of spending residents' days. PAP provides the content of the DSP and focuses on involving residents in activities that they find pleasant and also avoiding activities they find unpleasant. A PAP describes goals and ways to realize them.

Module 2 regards treatment by a psychologist and is complementary to Module 1 for NH residents who meet criteria for a depression diagnosis. If the communicative and cognitive abilities allow for talk therapy, this is initiated by the psychologist. The AiD program does not prescribe a specific therapy, but the manual contains precious memories therapy (Bohlmeijer et al. 2010) which is a form of life review therapy adapted for NH residents. If talk therapy is not possible, mediative therapy – in which the psychologist intervenes in the resident's social environment through educating and coaching the care team – is advised (Hamer 2003).

Module 3 regards pharmacological treatment. If treatment according to Modules 1 and 2 is not effective or if depression is very severe, the physician may consider prescribing antidepressants. For this, the NICE guideline dementia, which summarizes the most recent evidence and recommendations for treatment of depression in dementia, can be applied (https://www.nice.org.uk/guidance/cg42/evidence/full-guideline-including-appendices-17-195023341). It is important to consider that, in patients with dementia, there is no evidence in favor of pharmacological treatment of depressive symptoms and minor depression: the known trials are all negative, while research into effectiveness of antidepressants for major depression in dementia stays inconclusive. Therefore, pharmacological treatment should be prescribed with caution and, preferably, when other treatments have appeared to be ineffective. For residents with dementia, when the observed burden of depression is high, AiD suggests the prescription of antidepressants (selective serotonin reuptake inhibitors: sertraline, fluoxetine, citalopram) in combination with non-pharmacological strategies described above. Antidepressants with anticholinergic side effects should preferably be avoided. Effect and side effects (gastrointestinal and central nervous system related, dry mouth, dizziness/falls) should be monitored carefully. For severe major depression (with psychotic symptoms, suicidal thoughts, or refusal to eat), referral to a psychiatric hospital should be discussed with representatives of the resident. In these cases, electroconvulsive therapy may also be considered (Pellegrino et al. 2013).

The AiD trial showed that on dementia special care units, Module 1 was most effective and that on units for somatically frail residents Module 2 was. No evidence was observed for effects of Module 3, pharmacological treatment. In contrast, indications were found that it might have increased apathy (Leontjevas et al. 2013b).

13.2.3 Element 3: Monitoring and Evaluation

Element 3 has two goals: (1) timely detection of depressive complaints and (2) monitoring and evaluation of treatment in order to adapt it if necessary. If the element "assessment" shows no depressive complaints, AiD proposes to administer the observational scale of step 1 6 months later. Thus, through element 3, AiD is cyclic. This way, the care team remains alert regarding depressive symptoms. If there appear to be depressive complaints, further steps are necessary. If treatment is prescribed, a psychologist and/or physician make a treatment plan in accordance with element 2 and determine how and when to evaluate it. Ideally, this multidisciplinary evaluation takes place within 3 months after having set a diagnosis. As input for the evaluation, administering the assessment instrument of step 2 "screening" is advised as well as checking the diagnostic criteria of step 3 "diagnosing." During treatment, it is important to monitor both effects and feasibility of the proposed treatment options. All involved professionals have to be attentive to procedural hurdles and side effects when implementing treatment strategies and are responsible for informing each other and for trying to solve the encountered problems.

13.2.4 Apathy and Depression

It is also advisable to monitor apathy when managing depression. Apathy is characterized by diminished motivation in combination with a lack of goal-directed behavior, goal-directed cognition, and emotional affect, which leads to reduced interest and participation in the main activities of daily living, diminished initiative, early withdrawal from initiated activities, indifference, and flattening of affect (Marin et al. 1991; Starkstein et al. 2001; Robert et al. 2009). In NH residents with dementia, apathy is very common (Zuidema et al. 2009; Wetzels et al. 2010; Selbaek et al. 2013; van Reekum et al. 2005; Cipriani et al. 2014; Zwijsen et al. 2014). However, it is rarely considered a problem in that setting (Leone et al. 2013; Zwijsen et al. 2014), even though it has been found to be associated with a number of adverse outcomes, such as high caregiver burden, poor treatment response, reliance on caregivers to initiate activities of daily living, low quality of life, and more rapid cognitive and functional decline (van Reekum et al. 2005; Tagariello et al. 2009; Starkstein et al. 2006; Bakker et al. 2013; Mulders et al. 2016). The overlap of apathy with depression is evident, as loss of interest or pleasure is a principal symptom to diagnose depression, even when depressed mood is not present (APA 2000; Olin et al. 2002). However, various studies support the concept of apathy as a behavioral syndrome that can be discriminated from depression (Levy et al. 1998; Starkstein et al. 2008; Ishii et al. 2009). Recent studies show a combination of overlapping and different risk factors for apathy and depression after stroke (Withall et al. 2011; Yang et al. 2013). To be able to differ between depression and apathy, the diagnostic criteria for apathy in Alzheimer's disease and other neuropsychiatric disorders (DCA) (Barca et al. 2010) can be added to a diagnostic procedure for depression. Furthermore, the abbreviated Apathy Evaluation Scale (AES-10) was validated in the AiD trial (Leontjevas et al. 2012c) and can be administered next to screening instruments for depression.

Regarding treatment, as described above, the behavioral strategies applied in AiD activate not only residents with depressive features but can also be beneficial for apathy (Brodaty and Burns 2011), whereas pharmacological treatment of depression using antidepressants may induce apathy (Barnhart et al. 2004; Settle 1998). Thus, for monitoring and evaluation of treatment, measuring apathy – for instance, by using the AES-10 – is advised.

13.3 Requirements for Appropriate Treatment of Depression in NH Residents with Dementia

AiD was shown to have effects on depression, quality of life, and apathy. Moreover, it was considered relevant and feasible by the involved stakeholders (unit managers, physicians, and psychologists) (Leontjevas et al. 2012d). However, implementation of AiD during the AiD trial was not highly successful. For instance, treatment was not started in more than half of the indicated cases, and, while a DSP and PAP (Module 1) were applied more often in dementia units than in somatic units, treatment by a psychologist (Module 2) was executed almost three times less often in dementia units (Leontjevas et al. 2012d). Furthermore, element 3 (evaluation) was the least often implemented part of AiD in both unit types.

The reasons for suboptimal implementation reported by stakeholders shed light on requirements for adequate depression management. The stakeholders of the AiD trial mentioned several causes of suboptimal implementation in daily care, such as high workload, lack of time, difficulties in multidisciplinary collaboration or within the care team, staff changes and unfulfilled positions, low involvement of management, and reorganizations (Leontjevas 2012). High turnover of staff in the units not only resulted to additional expenditures but also compromised performing the program as planned. In 33 units that participated in the AiD trial, 22 physicians, 19 psychologists, and 11 unit managers changed their job during the intervention period (12 months on average). In 12 out of 33 units, more than 20% of the nursing staff that were educated by the researchers left the unit. It is not surprising, then, that the NH professionals mentioned frequent staff changes and shortage of (qualified) staff as an important barrier to carrying out the program. Supporting stable multidisciplinary staff and empowering personnel appear crucial for introducing care innovations. According to the professionals, implementation would have been facilitated if there were, in addition to less staff turnover, more investment in educational strategies and in activities for residents.

Furthermore, the suboptimal implementation of the evaluation element during the AiD trial calls for additional attention. When treatment strategies are not evaluated, depression may persist due to ineffective strategies that are not fine-tuned. Furthermore, when implementation is not evaluated, barriers to implementation may persist and prohibit the necessary changes. Both require a solid working routine with structurally planned evaluation meetings and room for discussion and treatment optimization.

Also, as mentioned by the stakeholders of the AiD trial when discussing the reasons of suboptimal implementation, adequate collaboration and allocation of stakeholders' roles is crucial. Implementing an innovation in NHs requires a *project leader*, preferably a local opinion leader, who coordinates the implementation process. *NH managers* have to be involved as well by approving and, more importantly, facilitating the implementation. NH managers who are able to empower their staff and who invest in their staff through acquiring a positive attitude toward change highly facilitate the implementation of care improvement programs. The *unit manager* is undoubtedly one of the key stakeholders who has to encourage implementation and create opportunities for nursing staff to be trained and to be involved in the intervention. Furthermore, *psychologists and physicians* have to initiate the intervention and specific treatment strategies and make sure treatment is being evaluated. Also, *nursing staff* needs to be involved in order to improve depression recognition but needs to be equipped to do so by education, feasible assessment instruments, and practical procedures. The final crucial stakeholders are the residents and their relatives. The involvement of relatives, friends, and other informal caregivers is also necessary for successful and tailored application of environmental treatment strategies, e.g., in facilitating and executing the pleasant activities plan (Verkaik et al. 2011). Therefore, the strategies that are used to implement the intervention should also be provided and tailored to the *residents and their relatives*. In order to improve effectiveness of activating strategies (AiD treatment Module 1), NH staff should be able to tailor the strategies to the needs and abilities of the resident.

Conclusion

Depression is a major problem in nursing homes and its recognition and treatment need improvement. This chapter describes a multidisciplinary approach to depression management in residents with dementia that was specifically developed for the nursing home setting. To date, not many evidence-based complex care interventions have been put into practice in a NH setting – a setting that shows high rates of reorganization, high staff turnover, low nursing staff education level, and a shortage of staff. Taking on the challenge of implementing care innovations is important for improving the quality of care and, through this, the quality of life of residents with dementia. Depression is treatable and AiD elements have been shown to help in detecting and treating this condition. This implies that it is possible to reduce the prevalence of depression in nursing home residents with dementia, that is, if we Act in case of Depression.

References

AGS/AAGP (2003) The American Geriatrics Society and American Association for Geriatric Psychiatry recommendations for policies in support of quality mental health care in US nursing homes. J Am Geriatr Soc 51:1299–1304

Alexopoulos GS, Abrams RC, Young RC et al (1988) Cornell scale for depression in dementia. Biol Psychiat 23:271–284

APA (2000) Diagnostic and statistical manual of mental disorder, 4th edn, Text Revision. American Psychiatric Association, Washington, DC

Bakker C, de Vugt ME, van Vliet D et al (2013) Predictors of the time to institutionalization in young- versus late-onset dementia: results from the Needs in Young Onset Dementia (NeedYD) study. J Am Med Dir Assoc 14:248–253

Banerjee S, Hellier J, Dewey M et al (2011) Sertraline or mirtazapine for depression in dementia (HTA-SADD): a randomised, multicentre, double-blind, placebo-controlled trial. Lancet 378:403–411

Barca ML, Selbaek G, Laks J et al (2008) The pattern of depressive symptoms and factor analysis of the Cornell Scale among patients in Norwegian nursing homes. Int J Geriatr Psychiatry 23:1058–1065

Barca ML, Engedal K, Laks J et al (2010) A 12 months follow-up study of depression among nursing-home patients in Norway. J Affect Disord 120:141–148

Barnhart WJ, Makela EH, Latocha MJ (2004) SSRI-induced apathy syndrome: a clinical review. J Psychiatr Pract 10:196–199

Bharucha AJ, Dew MA, Miller MD et al (2006) Psychotherapy in long-term care: a review. J Am Med Dir Assoc 7:568–580

Bohlmeijer E, Steunenberg B, Leontjevas R et al (2010) Dierbare Herinneringen: Protocol voor Individuele life-review therapie gebaseerd op autobiografische oefening. Universiteit Twente, Enschede

Brodaty H, Burns K (2011) Nonpharmacological management of apathy in dementia: a systematic review. Am J Geriatr Psychiatry 20:549–564

Brodaty H, Draper BM, Millar J et al (2003) Randomized controlled trial of different models of care for nursing home residents with dementia complicated by depression or psychosis. J Clin Psychiatry 64:63–72

Buettner LL, Fitzsimmons S (2002) AD-venture program: therapeutic biking for the treatment of depression in long-term care residents with dementia. Am J Alzheimers Dis Other Demen 17:121–127

Cipriani G, Lucetti C, Danti S et al (2014) Apathy and dementia Nosology, assessment and management. J Nerv Ment Dis 202(10):718–724

Coupland C, Dhiman P, Morriss R et al (2011) Antidepressant use and risk of adverse outcomes in older people: population based cohort study. BMJ 343:d4551

Gutzmann H, Qazi AZ (2015) Depression associated with dementia. Gerontol Geriatr 48(4):305–311

Hamer T (2003) Mediatietherapie. De beste stuurlui staan aan wal. In: Miesen B, Allewijn M, Hertogh C, Groot de F, Wetten van en M (eds) Leidraad Psychogeriatrie, deel B/C, Houten Bohn Stafleu Van Loghum, pp 414–437

Hyer L, Yeager CA, Hilton N et al (2008) Group, individual, and staff therapy: an efficient and effective cognitive behavioral therapy in long-term care. Am J Alzheimers Dis Other Demen 23:528–539

Ishii S, Weintraub N, Mervis JR (2009) Apathy: a common psychiatric syndrome in the elderly. J Am Med Dir Assoc 10(6):381–393

Jongenelis K, Pot AM, Eisses AM, Beekman AT, Kluiter H, Ribbe MW (2004) Prevalence and risk indicators of depression in elderly nursing home patients: the AGED study. J Affect Disord 83:135–142

Jongenelis K, Gerritsen DL, Pot AM et al (2007) Construction and validation of a patient- and user-friendly nursing home version of the Geriatric Depression Scale. Int J Geriatr Psychiatry 22:837–842

Konnert C, Dobson K, Stelmach L (2009) The prevention of depression in nursing home residents: a randomized clinical trial of cognitive-behavioral therapy. Aging Ment Health 13:288–299

Leone E, Deudon A, Bauchet M et al (2013) Management of apathy in nursing homes using a teaching program for care staff: the STIM-EHPAD study. Int J Geriatr Psychiatry 28(4):383–392

Leontjevas R (2012) Act in case of depression. PhD thesis

Leontjevas R, Gerritsen DL, Vernooij-Dassen M et al (2012a) Comparative validation of proxy-based Montgomery-Asberg depression rating scale and cornell scale for depression in dementia in nursing home residents with dementia. Am J Geriatr Psychiatry 20(11):985–993

Leontjevas R, Gerritsen DL, Vernooij-Dassen M et al (2012b) Nijmegen observer-rated depression scale for detection of depression in nursing home residents. Int J Geriatr Psychiatry 27(10):1036–1044

Leontjevas R, Evers-Stephan A, Smalbrugge M, Pot AM, Thewissen V, Gerritsen DL, et al (2012c) A comparative validation of the abbreviated Apathy Evaluation Scale (AES-10) with the Neuropsychiatric Inventory apathy subscale against diagnostic criteria of apathy. JAMDA 13(3):308.e1–6

Leontjevas R, Gerritsen DL, Koopmans RTCM, Smalbrugge M, Vernooij-Dassen (2012d) Proces evaluation to explore internal and external validity of the Act in case of Depression care program in nursing homes. JAMDA 13(5):488

Leontjevas R, Teerenstra S, Smalbrugge M et al (2013a) More insight into the concept of apathy: a multidisciplinary depression management program has different effects on depressive symptoms and apathy in nursing homes. Int Psychogeriatr 25(12):1941–1952

Leontjevas R, Gerritsen DL, Smalbrugge M et al (2013b) A structural multidisciplinary approach to depression management in nursing-home residents: a multicentre, stepped-wedge cluster-randomised trial. Lancet 381(9885):2255–2264

Levy ML, Cummings JL, Fairbanks LA et al (1998) Apathy is not depression. J Neuropsychiatry Clin Neurosci 10:314–319

Marin RS, Biedrzycki RC, Firinciogullari S (1991) Reliability and validity of the Apathy Evaluation Scale. Psychiatry Res 38(2):143–162

Mitchell AJ, Kakkadasam V (2011) Ability of nurses to identify depression in primary care, secondary care and nursing homes-A meta-analysis of routine clinical accuracy. Int J Nurs Stud 48:359–358

Mulders AJ, Fick IW, Bor H, Verhey FR, Zuidema SU, Koopmans RT (2016) Prevalence and correlates of neuropsychiatric symptoms in nursing home patients with young-onset dementia: the BEYOnD study. J Am Med Dir Assoc 17:495–500

Nelson JC, Devanand DP (2011) A systematic review and meta-analysis of placebo-controlled antidepressant studies in people with depression and dementia. J Am Geriatr Soc 59:577–585

Oestergaard S, Moldrup C (2011) Improving outcomes for patients with depression by enhancing antidepressant therapy with non-pharmacological interventions: a systematic review of reviews. Public Health 125:357–367

Olin JT, Katz IR, Meyers BS et al (2002) Provisional diagnostic criteria for depression of Alzheimer disease: rationale and background. Am J Geriatr Psychiatry 10:129–141

Pellegrino LD, Peters ME, Lyketsos CG et al (2013) Depression in cognitive impairment. Curr Psychiatry Rep 15(9):384

Proctor R, Burns A, Powell HS et al (1999) Behavioural management in nursing and residential homes: a randomised controlled trial. Lancet 354:26–29

van Reekum R, Stuss DT, Ostrander L (2005) Apathy: why care? J Neuropsychiatry Clin Neurosci 17(1):7–19

Robert P, Onyike CU, Leentjens AF et al (2009) Proposed diagnostic criteria for apathy in Alzheimer's disease and other neuropsychiatric disorders. Eur Psychiatry J Assoc Eur Psychiatrists 24:98–104

Selbæk G, Engedal K, Bergh S (2013) The prevalence and course of neuropsychiatric symptoms in nursing home patients with dementia: a systematic review. J Am Med Dir Assoc 14(3):161–169

Settle EC Jr (1998) Antidepressant drugs: disturbing and potentially dangerous adverse effects. J Clin Psychiatry 59(Suppl 16):25–30. discussion 40–22

Smalbrugge M, Pot AM, Jongenelis L et al (2006) The impact of depression and anxiety on well being, disability and use of health care services in nursing home patients. Int J Geriatr Psychiatry 21(4):325–332

Starkstein SE, Petracca G, Chemerinski E et al (2001) Syndromic validity of apathy in Alzheimer's disease. Am J Psychiatry 158:872–877

Starkstein SE, Jorge R, Mizrahi R et al (2006) A prospective longitudinal study of apathy in Alzheimer's disease. J Neurol Neurosurg Psychiatry 77:8–11

Starkstein SE, Mizrahi R, Power BD (2008) Depression in Alzheimer's disease: phenomenology, clinical correlates and treatment. Int Rev Psychiatry 20(4):382–388

Tagariello P, Girardi P, Amore M (2009) Depression and apathy in dementia: same syndrome or different constructs? A critical review. Arch Gerontol Geriatr 49:246–249

Teri L, Logsdon RG, Uomoto J et al (1997) Behavioral treatment of depression in dementia patients: a controlled clinical trial. J Gerontol B Psychol Sci Soc Sci 52(4):P159–P166

Thakur M, Blazer DG (2008) Depression in long-term care. J Am Med Dir Assoc 9(2):82–87

Verkaik R, Francke AL, van Meijel B et al (2011) The effects of a nursing guideline on depression in psychogeriatric nursing home residents with dementia. Int J Geriatr Psychiatry 26:723–732

Wetzels RB, Zuidema SU, de Jonghe JFM et al (2010) Course of neuropsychiatric symptoms in residents with dementia in nursing homes over 2-year period. Am J Geriatr Psychiatry 18(12):1054–1065

Withall A, Brodaty H, Altendorf A et al (2011) A longitudinal study examining the independence of apathy and depression after stroke: the Sydney Stroke Study. Int Psychogeriatr 23(2):264–273

Yang SR, Hua P, Shang XY et al (2013) Predictors of early post ischemic stroke apathy and depression: a cross-sectional study. BMC Psychiatry 13:164

Zuidema SU, de Jonghe JF, Verhey FR et al (2009) Predictors of neuropsychiatric symptoms in nursing home patients: influence of gender and dementia severity. Int J Geriatr Psychiatry 24(10):1079–1086

Zwijsen SA, Kabboord A, Eefsting JA et al (2014) Nurses in distress? An explorative study into the relation between distress and individual neuropsychiatric symptoms of people with dementia in nursing homes. Int J Geriatr Psychiatry 29:384–391

Delirium

14

John P. Gilmore and Kathryn A. Weigel

Abstract

Caring for the patient with dementia can be a difficult task requiring a heightened degree of empathy and understanding; however this difficulty can be further exacerbated when the patient experiences episodes of delirium. Care strategies for these two disorders of consciousness and cognition are often very different, and it is extremely important that they are not confounded; indeed when considering them individually, this is quite obvious. However when caring for the person who is experiencing delirium superimposed on dementia, we need an ever delicate approach to provide optimum care. It is vitally important that we do not excuse delirious episodes as part of the dementia process as it important not to diagnose delirium in the place of a deterioration in cognitive status because of dementia. This chapter presents some of the defining characteristics of delirium and differentiates it from dementia as well as identifying some of the precipitating and predisposing factors leading to delirium. It considers the impact and outcomes of delirium and delirium superimposed on dementia (DSD) and also considers some of the pharmacologic and non-pharmacologic management strategies for DSD, as well as interventions for the prevention of delirium.

Keywords

Delirium • Dementia • DSD • CAM • NH-CAM

J.P. Gilmore, RGN, BSc, Grad Dip, MSoc Sc (✉)
Canterbury Christ Church University, Canterbury, UK
e-mail: john.gilmore@canterbury.ac.uk

K.A. Weigel, MS, RN, GCNS
University of St. Francis, Joliet, IL, USA
e-mail: KWeigel@stfrancis.edu

© Springer International Publishing AG 2017
S. Schüssler, C. Lohrmann (eds.), *Dementia in Nursing Homes*,
DOI 10.1007/978-3-319-49832-4_14

14.1 Introduction

Delirium and dementia are amongst the most common causes of cognitive dysfunction and impairment in clinical and care settings, yet are very often unrecognised, undiagnosed or mistaken for each other (Fong et al. 2015). While dementia is characterised by chronic and progressive cognitive decline, delirium is a neuropsychiatric disorder classified by the *Diagnostic and Statistical Manual of Mental Disorders* (DSM-5) as a disturbance in attention, awareness and cognition that develops over a short period of time and fluctuates over the course of the day (American Psychiatric Association 2013). It may develop in many different settings, a person may already have delirium when they present to hospital or long-term care, or it may develop during their stay, and older people and people with dementia are at particular risk of developing delirium (NICE 2010). The limited literature on delirium, especially on experiences of delirium, is generally focussed on broad patient populations such as ICU, cardiac surgery, burns and palliative care (Partridge et al. 2013); very often in these studies, patients with pre-existing cognitive impairment, such as dementia, are excluded. Their relationship is further conflated in that experience of delirium is an independent risk factor for the subsequent development of delirium (Fong et al. 2015). Delirium and dementia commonly coincide, and indeed as mentioned pre-existing dementia is a significant risk factor for the development of delirium. Delirium which occurs in patients with dementia is referred to delirium superimposed on dementia (DSD), and it is a complex and common problem which can have serious complications and poor prognostic implications (Fick et al. 2002). Evidence suggests that DSD has a significant impact on rehabilitation and functional outcomes for those who experience it (Morandi et al. 2014). The experience of DSD can also be extremely traumatic for those affected, many of whom recall their delirious episodes and in turn experience distress (Morandi et al. 2015a), but this distress can also significantly impact family and caregivers (Morandi et al. 2015b). With the substantial increase of those older than 75 years in most developed countries, the phenomenon of DSD and its effect on cognitive function and well-being requires a considered and expert approach in order to effectively detect, manage and prevent it.

This chapter will discuss the distinguishing characteristics of delirium as well as the incidence, risks and outcomes delirium superimposed on dementia. We will further present strategies to detect, manage and prevent DSD.

14.2 Categorisation of Delirium

Originally delirium was considered solely to be manifested through a change in mental status, therefore a disorder of arousal (Inouye et al. 2014) someone could be in a hyperactive or aroused state or a more sedate or hypoactive state. However as delirium became more of a focus of clinicians and through more advanced observation and interaction, it became apparent that delirium was also characterised by a change in clarity of thought and attention. It is now accepted widely that delirium is primarily as a disorder of cognition, with attentive and global cognitive impairment as the key features (Inouye et al. 1990).

Delirium is still however manifested in two broad psychomotor forms, hyperactive delirium and hypoactive delirium. Hyperactive delirium is usually identified quite quickly, as patients who present with hyperactive delirium can be outwardly confused and disruptive; we often see this form in patients who are concurrently withdrawing from alcohol or other drugs. Hypoactive delirium is especially prevalent in older patients, this form is less obviously noted and very often the patient is more sedate and withdrawn, and generally hypoactive delirium is associated with worse outcomes (Marcantonio 2012). It should also be noted that very often patients will present with a mixed delirium, where they fluctuate from hyperactive to hypoactive delirium throughout the day or the duration of the disorder. While the outward presentations of the different types of delirium are quite distinct, EEG tracings do not differ significantly (Koponen et al. 1989).

14.3 Distinguishing Delirium from Dementia

Delirium and dementia are very often considered to be mutually exclusive and distinct conditions; however it is important to acknowledge and understand the linkages between them. A good grasp of the interface between delirium and dementia could in fact deepen our understanding and advance both our conceptualisation and treatment approach to each (Fong et al. 2015). It is important not to confound them, they are indeed distinct and while this chapter shows the strong linkages, the DSM-5 asserts caution stating that dementia should not be diagnosed in the face of delirium and delirium should not be diagnosed when symptoms are better accounted for by pre-existing, established or evolving dementia (American Psychiatric Association 2013). In practice however it can be difficult to distinguish. When you ask healthcare practitioners to identify the symptoms of either condition, you are likely to get a very similar list, confusion, agitation, hallucinations and inappropriate mood. Indeed there is a blurred division when you consider the phenomena of persistent delirium, which can last for months or even years (Cole et al. 2003) along with reversible dementia. Even the most experienced clinicians can find it difficult to differentiate between the two diagnoses, and the differentiation may ultimately depend on an acute change from the patient's baseline, which sometimes may not be known. This supports the central role family and carers can play in the recognition and diagnosis of DSD (Morandi et al. 2015b). Despite these complexities and anomalies, typically there are certain features which differentiate the conditions. Firstly, in the phasing of onset, as declared in the NICE guidelines (2010), delirium has an acute onset, usually over a matter of hours or days; in contrast to this, we know that dementia is more progressive and develops over months or years. Another key element of delirium is that the altered cognition and consciousness fluctuate over the course of the day, with periods of lucidity and delirium occurring in close proximity; in dementia these cognitive behaviours typically remain intact until the later, advanced stages (Fong et al. 2015). A useful way to conceptualise delirium is as an acute brain organ dysfunction, a multifactorial syndrome comparable in that way to acute heart or kidney failure. Very often the diagnosis is only made retrospectively after there is a resolution of symptoms and a return to normal functioning, and this obviously makes it more difficult to establish the precipitating factors. It is suggested that where there is an acute change in mental status, it should be treated as delirium until proven otherwise (Fong et al. 2015).

14.4   Incidence

Reporting of delirium is poor and so it can be difficult to accurately estimate its prevalence (NICE 2010); however all studies examining delirium rates in hospital and community care settings show a significant proportion of patients experiencing delirium. Inouye et al. (2014) suggest that as much as 50% of those over the age of 65 admitted to hospital will suffer from delirium. Morandi et al. (2015a) highlight that the prevalence rates of DSD range between 22% and 89% in both community and hospital settings.

14.5   Causes

While delirium can indeed be caused by a single factor or event, most often in elderly people, the causation is multifactorial (Inouye and Charpentier 1996). It is likely that each individual episode of delirium has a unique set of component contributors and it may be more helpful to broadly consider the predisposing factors and the precipitating factors (see Table 14.1).

Indeed the development of delirium is very often contingent on a complex interrelationship between these predisposing risks and precipitating factors, where those already vulnerable, perhaps because of having a number of predisposing factors, are exposed to a single (or multiple) precipitating factor(s). For example, a patient with dementia or other cognitive impairment may only develop delirium if

Table 14.1 Predisposing and precipitating factors for the development of delirium

Predisposing factors	Precipitating factors
Dementia	Drugs
Other cognitive impairment	Physical restraints
History of delirium	Urinary catheter
Functional impairment	Infection
Visual impairment	Electrolyte imbalance
Hearing impairment	Metabolic acidosis
Comorbidity or severity of illness	Iatrogenic event
Depression	Surgery
History of transients ischemia or stroke	Trauma
Alcohol	Coma
Older age	

Reproduced from Inouye et al. (2014)

they or when they are physically restrained to stop them wandering, are given a sedative agent at night-time or develop a urinary infection. It is extremely important to distinguish the predisposing elements here, often which we cannot control, from the much more controllable precipitating factors in order to provide adequate care and treatment.

14.6 Pathophysiology

Given the complex multifactorial causation and the probability that each individual episode of delirium has, a unique set of contributors, to isolate a single mechanism of delirium, is practically impossible. There is evidence amassing however highlighting how different sets of biological factors interacting can lead to acute cognitive dysfunction by interfering with large-scale neuronal networks. These include inflammation, metabolic imbalance, neurotransmitter derangement, physiological stressors, electrolyte imbalance and genetic abnormalities (Watt et al. 2013). We know that although delirium can occur at any age, children and older people are particularly vulnerable (Inouye et al. 2014); children obviously have less developed neuronal networks, and in older people they are more likely to have age-related damage to these networks, and so this further points favourably to the hypotheses that neuronal networks play a key role in the pathophysiology of delirium.

14.7 Diagnosis

The high prevalence and complex presentation of delirium means it is important that appropriate tools are used to aid in its diagnosis. Delirium is often unrecognised and easy to overlook (Inouye et al. 2014), and as mentioned above it is important not to class all confused or inappropriate behaviour as delirium, as much as it is important not to excuse delirious behaviour because the patient has an underlying cognitive impairment, psychiatric history or dementia. While some potential has been explored for the use of EEG of CT/MRI neuroimaging for the diagnosis of delirium, it shows low yield in unselected patients (Agency for Healthcare research and Quality 2013). There are a number of validated tools which can be applied to diagnose delirium. The NICE guidelines (2010) recommend using the DSM criteria as a basis for clinical assessment or alternatively using the Confusion Assessment Method (CAM) (Inouye et al. 1990). CAM is a 5-min questionnaire by which the present severity and fluctuation of nine delirium features are identified (Wong et al. 2010). The features tested are acute onset, inattention, disorganised thinking, altered level of consciousness, disorientation, memory impairment, perception disturbances, psychomotor agitation or retardation and altered sleep wake cycle. Based on the DSM criteria for delirium, the questionnaire is in the form of the algorithm and is quick and easy to administer. The step-by-step process first establishes the essential features which are sudden onset and fluctuating course as well as inattention. The latter part features a test to establish either disorganised thinking or altered level of consciousness. So essentially if you have the first two features and either (or both) of the latter, you are diagnosed as CAM positive and delirious. CAM is by far the most widely used assessment tool for delirium (Inouye et al. 2014) and has been adapted for use in several specialist settings such as ICU and emergency departments. CAM has also been adapted for use in nursing home patients (Dosa et al. 2007). The NH-CAM rearranges the minimum data set items which were previously used to identify delirium in nursing homes into a similar structure as the original CAM (Fig. 14.1). Other tools used include the Clinical Assessment of Confusion (Vermeersch 1990), the Global Attentiveness Rating (O'keefe and Gosney 1997) and the Delirium Observation Screening Scale (Schuurmans et al. 2003); however given its simplicity, efficiency, adaptability and efficacy, the best evidence supports the use of CAM (Wong et al. 2010). As with any tool, the quality of outcome is dependent on the ability of the user, and so it is important that adequate training is engaged to use such tools. Another important factor, especially in those with pre-existing cognitive impairment or dementia, is establishing their baseline cognitive ability. Families and carers can play a vital role in the diagnosis of delirium, and in fact the CAM has further been adapted to allow for families and carers to assess for signs of delirium CAM-ICU (Steis et al. 2012).

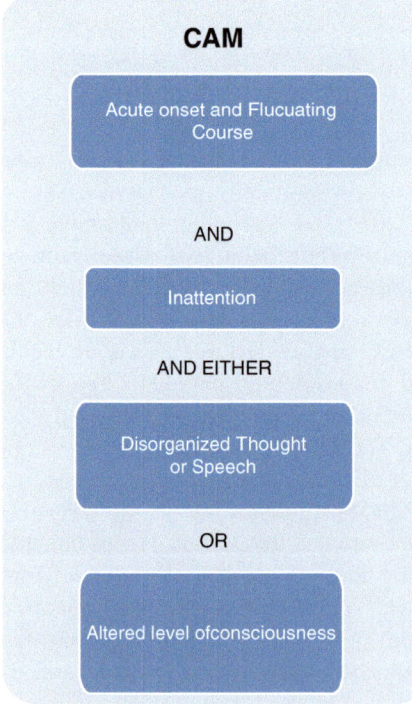 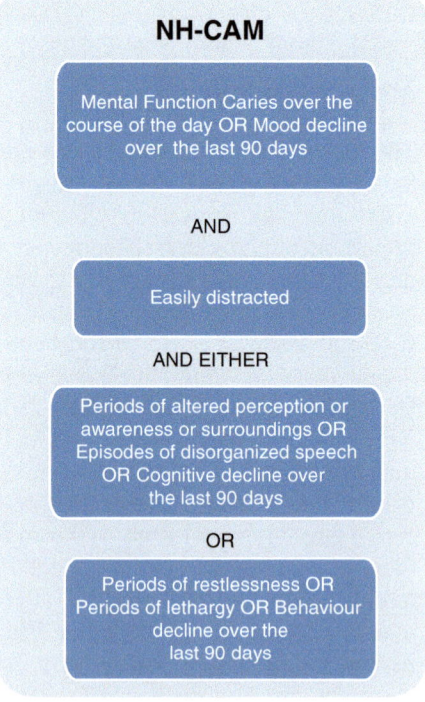

Fig. 14.1 Comparison of CAM and NH-CAM

14.8 Outcomes

Independently both dementia and delirium have a large impact effecting length of stay in hospital, healthcare costs, morbidity, mortality and loss of functional independence. These effects are amplified when DSD is considered; however, unfortunately the consequences of DSD remain a relatively neglected research area (Fick et al. 2005). While there is conflicting evidence in the data around DSD and mortality, there are strong suggestions that it can significantly add to risk of death (Bellelli et al. 2007). It has however been well established that delirium, as a stand-alone factor, has a significant impact on mortality (McCusker et al. 2002). DSD also has been found to have a significant impact on rehabilitation, mobility and functional independence. Morandi et al. (2014) have signified that DSD needs to be recognised by clinicians as a prognostic factor in rehab, reporting a significant negative effect on functional outcomes, as well as leading to institutionalisation of patients. A further study by Morandi et al. (2015a) considered the psychological and emotional impact of DSD on patients. The study reported increased anxiety, depression and low mood amongst people who had experienced DSD. O'Malley et al. (2008) found that the experiences of patients who had delirium could be grouped into three main themes, incomprehension and feelings of discomfort, the need to keep distance and to protect oneself, and interventions which diminish suffering. Delirium and DSD can also have a profound effect on family, caregivers and healthcare staff; an important note to take from Morandi et al. (2015b) is that while there were elements of distress in both the informal caregivers and healthcare staff, it was substantially higher in the informal carers.

14.9 Management of DSD

Determining and correcting the underlying cause of delirium is the primary intervention in managing DSD, but the symptoms of delirium must be managed until the delirium is resolved. In general, the management of DSD can be classified into the two categories of non-pharmacologic and pharmacologic interventions. Non-pharmacologic interventions are preferred as first-line approaches because the medications used to treat the symptoms of delirium may actually exacerbate or prolong its course.

14.9.1 Non-pharmacological Interventions

Non-pharmacologic interventions are aimed at eliminating and/or decreasing the extrinsic risk factors associated with the development of delirium as well as decreasing the intensity and length of delirium symptoms and focus on modifications of the environment and interactions with the patient. Adequate night-time sleep needs to be assured and can be optimised through minimal frequency of vital sign assessment overnight in stable patients, early morning phlebotomy scheduled for later morning and reduction of noise, light and staff activities during the night. Sensory deficits must be accommodated, and associated modifications include the use of large clocks and posting of orientation boards with current date and names of assigned staff, adjusting approaches to the patient to accommodate type of visual and/or hearing impairment (e.g. approach from unaffected side if unilateral deficit) and communicating with a slow, calming voice at appropriate loudness level and facing the patient at eye level. Although there is little documented research examining these interventions, their use has become standard practice due to experience, common sense and lack of adverse effects (American Psychiatric Association 2010). As noted in the NICE guidelines (2010) regarding the prevention of delirium, the issues of hydration, nutrition, oxygenation, pain, mobility and/or immobility, infection, and the effects of medications must also be addressed in the management of delirium.

The interactions of all staff and family members with the patient are of paramount importance, and it is vital that all are educated regarding the risks, signs, symptoms and management of delirium. It is equally important that family members be supported and involved in the interdisciplinary plan of care from the outset (NICE 2010). Reassurance of safety, validation, redirection of attention to non-threatening topics, engaging in pleasant conversations or activities and maintaining interactions with the resident throughout the day to minimise under-stimulation or overstimulation are necessary. If the presence of family members is calming, it may minimise symptoms and improve sleep quality and should be encouraged; but, if the presence of family members causes or increases agitation, it will only exacerbate symptoms and should be discouraged and/or minimised.

The use of physical restraints is contraindicated due to association with increased agitation, increased risk of injury, increased risk of death and prolongation of delirium (Evans et al., 2003). If absolutely necessary, physical restraints should be used only for a very short term in only the most severe cases of psychomotor agitation where there is significant risk of injury to the resident or staff and only after all other alternatives have been exhausted (Salzman et al. 2008).

14.9.2 Pharmacological Interventions

Pharmacologic interventions may sometimes be required in addition to non-pharmacologic interventions in cases where the patient's agitation is very severe and/or when the patient or staff is at risk for harm. If pharmacological intervention is absolutely indicated, evidence and published guidelines recommend the use of first-generation antipsychotics, such as haloperidol or chlorpromazine (American Psychiatric Association 2010). Second-generation antipsychotics, such as risperidone, quetiapine and olanzapine, and anxiolytics, such as benzodiazepine, may be suggested, but these medications are not recommended as first-line pharmacological interventions. The US Food and Drug Administration has, in fact, administered black box warnings for the use of atypical antipsychotics, benzodiazepines have been shown to increase the risk of delirium, and current research has shown an association with as much as a two-fold increase in mortality for individuals with Alzheimer's dementia receiving atypical antipsychotics (Clegg and Young 2011, Musicco et al. 2011). Any of these medications should be used only when absolutely necessary, after careful and thorough review of the patient's record and in the lowest dose for the shortest duration possible. Assessment for development of extrapyramidal symptoms (EPS), increased risk of falls, sedation and development or exacerbation of cardiac abnormalities must be ongoing, and all staff and family members must be updated regarding the patient's status. Consideration of the type of dementia and comorbidities is imperative. The use of antipsychotics is inappropriate for individuals with Lewy body dementia or Parkinson's disease with dementia, and the use of these and other psychotropic medications can be inappropriate in the presence of other conditions or diseases (NICE 2010).

14.9.2.1 Prevention of Delirium

While there is an onus on healthcare providers to be diligent in the screening and treatment of delirium, it is, by in large, preventable. By being more aware of the predisposing and precipitating factors as mentioned above (Inouye 2014), caregivers and healthcare providers are equipped to act promptly in the prevention and early treatment of delirium. NICE (2010) identify 13 recommendations for the prevention of delirium in at-risk patients (see Table 14.2).

Table 14.2 Recommendations

1. Ensure that persons at risk for delirium are cared for by a team of healthcare professionals who are familiar with the person at risk. Avoid moving persons within and between wards or rooms unless absolutely necessary
2. Give a tailored, multicomponent intervention package. Within 24 h of hospitalisation, assess persons at risk for clinical factors contributing to delirium. On the basis of the results of this assessment, provide a multicomponent intervention tailored to the person's individual needs and care setting
3. The tailored, multicomponent intervention package should be delivered by a multidisciplinary team trained and competent in delirium prevention
4. Address cognitive impairment or disorientation by providing appropriate lighting and clear signage; ensuring that a clock (consider providing a 24-h clock in the critical care unit) and a calendar are easily visible to the person at risk; talking to the person to reorient them by explaining where they are, who they are and what your role is; introducing cognitively stimulating activities (e.g. reminiscence); and facilitating regular visits from family and friends
5. Address dehydration and constipation by ensuring adequate fluid intake to prevent dehydration by encouraging the person to drink – consider offering subcutaneous or intravenous fluids, if necessary, and taking advice when managing fluid balance in persons with comorbid conditions (e.g. heart failure or chronic kidney disease)
6. Assess for hypoxia and optimise oxygen saturation, if necessary, as clinically appropriate
7. Address infection by looking for and treating infection, avoiding unnecessary catheterisation and implementing infection-control procedures in line with the NICE clinical guideline on infection control

(continued)

Table 14.2 (continued)

8. Address immobility or limited mobility through the following actions: encourage persons to mobilise soon after surgery and walk (provide appropriate walking aids that are accessible at all times) and encourage all persons, including persons who are unable to walk, to carry out active, range-of-motion exercises
9. Address pain by assessing for pain; looking for nonverbal signs of pain, particularly in persons with communication difficulties (e.g. persons with learning difficulties or dementia or persons on a ventilator or who have a tracheostomy); and initiating and reviewing appropriate pain management in any person in whom pain is identified or suspected
10. Carry out a medication review for persons receiving several drugs, taking into account both the type and the number of medications
11. Address poor nutrition by following the advice given in the nutrition support in adults section in the NICE clinical guideline 32 and ensuring that dentures fit properly in persons who have them
12. Address sensory impairment by resolving any reversible cause of the impairment, such as impacted ear wax, and ensuring hearing and visual aids are available to and used by persons who need them, and check that such aids are in good working order
13. Promote good sleep patterns and sleep hygiene by avoiding nursing or medical procedures during sleeping hours, if possible; scheduling medication rounds to avoid disturbing sleep; and reducing noise to a minimum during sleep periods

Reproduced from O'Mahony et al. (2011)

Conclusion

With our global ageing populations and the increased demands for enhanced and supported care, it is likely that the issue of delirium will continue to intensify in nursing home settings. There is a great need for more research, information and communication about delirium, to embed good care practice and preventative measures, as well as to ensure prompt recognition and appropriate treatment.

References

Agency for Healthcare Research and Quality (2013) National quality clearinghouse measure: delirium: proportion of patients meeting diagnostic criteria on the confusion assessment method (CAM). http://www.qualitymeasures.ahrq.gov/content.aspx?id=27635. Accessed 16 June 2016

American Psychiatric Association (2010) Practice guidelines for the treatment of patients of patients with delirium. APA, Washington DC

American Psychiatric Association (2013) Diagnostic and statistical manual of mental disorders, 5th edn. APA, Washington, DC

Bellelli G, Frisoni GB, Turco R et al (2007) Delirium superimposed on dementia predicts 12-month survival in elderly patients discharged from a postacute rehabilitation facility. J Gerontol A Biol Sci Med Sci 62(11):1306–1309

Clegg A, Young JB (2011) Which medications to avoid in people at risk of delirium: a systematic review. Age Ageing 40(1):23–29

Cole M, McCusker J, Dendukuri N et al (2003) The prognostic significance of subsyndromal delirium in elderly medical inpatients. J Am Geriatr Soc 51(6):754–760

Dosa D, Intrator O, McNicoll L et al (2007) Preliminary derivation of a nursing home confusion assessment method based on data from the minimum data set. J Am Geriatr Soc 55(7):1099–1105

Evans D, Wood J, Lambert L (2003) Patient injury and physical restraint devices: a systematic review. J Adv Nurs 41:274–282

Fick DM, Agostini JV, Inouye SK (2002) Delirium superimposed on dementia: a systematic review. J Am Geriatr Soc 50(10):1723–1732

Fick DM, Kolanowski AM, Waller JL, Inouye SK (2005) Delirium superimposed on dementia in a community-dwelling managed care population: A 3-year retrospective study of occurrence, costs, and utilization. J Gerontol B Psychol Sci Soc Sci 60:748–753

Fong TG, Davis D, Growdon ME et al (2015) The interface between delirium and dementia in elderly adults. Lancet Neurol 14(8):823–832

Inouye SK, Charpentier PA (1996) Precipitating factors for delirium in hospitalized elderly persons. Predictive model and interrelationship with baseline vulnerability. JAMA 275(11):852–857

Inouye SK, Van Dyck CH, Alessi CA et al (1990) Clarifying confusion: the confusion assessment method. A new method for detection of delirium. Ann Intern Med 113(12):941–948

Inouye SK, Westendorp RG, Saczynski JS (2014) Delirium in elderly people. Lancet 383(9920):911–922

Koponen H, Hurri L, Stenbäck U et al (1989) Computed tomography findings in delirium. J Nerv Ment Dis 177(4):226–231

Marcantonio ER (2012) Postoperative delirium: a 76-year-old woman with delirium following surgery. JAMA 308(1):73–81

McCusker J, Cole M, Abrahamowicz M et al (2002) Delirium predicts 12-month mortality. Arch Intern Med 162(4):457–463

Morandi A, Davis D, Fick DM et al (2014) Delirium superimposed on dementia strongly predicts worse outcomes in older rehabilitation inpatients. J Am Med Dir Assoc 15(5):349–354

Morandi A, Lucchi E, Turco R et al (2015a) Delirium superimposed on dementia: a quantitative and qualitative evaluation of patient experience. J Psychosom Res 79(4):804–812

Morandi A, Lucchi E, Turco R et al (2015b) Delirium superimposed on dementia: a quantitative and qualitative evaluation of informal caregivers and health care staff experience. J Psychosom Res 79(4):272–880

Musicco M, Palmer K, Russo A et al (2011) Association between prescription of conventional or atypical antipsychotic drugs and mortality in older persons with Alzheimer's disease. Dement Geriatr Cogn Disord 31:218–224

National Institute for Clinical Excellence (NICE) (2010) Delirium: diagnosis, prevention and management accessed at www.nice.org.uk/nicemedia/live/13060/49908/49908.pdf. Accessed on 13 June 2016

O'Keeffe ST, Gosney MA (1997) Assessing attentiveness in older hospital patients. J Am Geriatr Soc 45(4):470–473

O'Mahony R, Murthy L, Akunne A et al (2011) Synopsis of the National Institute for Health and Clinical Excellence guideline for prevention of delirium. Ann Intern Med 154:746–751

O'Malley G, Leonard M, Meagher D et al (2008) The delirium experience: a review. J Psychosom Res 65(3):223–228

Partridge JS, Martin FC, Harari D et al (2013) The delirium experience: what is the effect on patients, relatives and staff and what can be done to modify this? Int J Geriatr Psychiatry 28(8):804–812

Salzman C, Jeste DV, Meyer RE et al (2008) Elderly patients with dementia-related symptoms of severe agitation and aggression: consensus statement on treatment options, clinical trials methodology, and policy. J Clin Psychiatry 69(6):889–898

Schuurmans MJ, Shortrifge-Baggett LM, Duursma SA (2003) The delirium observation screening scale. Res Theory Nurs Pract 17(1):31–50

Steis MR, Evans L, Hirschman KB et al (2012) Screening for delirium using family caregivers: convergent validity of the Family Confusion Assessment Method and interviewer-rated Confusion Assessment Method. J Am Geriatr Soc 60(11):2121–2126

Vermeersch PE (1990) The clinical assessment of confusion. Appl Nurs Res 3(3):126–133

Watt D, Budding DE, Koziol LF (2013) Delirium In: Noggle CA, Dean RS (eds) The neuropsychology of psychopathology. Springer, New York

Wong CL, Holroyd-Leduc J, Simel DL et al (2010) Does this patient have delirium? The value of bedside instruments. JAMA 304(7):779–786

Dementia Care in Nursing Homes Requires a Multidisciplinary Approach

15

Jos Schols and Tinie Kardol

Abstract

Dementia care in nursing homes involves care for very frail and disabled older residents, suffering from complex problems in various domains of life. These problems require an integrated approach, focusing on the resident as a human being with a disease who needs high-quality professional care which contributes to his or her quality of life and also supports the family and other informal care-givers. To enable an integrated approach, multidisciplinary teamwork is necessary. Offering care from a multidisciplinary approach puts challenges on the organization of care, more specifically on the share each healthcare professional gets in the care process, on the related mutual agreements between different healthcare professionals and on their mutual communication. In the near future, more attention must be paid as well to the equal role that residents and family caregivers themselves may play in this process of multidisciplinary care.

Keywords

Nursing home • Multidisciplinary approach • Multidisciplinary team • Resident • Dementia

J. Schols, MD, PhD (✉)
Department of Health Services Research, School Caphri, Maastricht University, Maastricht, The Netherlands
e-mail: jos.schols@maastrichtuniversity.nl

T. Kardol, PhD
Department of Educational Sciences and Psychology, Free University of Brussels (VUB), Ixelles, Belgium

© Springer International Publishing AG 2017
S. Schüssler, C. Lohrmann (eds.), *Dementia in Nursing Homes*,
DOI 10.1007/978-3-319-49832-4_15

15.1   Introduction

Dementia care in nursing homes represents care for very frail and disabled residents, suffering from complex problems in various domains, including the physical, psychological and social domain. These problems require an integrated approach, not primarily targeting the disease but focusing on the resident as a human being with a disease and also supporting the family and other informal caregivers (Boyd et al. 2005, Schols et al. 2004). Ideally, this approach gets stature through a coherent and coordinated care supply, which is provided by multiple disciplines within a healthcare facility and/or in alignment with disciplines of other healthcare organizations. To enable an integrated approach, multidisciplinary teamwork is necessary. Offering care from a multidisciplinary approach puts challenges on the organization of care, more specifically on the share each healthcare professional gets in the care process, on the related mutual agreements between different healthcare professionals and on their mutual communication. In the eyes of the residents and their family caregivers, integrated care actually is taken for granted (Institute of Medicine 2001). They do find it most normal that healthcare professionals, who are involved in the care of a particular resident, know each other's activities, so as to ensure that the care will be offered coherently. In short, in their eyes, this should simply be standard care (Huyse et al. 2010). Nevertheless, daily care practice is often still unbendable, and in many cases care provision occurs rather fragmented, both in and outside healthcare institutions.

In this chapter the following issues will be addressed:

- The necessity of integrated multidisciplinary care for nursing home residents with dementia.
- Theoretical aspects of multidisciplinary care.
- The Dutch nursing home as interesting example.

A multidisciplinary approach in fact is relevant for many issues and problems that occur in the nursing home setting and that are discussed in this book. Therefore, this chapter has a more general and descriptive character.

15.2   The Necessity of Integrated Multidisciplinary Care for Residents with Dementia

Nursing home residents with dementia are mostly old to very old persons, who seldom suffer from dementia alone. Often they show a complex geriatric profile consisting of considerable comorbidities, disabilities, handicaps and polypharmacy and also challenging care problems such as malnutrition, falls, pressure ulcers, incontinence, use of restraints and not to forget behavioural problems ranging from apathy towards agitation and/or aggression.

Such a profile is challenging to cope with in the traditional healthcare model which is mainly single disease oriented and based on disease-specific guidelines, coming forward from the strongly promoted evidence-based approach that is based upon the paradigm of the randomized controlled trial. In fact, this approach causes fragmentation of care because it asks for homogeneous patient groups and not for multimorbid heterogeneous ones (Boyd et al. 2005).

Nursing home residents suffering from dementia are already far beyond this single disease status. Their complex polyvalent problems require multifaceted activities of multiple care providers and professionals (Hertogh et al. 1996, von Korff et al. 2009). These activities do start already before their admission to the nursing home and have to be aligned directly with the preferences of the person with dementia and his or her family caregivers who also are involved from the beginning of the dementia process. This complex care process puts demands on the collaboration, communication, coordination and continuity of care inside and outside the nursing home and of course in the transitional phase as well; not to forget the difficult cure – care decisions that often have to be made during their total care trajectory (Goodman et al. 2016).

Residents with dementia therefore represent complex patients. Offering tailored care to them in both the home situation and the nursing home, during their total 'patient journey', has become increasingly difficult during the years, as healthcare systems of many countries have become rather fragmented and highly differentiated. These difficulties are also experienced by the family caregivers and professional caregivers.

In the Nursing Home
Nursing home residents with dementia are quite old and very care dependent, and they often show complex behavioural problems as well. The challenge is to offer these residents adequately integrated nursing, treatment and welfare services in the nursing home environment, in such a way that these services contribute to their well-being and quality of life, by also taking into account their former lifestyle and supporting family connections.

In most countries, nursing home care is basically offered by employed nurses and welfare workers and additionally by regularly or on demand visiting physicians (mostly general practitioners) and paramedical professionals, including physiotherapists, occupational therapists, speech therapists and dieticians. In some countries, including the Netherlands, physicians and paramedical professionals are employed by the nursing home organization itself (Schols et al. 2004). In nursing homes of most Western countries, it is nowadays rather standard to make an integrated care plan for (= together with) every resident and his or her primary family caregivers. This care plan is made after assessing the relevant biopsychosocial factors of the resident and consists of tailored nursing, treatment and welfare activities that have to be executed in a collaborative, multidisciplinary model by different disciplines, of which the outcome and follow-up are monitored regularly (Smith and Clarke 2006). The quality of care related to this institutional care model is not only dependent on the quality of the individual professionals but also on both the effectiveness and embedding of the 'multidisciplinary care model' itself. *Effectiveness* refers to adequate planning of the care and welfare processes and the way these processes are supported by adequate communication and shared decision-making within the team and with the resident and his or her family. Effectiveness also refers to the overall governance of the care processes. *Embedding* means that the care model must be embedded in an appropriate living environment. Nowadays, most nursing homes want to offer their residents with dementia a rather homelike environment to live in, to enable the residents to live their lives as much as they were used to (Huyse et al. 2010).

15.3 Theoretical Aspects of Multidisciplinary Care

This section describes some relevant theoretical aspects of multidisciplinary care provision without aiming to be complete.

Multidisciplinary collaboration is not a new phenomenon in healthcare. In various settings, including nursing homes, collaboration between, for instance, physicians and nurses exists already for a very long time. However, in the past this collaboration was mainly based on hierarchy and differences in power (Fewster-Thuent and Velsor-Friedrich 2008). Throughout the years, one has been looking for new, more egalitarian forms of multidisciplinary collaboration. In these efforts, the main problems of multidisciplinary collaboration involve problems in the relation between disciplines (and persons!), the preservation of professional autonomy and the relation with the own professional background, the different discipline-related languages and jargons and also the issue of team leadership. Moreover, in larger healthcare organizations, different multidisciplinary teams within an organization may sometimes develop towards too autonomous functioning and getting 'lost' from the total organization. What remains, however, is the consensus that a multidisciplinary approach is to prefer above a monodisciplinary one for residents with complex problems, meaning problems that show a component complexity, a coordinative complexity and an ambiguity (Stoffels 2008, Jonge et al. 2006, Huyse et al. 2006). *Component complexity* means that more than one medical or nursing or psychosocial domain is involved. *Coordinative complexity* involves that there is also a dynamic interaction between these domains and that intervention on one domain can interfere with problems in other domains. *Ambiguity* (for instance, in ethical dilemmas) means that insufficient or inconsistent evidence-based information is available and that consensus and therefore adequate and rather intense communication are needed to achieve the best possible solution for daily practice. Offering tailored care to residents with such complex problems ultimately is the main goal and common interest of a collaborative approach, which has to lead to a win-win situation for the residents and the professionals (Firth-Gozens 1998).

15.3.1 The Process of Collaboration

Teamwork in healthcare is more difficult to manage than in commercial environments because every team member has its own professional background with historically included ideas about professional autonomy and responsibility (Firth-Gozens 2001). Despite this, some central norms have been described in literature for the allocation of responsibilities in hospitals, which also may apply for nursing homes (Mitchell et al. 2008, Xyrichis and Lowton 2008, Opie 1997):

• For a resident and his or her family, it must be clear who is the contact point for questions about the care and treatment.
• It must be clear who is responsible for monitoring the total care trajectory of the resident.
• All care professionals involved must make appointments about their separate but complementary tasks and responsibilities in the care for the resident.
• All necessary resident data must be available in a paper or digital record that can be accessed by the professionals involved.
• If the complexity of the resident's problems increases, additional appointments have to be made, based on relevant risk analyses.

In addition, the process of collaboration itself indeed has consequences for professional autonomy. Professional responsibility is closely linked to expression and feelings of professional autonomy (Opie 1997). Whether a change in professional autonomy will be experienced as a problem depends also on the personality traits of the professional involved. Moreover, personality traits as such may influence the process of teamwork. For instance, introvert persons may feel barriers to collaborate in a team with many extrovert persons. Diversity within a team can be threatening; many people like to work in a team with people that match more to their own character and style. Gender and culture differences may also play a role in the way multidisciplinary care can be executed successfully.

Anyhow, good multidisciplinary teamwork requires a transparent decision process, and the ability of all team members to self-reflect on their professional behaviour and to undergo mutual feedback forms a positive attitude.

From the perspective of nurses, data are available about collaboration in healthcare as well. The traditional, hierarchically oriented, relationship between physicians and nurses always has offered less space for an equal work relationship. Next to this already mentioned phenomenon, nurses often express both lack of time and lack of clarity about the role of doctors versus nurses in the care for the residents. In addition, this lack of clarity is also difficult for the residents and their family themselves. Despite this, more recently a trend has become visible in which higher educated nurses and nurse practitioners more often get a coordinating role in multidisciplinary collaborative care models (Fewster-Thuent and Velsor-Friedrich 2008).

15.3.2 Collaborative Competences in Daily Practice and Education

Success of multidisciplinary teamwork does not only depend on the main goal related to optimizing integrated care for the residents and on the common interests of the team members themselves; it also will benefit from goals that have been set for the collaboration process itself.

It is important to realize that 'collaboration' can be learned and therefore educational institutes, schools and universities in fact have a role in this. Multidisciplinary care provision should get more attention in the regular medical and nursing studies and might be facilitated also by using innovative educational activities taking place across the borders of different disciplines.

Collaboration is one of the competence domains of the CanMEDS model which mentions the following characteristics of a well-functioning collaborative model (The Royal College of Physicians and Surgeons of Canada 2005):

- Building up an efficient and effective multidisciplinary team.
- Working together effectively with patients, family caregivers and other professionals in society and healthcare.
- Providing tailored information, leadership, consultative activities and participating in multidisciplinary team meetings.

If motivated and open for self-reflection, professionals can learn how to work in a multidisciplinary way. This starts with the overall awareness of the importance of adequate multidisciplinary collaboration. Next to this, knowledge of the roles of different team members and of various models of multidisciplinary collaboration is important.

The following skills can be learned and practised (Boenink et al. 2010):

- Negotiating, expression of professional leadership and being accountable for one's own activities.
- (Shared) decision-making and conflict management.
- Allocating of tasks and responsibilities and testing the subsequent effects.
- Effective consultation with respect to collaboration dynamics.
- Joint education.

15.3.3 Quality of Multidisciplinary Care

Above all, multidisciplinary care is a matter of cooperation and teamwork. While in various sectors of the society it has been shown that effective teams improve results of products and services, this is not so obvious for healthcare settings, including nursing homes. There is hardly any good research available and it is not yet clear what is meant by effective teams. There is some evidence that factors including a common vision and concrete targets, an accepted division of responsibilities and roles, clear communication, mutual trust and a sense of acceptance and security and also adequately connecting leadership may determine the success of a team (Bosch 2009, Ouwens et al. 2008). However, to get a complete picture of the quality of multidisciplinary care, all relevant dimensions of quality should be measured at both the level of the care provision itself and the level of the residents themselves. These dimensions involve amongst others: the accessibility of care, team cooperation, coordination of care, communication and approach of residents. There are still hardly any validated instruments available that can measure all these quality dimensions in connection to each other for multidisciplinary care (Ouwens et al. 2005, Minkman et al. 2009).

Implementation of evidence-based guidelines is an important way to strengthen quality of care (Boyd et al. 2005, Miller and Petrie 2000). Nevertheless, there are large disadvantages in application of the current guidelines for residents with multimorbidity and problems in multiple domains, including nursing home residents. Patients with complex problems and older persons are often excluded from the clinical trials on which these guidelines are based, and therefore extrapolation of the trial results to these patients is not possible. The application of multiple guidelines at the same time in residents with multimorbidity may lead to a situation in which the recommendations of one guideline can be contrary to the recommendations of another guideline and as such hamper the provision of safe integrated care. Especially, the interaction between somatic and psychosocial diseases within both the social and care context of a complex patient, such as a nursing home resident, requires a holistic approach. In such a situation, the multidisciplinary team should focus primarily on the individual residents instead of focusing on evidence-based guidelines for disease-specific patient groups. It must be stressed that to improve the quality of multidisciplinary care in healthcare, including the nursing home setting, it is very important that in the near future adequate multidisciplinary guidelines will be developed that can be tailored more to the heterogenic profile of people with these complex problems.

Another current barrier for the quality of multidisciplinary care in long-term care settings that needs more attention is the often present fragmentation of care within the care institute, especially the curtains between physicians and nurses and also the curtains between the professional and managerial perspectives. Moreover, residents and their family caregivers or legal representatives are seldom involved as partners in the actual care process. It will be clear that adequate quality of integrative collaborative care will not be achieved in such a situation.

Nursing home residents, being representatives of complex patients, require a multidisciplinary approach by using the concept of case and care complexity. This means that the integral care process starts with an overall comprehensive assessment of the problems and care needs in all domains to subsequently target the multicomponent, multidisciplinary and adequately monitored intervention strategy. The distinction between case complexity and care complexity enables to determine which knowledge, competences and disciplines are needed to tackle the problems adequately together and also determines both the relevance of adequate medical and nursing governance of the multidisciplinary care process (Schols et al. 2004, Hertogh et al. 1996, Jonge et al. 2006).

15.4   The Dutch Nursing Home as Interesting Example

There are differences between the Western countries with regard to the organization of care for the elderly in general and in nursing home care in particular. In this chapter the focus is on Dutch nursing homes because in principle they have an organizational structure that may facilitate optimal multidisciplinary care for their residents (Schols et al. 2004).

In 2016, there were approximately 345 nursing homes in the Netherlands with about 63,000 beds (27,000 in somatic wards, primarily for residents with somatic diseases, i.e. physical problems, and 36,000 in psychogeriatric wards for residents with dementia). Because older persons with chronic physical diseases nowadays have increasing possibilities to age in their own place for a longer time, it is expected that in the near future most beds will be designated for psychogeriatric residents (= residents with dementia). Psychogeriatric wards of Dutch nursing homes are buildings that, with their corridors, colours and closed-door systems, are adapted for residents with loss of orientation because of dementia. In the last two decades, these wards have gradually lost their hospital-like expression, and considerable efforts have been done to make the nursing home for these residents more homelike. In the meantime, also the phenomenon of small-scale living for this target group has been introduced nationwide (Verbeek et al. 2012).

Approximately 60,000 new residents are admitted to Dutch nursing homes every year (40,000 somatic and 20,000 psychogeriatric residents). These residents are characterized by advanced age (>80 years), although also younger people can be admitted to a nursing home, for example, residents with young-onset dementia. The man to woman ratio is 1:2. The most common causes of morbidity in somatic residents are cerebrovascular accidents (26%), other neurologic disorders (e.g. Parkinson's disease, 7%), problems affecting mobility (30%; fractures constitute 25% of this amount, with more than half being hip fractures; the remaining 5% are locomotor disorders) and malignancies (8%). The most frequent diagnosis in psychogeriatric residents involves the dementia syndrome (85%), with Alzheimer's disease being the most frequently occurring type.

Most somatic residents are admitted from the hospital (65%) or by their family physician (26%); psychogeriatric residents primarily come from their own homes (53%), from residential homes (23%) or from hospitals (20%) (Schols et al. 2004, with updated figures).

The nursing home today is far from the ultimate living environment for the resident. For a substantial part of the somatic residents (51%), nursing homes today have a specific geriatric rehabilitation function. After their rehab programme, these residents can return home again or to an assisted living facility. The rest of the somatic residents and most psychogeriatric residents (>90%) remain in the nursing home until their death.

The types of care offered by nursing homes include institutional long-term care, geriatric rehabilitation, respite care, palliative (or hospice) care and crisis intervention. Psychogeriatric residents are usually admitted for institutional long-term care. Most nursing homes additionally offer day care services as a way of respite care for family caregivers or other informal caregivers of older people with long-lasting physical diseases and/or dementia, thereby enabling these people to stay longer at home (Schols et al. 2004, Hertogh et al. 1996).

15.4.1 The Multidisciplinary Care Concept of Dutch Nursing Homes

Nursing home care in the Netherlands is executed by multidisciplinary care teams employed by the nursing homes themselves. The nursing home team consists, next to physicians and nurses, of physiotherapists, occupational therapists, speech therapists, dieticians, psychologists, social workers, pastoral workers and recreational therapists. This allows for the multidisciplinary setting to provide adequate continuous long-term care. Nursing and treatment are based on each resident's personal needs and wishes and on an integration of relevant cure and care. In agreement with the resident and his or her relatives, an integrated care plan is defined after admission and of course after a thorough multidisciplinary assessment of the resident's problems. The role and tasks of each team member follow from this. In addition to medical care, the nursing home physician is responsible for providing substantial directions for the total care, while the first responsible nurse on the ward is responsible for the daily coordination of the execution of the multidisciplinary care plan. On the basis of this plan, the effectiveness of the care is evaluated regularly within the team and with the resident and/or the family relatives; and, if necessary, the care plan is revised. This multidisciplinary, cyclically evaluated systematic approach characterizes the delivery of care in Dutch nursing homes (Schols et al. 2004, Hertogh et al. 1996).

Two short cases will illustrate the multidisciplinary approach more clearly.

Case 15.1
A female resident, age 89, is staying in the nursing home for 12 months since she got a stroke at home, making her completely care dependent. She also suffers from diabetes mellitus and depression. Adequate communication is possible because she does not suffer from aphasia. During the last few months, she shows unintentional weight loss, and if this would be neglected, gradually a risk of malnutrition would occur. Of course the nursing home team will be alerted by this. In most cases, the daily caring nurses are the first who observe a reduced food intake or problems with eating and drinking. Subsequently they alert the nursing home physician (NHP), who first will look for possible medical reasons for the unintentional weight loss, including the status of her diabetes. At the same time, the NHP will consult the dietician, speech therapist, occupational therapist and physiotherapist, to, respectively check the actual food and fluid intake and problems with meal preferences (dietician) and also problems related to dysphagia (speech therapist), self-ability to eat

and drink (occupational therapist) and mobility problems (physiotherapist). The dentist who regularly visits the nursing home checks her oral status, and finally the psychologist undertakes actions to explore additional problems related to her mood and cognition. Of course, during this trajectory a close communication takes place with the resident herself and her close family relatives. This approach enables the team to get a complete picture of the problem, and a multifactorial intervention plan can be developed, tailored to the preferences and prognosis of the resident.

In this case it appeared that the resident was very unhappy and sad with her care-dependent status; she felt that the meaning of her life had gone. In addition, she did not like to eat and drink while sitting in front of two other residents who were even more care dependent and who ate in a very indecent way. Finally, her dentures were not fitting well any more. The nutrition problem was solved after she got personal support by the psychologist for a certain period. Moreover she got a daily activity programme that fitted better in her former lifestyle, she was given another place in the living room during mealtimes and her dentures were adapted to improve the chewing function. Of course, she was followed up thereafter and regularly discussed in the multidisciplinary team meetings, to see whether the execution of the care plan was according to the appointments and agreements made before.

Case 15.2

A male resident, age 84, suffering from Alzheimer's dementia, slight Parkinsonism, arthrosis and hearing difficulties is staying in the nursing home for 3 months. In the nursing home, every day he is wandering all the time until exhaustion; he is continuously seeking around and also shows long periods of prolonged shouting at everyone. If the nurses try to calm him down, he reacts verbally agitated and sometimes also aggressive to them. Finally, the nurses do not know anymore what to do, and they ask the nursing home physician (NHP) whether she can prescribe him a neuroleptic (haloperidol) to calm him down and to relieve them from this problem. They also want the NHP to approve that they tie him up during parts of the day with a belt in his chair, because they are afraid he would fall very soon because of his constant wandering.

Of course, these are possible and maybe also feasible solutions for the nurses, but the NHP doubts whether this strategy would really benefit the resident. Maybe it would do him more harm by making him dull and groggy, aggravating his Parkinsonism and additionally increasing his fall risk even more.

So, after she has looked for possible intervening medical problems and having asked the speech therapist to check the well functioning of the resident's hearing aid, she decides to consult the psychologist of the nursing home team to explore more in depth, together with the rest of the nursing team, the background and possible reasons of the resident's behaviour. This process requires a thorough and integral exploration of his challenging behaviour, including questions like how does the concrete wandering and shouting behaviour look like, how long is this behaviour present, was it already present in the past before nursing home admission, when does it occur during day or night, what are the triggers, what can we learn from the family, etc.

In addition, it is also important to know whether there are factors that work alleviating. Are there any physical or social activities that calm him down during the day, which make him more calm and create a situation in which his wandering and resting behaviours are more in balance? In this process, many contacts take place with close family relatives, to actually learn from them and their perceptions of the problem. Attention is also paid to the sorrows of the nurses regarding possible fall incidents.

In this case, the nurses, psychologist and NHP are the team members who, together with the family relatives, are mostly involved in finding a solution for the resident's behavioural problem and to make both mutual appointments on the strategy that will be followed as well as to get agreement on the risks that will be taken to prevent that the resident will be restricted in his daily activities unnecessarily. Mostly, the ultimately chosen strategy is a multifactorial one, including a variety of non-pharmacological interventions and prevention of avoidable use of psychotropic drugs.

This multidisciplinary care approach is really helpful to tackle the complex problems of nursing home residents, to ultimately offer them the right and tailored living, welfare and care services. Although there is still little evidence, some literature supports that this care approach may lead to a lower prevalence and incidence of relevant care problems such as pressure ulcers, malnutrition, falls and unnecessary use of physical and/or chemical restraints and that it also prevents unnecessary hospital admissions (Halfens et al. 2013, Gulpers et al. 2011). It will be clear that these outcomes may contribute to a better quality of care and reduction of healthcare costs.

15.4.2 Employing the Multidisciplinary Team in a Setting in which Learning Is Leading

Why has the Dutch nursing home sector chosen for a model in which all professionals of the multidisciplinary team are employed by the nursing home itself and not for a situation in which the nursing home is visited by many different consulting professionals?

The following reasons can be mentioned (Schols et al. 2004):

- Nursing home residents need more and longer medical and paramedical consultations.
- The complex problems of these residents require more continuity of care and also more proactive and preventive interventions.
- Family physicians, other consulting medical specialists and paramedical professionals from community healthcare services often have inadequate time, affinity or experience to give these residents the continuous attention they need.
- Medical, paramedical and psychological care in nursing homes is not a job that can be done fast and simply on the side of main general practice medicine, hospital medicine or community care.
- By using their own physicians, psychologists and paramedical personnel, nursing homes can achieve logistic and organizational advantages contrary to the situation in which a nursing home is visited by many different consulting professionals.
- Professionals employed by the nursing home itself or working within a closed staff model seem to be more committed and knowledgeable about long-term care practice and are more continuously available.
- The nursing staff will get more uniform and testable instructions, and the implementation of a well-considered quality system of care will be facilitated.

Finally, it is expected that such an employment model may facilitate the concrete multidisciplinary care approach in a much easier and controllable way.

In this respect it is also understandable that nursing home medicine (nowadays called elderly care medicine) in the Netherlands has been recognized as a distinguished specialty. Actually, this means acknowledgement of the fact that nursing home residents need specific and continuous medical care and that the competency in nursing home medicine requires specific training and experience in handling complex medical care in a highly regulated, multidisciplinary care context, that accommodates both post-acute and long-term care. The acknowledgement of nursing home medicine as a specific discipline has provided the nursing home physician an identity and a position between the family physician and the hospital (clinical) geriatrician.

In the last two decades, Dutch nursing homes pay more and more attention to quality of care with regard to staffing, resident participation and services provided. This attention is encouraged by various policy measures that start from the vision that institutions must take responsibility for quality themselves, meaning that legislation defines responsibilities rather than outcome requirements. Subsequently, the execution of these responsibilities is supervised by an autonomous department of the Ministry of Health, Welfare and Sport, the Health Care Inspectorate, which visits the nursing homes regularly to monitor this. Since 1990, an increasing number of multidisciplinary guidelines have become available to additionally support the multidisciplinary approach to nursing home care, and most nursing home organizations have implemented a well-considered quality system of integral care with incorporation of these more feasible guidelines (Schols et al. 2014).

An increasing number of nursing homes is currently also participating in one of the academic collaborative centres on elderly care that are present around six universities in the country. Participation in these centres bridges the gap between nursing home research and daily practice of nursing home care and eventually contributes to a better care, benefitting the residents (Verbeek et al. 2013).

15.4.3 Future Developments in Dutch Multidisciplinary Nursing Home Care

In the near future, more attention will be paid to the equal role that residents and family caregivers themselves may play in the daily care process. Striving for more personalized care and shared decision-making are the main goals in this respect, and this will require even more attention for the dialogue with the resident and the family.

This is extra important because, in the near future, nursing home residents will enter the nursing home in more advanced stages of their diseases, after having tried first to stay home as long as possible. At that moment, their condition at admission will be more complex and their length of stay in the nursing home automatically shorter as well. This will make that important end-of-life questions will raise already shortly after admission, asking for a close contact and cooperation between the resident, the family and the care professionals in the nursing home.

Regarding the functioning of the professional team members, more attention will be paid to additionally improving and strengthening of the multidisciplinary care performance by paying specific attention to working in a more interdisciplinary way. From a team point of view, this may lead to a situation in which professionals not primarily act in a cumulative way, but actually look and act beyond the borders of their own discipline. Then multidisciplinary care will ultimately lead to a win-win situation in which '1 + 1 ≠ 2' but '1 + 1 = 3', representing both the 'added value' of multidisciplinary and interdisciplinary collaboration and the fact that the care indeed will become real integrated care.

Nowadays, also a new trend has become visible in which Dutch nursing homes increasingly perform care activities for old, sick and functionally impaired patients in the community. This phenomenon has been originated by the following factors:

- The demographic increase of (frail) elderly in the community.
- The growing costs of chronic care and the shortage of nursing home beds.
- The phenomenon of hospitals that focus more and more on acute, short-term care.
- The wish of many frail elderly and patients with chronic diseases and disabilities to receive care as long as possible where they live, in the community.

The trend towards *ageing in place* involves challenges for community care services which have to deal with increasingly complex care problems of older people at home, including people suffering from dementia. As a consequence, Dutch nursing homes today also stress their contribution to the community-based care for older people, making the relationship of nursing home professionals to family physicians, community nurses and others extra important. In this way, in the community, a model of 'shared care' can be realized and tailored to the frail older person's individual needs and wishes. It will be clear that, by bringing in this complementary outreaching nursing home care, also relevant aspects and benefits of the intramural multidisciplinary approach can be extended towards the community healthcare services.

In other Western countries, demographic developments and changing care trends will also lead to comparable changes in the concepts of care and the healthcare system. This will require further elaboration of the concept of shared care between community care and institutional care.

For this purpose, the Dutch experience might be helpful as well.

References

Boenink AD, Slootweg IA, Schols JMGA (2010) Theory and models of multidisciplinary collaboration. In: Leentjens AFG, Gans ROB, Schols JMGA, van Weel C (eds) Manual of multidisciplinary care (Dutch). De Tijdstroom, Utrecht

Bosch M (2009) Organizational determinants of improving health care delivery. Dissertation, UMC St. Radboud Nijmegen, Nijmegen, The Netherlands

Boyd CM, Darer J, Boult C et al (2005) Clinical practice guidelines and quality of care for older patients with multiple comorbid disease. Implications for pay per performance. JAMA 294:716–724

de Jonge P, Huyse FJ, Stiefel FC (2006) Case and care complexity in the medically ill. Med Clin North Am 90:679–692

Fewster-Thuent L, Velsor-Friedrich B (2008) Interdisciplinary collaboration for health care professionals. Nurs Adm Q 32:40–48

Firth-Gozens J (1998) Celebrating teamwork. Qual Health Care 7(Suppl):S3–S7

Firth-Gozens J (2001) Multidisciplinary teamwork: the good, bad and everything in between. Qual Health Care 10(2):65–66

Goodman C, Dening T, Gordon AL et al (2016) Effective health care for older people living and dying in care homes: a realist review. BMC Health Serv Res 16(1):269. doi:10.1186/s12913-016-1493-4

Gulpers MJ, Bleijlevens MH, Ambergen T et al (2011) Belt restraint reduction in nursing homes: effects of a multicomponent intervention program. J Am Geriatr Soc 59(11):2029–2036. doi:10.1111/j.1532-5415.2011.03662.x

Halfens RJ, Meesterberends E, van Nie-Visser NC et al (2013) International prevalence measurement of care problems: results. J Adv Nurs 69(9):e5–17. doi:10.1111/jan.12189

Hertogh CMPM, Deerenberg-Kessler W, Ribbe MW (1996) The problem-oriented multidisciplinary approach in Dutch nursing home care. Clin Rehabil 10:135–142

Huyse FJ, Stiefel FC, de Jonge P (2006) Identifiers, or 'red flags', of complexity and need for integrated care. Med Clin North Am 90:703–712

Huyse FJ, van Weel C, Latour CHM (2010) The necessity of integrated care in complex patients (Dutch). In: Leentjens AFG, Gans ROB, Schols JMGA, van Weel C (eds) Manual of multidisciplinary care (Dutch). De Tijdstroom, Utrecht

Institute of Medicine (2001) Crossing the quality chasm: a new health system for the 21th century. Committee on Quality of Health Care in America. National Academy press, Washington, DC

Miller J, Petrie J (2000) Development of practice guidelines. Lancet 355(9198):82–83

Minkman M, Ahaus K, Fabbricotti I et al (2009) A quality management model for integrated care: results of a Delphi and Concept Mapping study. International J Qual Health Care 21:66–75

Mitchell GK, Tieman JJ, Shelby-James TM (2008) Multidisciplinary care planning and teamwork in primary care. Med J Aust 188(8 Suppl):S61–S64

Opie A (1997) Effective teamwork in health care: a review of issues discussed in recent research literature. Health Care Anal 5(1):62–70

Ouwens M, Wollersheim H, Hermens R et al (2005) Integrated care programmes for chronically ill patients: a reviewof systematic reviews. International J Qual Health Care 17:141–146

Ouwens M, Hulscher M, Akkermans R et al (2008) The team climate inventory: application in hospital teams and methodological considerations. Qual Saf Health Care 17:275–280

Schols JMGA, Crebolder HFJM, van Weel C (2004) Nursing home and nursing home physician: the Dutch experience. JAMDA 5(3):207–212

Schols JMGA, Frijters DHM, Kempen GIJM et al (2014) Quality monitoring of long-term care in the Netherlands. In: Mor V, Leone T, Maresso (eds) Regulating long-term care quality; an international comparison. Cambridge University Press, Cambridge, UK

Smith GC, Clarke D (2006) Assessing the effectiveness of integrated interventions: terminology and approach. Med Clin North Am 90:533–548

Stoffels AMR (2008) Cooperation among medical specialists: 'pain'or 'gain'. Dissertation, Rijksuniversiteit Groningen, Groningen, The Netherlands

The Royal College of Physicians and Surgeons of Canada (2005) CanMEDS 2005 Framework. http://www.royalcollege.ca/portal/page/portal/rc/common/documents/canmeds/framework/the7_canmeds_roles_e.pdf. Assessed July 2016

Verbeek H, Zwakhalen SM, van Rossum E et al (2012) Small-scale, homelike facilities in dementia care: a process evaluation into the experiences of family caregivers and nursing staff. Int J Nurs Stud 49(1):21–29. doi:10.1016/j.ijnurstu.2011.07.008

Verbeek H, Zwakhalen SM, Schols JM et al (2013) Keys to successfully embedding scientific research in nursing homes: a win-win perspective. J Am Med Dir Assoc 14(12):855–857. doi:10.1016/j.jamda.2013.09.006

Von Korff MR, Scott KM, Gureje O (eds) (2009) Global perspectives on mental-physical comorbidity. Cambridge University press, Cambridge

Xyrichis A, Lowton K (2008) What fosters or prevents interprofessional teamworking in primary and community care? Int J Nurs Stud 45(1):140–153

The Prevention and Reduction of Physical Restraint Use in Long-Term Care

16

Jan Hamers

Abstract

In the year 1999, the appeal to reduce the use of physical restraints in persons with dementia living in institutionalized long-term care settings was sharply criticized by nursing home staff in the Netherlands. At that time, it was argued that the use of physical restraints such as waist belts and two-sided full-enclosed bedrails was needed to provide safe care in residents suffering from cognitive impairment, such as dementia. Physicians and nurses demonstrated, showing individual cases of residents with severe injuries after falls, that the use of restrictive physical restraints in nursing homes was legitimate. How different is this in 2017? Nowadays, the large majority of nursing home staff does not assess the use of belts and other restrictive physical restraints as adequate anymore. Like in many countries, in the Netherlands, the use of physical restraints is an indicator of poor quality of care in institutionalized long-term care settings now. This is the result of more than 15 years of scientific research and dissemination and implementation of research results in clinical practice and healthcare policy. In this chapter, an overview of this research process conducted in *the Living Lab in Ageing and Long-Term Care* (Verbeek et al. 2013) will be presented. The Living Lab is a structural collaboration between Maastricht University, Zuyd University of applied sciences and long-term care organizations providing care for persons with dementia.

Knowing that many older persons suffering from cognitive impairment do not have a formal diagnosis of dementia, this chapter focuses on persons with cognitive impairment in general and dementia in particular. After a description of physical restraints in institutionalized long-term care, its prevalence, determinants, and consequences, we will describe the effects of an approach named EXBELT, aiming at the prevention and reduction of physical restraints in persons with dementia living in institutionalized long-term care settings. This chapter

J. Hamers, PhD, RN, FEANS
Department of Health Services Research, Research School Caphri, Maastricht University, Maastricht, The Netherlands
e-mail: jph.hamers@maastrichtuniversity.nl

© Springer International Publishing AG 2017   219
S. Schüssler, C. Lohrmann (eds.), *Dementia in Nursing Homes*,
DOI 10.1007/978-3-319-49832-4_16

will be concluded with the use of physical restraints in persons with cognitive impairment living in the community, as aging in place is highly on the agenda in many countries.

Keywords
Physical restraints • Involuntary treatment • Nursing home • Home care • Dementia

16.1 Physical Restraints

In a recent study (Beerens et al. 2014), physical restraint use (belt restraints, locked chair/table, deep/overturned chair, bedrails) in persons with dementia was assessed in eight European countries and resulted in an average prevalence number of 31%. However, the variety between countries was very wide, ranging from 6% to 83%. These results are in line with earlier studies, showing a wide variety in prevalence numbers of physical restraints in institutionalized long-term care facilities such as nursing homes, ranging from about 6% to 70% (e.g., Hamers and Huizing 2005; Heinze et al. 2012; Schüssler et al. 2014). This variety in prevalence numbers is partly attributed to the use of different methods and definitions of physical restraint. To illustrate, some studies have excluded bedrails as a measure of physical restraint. Others have included sensor alarms that by some authors are not viewed as a restraint measure. As a result, prevalence rates of different studies are difficult to compare, and consensus on a consistent definition of physical restraints is needed.

Therefore, an international group of 48 experts consisting of researchers and clinicians from 13 countries (Australia, Belgium, Canada, Finland, Germany, Hong Kong, the Netherlands, Norway, Spain, Sweden, Switzerland, the United Kingdom, the United States) who have made sustained contribution to research and clinical application in the field of physical restraint in clinical care has agreed upon a new definition of physical restraint recently (Bleijlevens et al. 2016). They define physical restraint as *"any action or procedure that prevents a person's free body movement to a position of choice and/or normal access to his/her body by the use of any method, attached or adjacent to a person's body that he/she cannot control or remove easily"* (Bleijlevens et al. 2016). Examples of physical restraints are the use of two-sided full-enclosed bedrails, waist belts, overturned geriatric chairs, and chairs with a locked tray table.

16.2 Determinants and Consequences of Restraint Use

The opinion of many people is that the use of physical restraints is a result of shortages in nursing home staff, or other organizational characteristics are debatable. Although Wagner et al. (2012), conducting secondary analyses using

OSCAR data, found an association between decreased likelihood of deficiency citations for physical restraints (indicating better quality of care) and higher RN staffing levels, this was not supported by observational studies (e.g., Engberg et al. 2008; Heinze et al. 2012) investigating associations of organizational characteristics and restraint use. For instance, Huizing et al. (2007) examined objective and subjective measures of workload, social support, sickness absence, and FTE ratio and found no associations with restraint use (as assessed by blinded independent raters) in persons with cognitive impairment, including dementia. They even reported more restraint use, when more staff was available (Huizing et al. 2007).

Residents' characteristics are the most important determinants of physical restraint use in persons with cognitive impairment. Poor cognitive status, poor mobility, and dependence in activities of daily living seem to be important predictors of restraint use (e.g., Capezuti 2004; Hofmann and Hahn 2013; Kirkevold et al. 2004; Meyer et al. 2008; Pellfolk et al. 2012). The most important reason to use physical restraint is to increase the residents' safety. The assumption is that the use of physical restraints will prevent falls and severe injuries (e.g., fractures) as a result from falls (Hamers et al. 2004; Pellfolk et al. 2012). However, it is known that the use of physical restraints has many negative consequences. Some residents will become incontinent as a result of being restrained; they cannot go to the toilet independently. Other residents will develop apathetic or aggressive behavior, as they are willing to free themselves from a belt restraint. In a study by Castle (2006), it was concluded that belt restraints led to a decrease in cognitive performance, an increase of depression, and a decrease of social engagement. Furthermore, restraining a person will negatively affect the person's muscle strength and balance, increasing the risk of falls and creating a vicious circle (Hamers et al. 2009). Finally, it has been reported that the use of physical restraints can result in injuries and even fatal accidents, just because people want to free themselves. It is evident that physical restraint use in older people does not contribute to better health or quality of life. Therefore, restraint use should be prevented and reduced in institutional long-term care settings.

16.3   Approaches Aiming at the Reduction of Physical Restraints

During decennia, in most countries, nursing home staff has been educated that the use of physical restraints is an adequate care in order to prevent harm in nursing home residents with cognitive impairment. This may explain why the development of training programs has been the main approach in order to reduce the use of physical restraints (e.g., Kuske et al. 2009; Lai et al. 2006; Huizing et al. 2009a, b; Testad et al. 2005). Some approaches are elaborated by introducing a nurse specialist who acts as a consultant aiming at the further reduction of restraints in complex individual cases (Capezuti et al. 2007; Evans et al. 1997; Huizing et al. 2009a, b).

Different research designs (ranging from chart reviews to randomized clinical trials) have been employed to evaluate the effectiveness of the different approaches. Controlled studies report negative results ("the approach is not effective") more often than uncontrolled studies. In general, training programs aiming at the reduction of physical restraints seem to improve the knowledge of nursing staff regarding restraint use, its determinants and consequences, and the need to prevent restraint use (Kuske et al. 2009; Mac Dermaid and Byrne 2006). However, educational programs are insufficiently effective in reducing the use of physical restraints (Kuske et al. 2009; Testad et al. 2005; Möhler et al. 2012). This was also found in a study by our research group in the Netherlands; a randomized controlled study by Huizing et al. (2009a) using an intensive educational training program in combination with a nurse specialist showed no effect in preventing or reducing the use of physical restraints in nursing home residents with cognitive impairment (most suffering from dementia). Different explanations were brought up for this negative outcome. First, nursing staff said that they experienced no or insufficient support from the nursing home management by emphasizing the need to reduce physical restraints. Furthermore, nursing staff said that direct staff members who did not attend the training program were hindering initiatives to reduce restraints. Finally, alternative measures (e.g., infrared warning alarm, physical exercises by physiotherapist) were insufficiently available. These results have led to the further development of an approach in the Living Lab in Ageing and Long-Term Care (Verbeek et al. 2013) aiming at the reduction of physical restraints in persons with cognitive impairment living in long-term care facilities: "EXBELT."

16.4   EXBELT

The EXBELT approach comprises four key components (Gulpers et al. 2011):

1. Implementation of an institutional policy change, including:
   (a) Prohibition of the use of belt restraint for newly admitted residents and initiating belt restraint use for already admitted residents and overall reduction of current use of belt restraint.
   (b) Written and oral communication regarding the forthcoming policy change provided by the nursing home management to all members of nursing home staff and to residents' relatives. The policy change is announced to nursing home staff and legal representatives of the residents in a formal letter and announcements in internal newspapers and in group meetings aimed at the legal representatives of the residents.
   (c) Oral communication regarding the policy change provided by the nurse specialists during the educational program to the nursing home staff.
2. Education: An intensive educational intervention program providing information about physical restraints and fall prevention, the negative aspects of physical restraint use, staff attitudes toward physical restraint use, how to make decisions regarding alternative interventions, and the use of resident-centered interventions. The educational program is offered to nursing home staff

(physicians, nurses, paramedical staff, psychologists, and ward managers). Each meeting lasts approximately 3 h during nursing home staff's working hours. A 90-min educational session, summarizing the content of the 9 h of education, is provided separately to members of the nursing staff who cannot attend the program sessions.

3. Consultation: A nurse specialist who delivers the educational program also provides on-site consultation from the start of the educational program to individual nurses regarding challenges in reducing restraints. The nurse specialists are available on demand, with each ward receiving at least two consultations.

4. Availability of alternative interventions: Nursing home managers provide resident-centered alternative interventions, such as hip protectors, infrared alarm systems, balance training, exercise, special pillows, and adjustable low-height beds. The nurse specialist who provides on-site consultation facilitates decision-making regarding alternative interventions and encourages the use of alternative interventions (Gulpers et al. 2011).

16.4.1 Effectiveness of EXBELT

The effectiveness of EXBELT has been evaluated using a quasi-experimental study design (Gulpers et al. 2011, 2012), including 26 wards from 13 psychogeriatric nursing homes. These psychogeriatric nursing homes provide care for older persons with cognitive impairment; the majority of the residents are suffering from dementia. EXBELT was introduced on 15 wards (EXBELT group, 317 residents); 11 wards (control group, 201 residents) received care as usual. Assessments of the main outcome (belt restraints) and secondary outcomes (other types of physical restraints) were conducted by blinded independent raters who visited each of the 26 wards unannounced four times in a 24-h period (morning, afternoon, evening, and night). The assessments were done at baseline and 4 and 8 months later. In a separate study, the long-term effects of EXBELT have been examined (Gulpers et al. 2013). Therefore, similar assessments of primary and secondary outcomes have been conducted 24 months after baseline. Alongside the effect evaluation, a process evaluation has been conducted (Bleijlevens et al. 2013).

16.4.1.1   Restraint Reduction
At baseline, belt restraints were used in 19% of the residents on the control wards and in 17% of the residents on the wards where EXBELT was introduced. Eight months after baseline, the use of belt restraints was reduced with 50% in the EXBELT group, while there was no reduction in the control group ($p = 0.005$) (Gulpers et al. 2011). Furthermore, there were also differences in the use of other type of restraints. For example, in the EXBELT group, less bedrails ($p = 0.001$) were used than in the control group. The two groups did not differ with regard to the use of psychotropic medication and the number of falls (Gulpers et al. 2011). Remarkably, no alternative measures were used in half of the residents where belt restraints were stopped. The alternatives mostly used were the use of low beds and sensor pads.

16.4.1.2   Restraint Prevention

Even more important results were reported regarding the prevention of belt restraints. Eight months after follow-up, in the EXBELT group, no belt restraints (0%) were used in new residents, while restraints were used in 20% of newly admitted residents in the control group ($p = 0.03$) (Gulpers et al. 2012). Although the number of other restraints was lower in the EXBELT group, this was not statistically significant. The two groups did not differ with regard to the use of psychotropic medication and the number of falls (Gulpers et al. 2012).

The process evaluation showed that the EXBELT intervention was implemented according to the protocol. However, the nursing staff said that the instructions regarding the announcement of the policy change could be improved and that the nurse specialist could act even more proactively (Bleijlevens et al. 2013).

16.4.1.3   Long-Term Effects

Two years after baseline, the prevalence of belt restraints had been further reduced in the EXBELT group, while the use in the control group remained almost unchanged ($p = 0.036$). If we include all residents living on the EXBELT and control wards 2 years after baseline, the prevalence numbers of belt restraints in both groups are 3% and 13% ($p < 0.001$), respectively (Gulpers et al. 2013). However, the study on long-term effects also learned that physical restraints are not reduced or prevented automatically. The positive outcomes of the EXBELT approach did not inspire the control wards to change their policy regarding the use of physical restraints. Two years after the EXBELT study was started, clinical restraint practice on these wards did not change!

16.4.2 Conclusions: Restraint Reduction and Prevention

The EXBELT approach has shown to be effective in the prevention and safe reduction of belt and other restraints in institutionalized long-term care facilities providing care for persons with dementia or other cognitive impairment, and the implementation of EXBELT has proven to be feasible. However, it should be emphasized that in many countries, researchers have been working on approaches aiming at the reduction of physical restraints in this vulnerable group (e.g., Evans et al. 1997; Koczy et al. 2011; Köpke et al. 2012; Kwok et al. 2012; Milke et al. 2008;Möhler et al. 2012; Pellfolk et al. 2010; Testad et al. 2010). All roads lead to Rome is a saying that can be applied here: there is no single approach for reducing restraints, but we can all learn from different approaches and tailor them to specific settings and countries.

However, the EXBELT studies have learned that the implementation of effective approaches is badly needed to change clinical practice and that the reduction of restrictive physical restraints must remain on the agenda!

16.5 New Challenges: Physical Restraint Use in the Community

With the graying of the society, "the aging in place" policy in many countries, and the increase of older persons with cognitive impairment, mainly dementia, there is a new challenge: prevention of physical restraint use in the community. Although information on restraint use in older persons receiving home care is scarce, there are strong indications that physical restraints are used in the community. Four out of five nurses in Dutch home care reported having applied physical restraints such as bedrails or chairs with a locked table (De Veer et al. 2009). A Japanese study reported that 41% of the home care providers had observed restraint use at home (Kurate and Ojima 2014), and in a qualitative study in Belgium, nurses providing home care also stated that physical restraints were frequently used (Scheepmans et al. 2014). It is worth noting that all these studies reported that family caregivers initiated the use of restraints, which is in contrast to institutional long-term care where professional staff mostly decide upon the use of restraints (Kurate and Ojima 2014; Scheepmans et al. 2014). The first prevalence figures concerning the use of physical restraints (belt restraints, locked chair/table, deep/overturned chair, bedrails) in the community reported in eight European countries show an overall use of physical restraints in 10% of about 1200 persons with dementia. However, the variety was large, ranging from 3% in the Netherlands to 20% in Germany (Beerens et al. 2014).

Recently, Hamers et al. (2016) conducted a prevalence study on the use of involuntary treatment in a sample of 837 older persons with cognitive impairment, including dementia, living in their own homes and receiving professional home care. Involuntary treatment is defined as a treatment that professional and family caregivers provide without the consent of the person receiving the treatment (Hamers et al. 2016). Involuntary treatment includes the use of physical restraints (e.g., waist belts), psychotropic medication (e.g., antipsychotics), and nonconsensual care (e.g., forced hygiene) (Hamers et al. 2016). Involuntary treatment was used in 39% of the total sample. The most common were nonconsensual care (79%; e.g., concealing medication in food, forcing hygiene) and psychotropic medication (41%). In 7% of the sample, physical restraints (e.g., deep or overturned chair, bilateral full-enclosure bedrails) were used. The family of the person with cognitive impairment most often requested the use of involuntary treatment (Hamers et al. 2016).

Family caregivers who want to minimize the risk of harm or injury may perceive physical restraints as the only way to prevent falls or injuries or to control behavioral symptoms in persons with cognitive impairment. However, family and professional caregivers do not always realize that restraints have negative effects on persons with cognitive impairment and, for example, may increase the risk of falling with injury (Hamers et al. 2016). To prevent inappropriate use of involuntary treatment at home, (development of) services and programs aiming to support family and professional caregivers should be invested in (Hamers et al. 2016). As we can learn from research in long-term care facilities, education and consultation are necessary to increase knowledge of the consequences of involuntary treatment but are in themselves not sufficient to change caregiver behavior. Looking at the EXBELT approach, policy changes and a strong focus on helping families and professional caregivers understand behavioral communication of the person with cognitive impairment and responding more appropriately to the needs being thus expressed are essential components of an approach to reduce and prevent involuntary treatment in general and physical restraints in particular.

Conclusion

Despite the fact that the use of physical restraints is an indicator of poor quality of care, restraint use is still prevalent in persons with dementia and other cognitive impairment living in institutionalized long-term care. Effective approaches are available to safely reduce and prevent restraint use, such as waist belts and bedrails. However, these approaches are not automatically implemented in clinical practice. Furthermore, we are facing a new challenge in long-term care. With the increase of older persons with dementia and other cognitive impairment in the community, there is an increasing risk on involuntary treatment, including the use of physical restraints at home. Therefore, the reduction and prevention of restraint use in persons with dementia should stay on the agenda.

References

Beerens HC, Sutcliffe C, Renom-Guiteras A et al (2014) Quality of life and quality of care for people with dementia receiving long term institutional care or professional home care: the European RightTimePlaceCare study. J Am Med Dir Assoc 15:54–61

Bleijlevens MHC, Gulpers MJM, Capezuti E, Van Rossum E, Hamers JPH (2013) Process evaluation of a multi-component intervention program (EXBELT) to reduce belt restraints in nursing homes. J Am Med Dir Assoc 14:599–604

Bleijlevens MH, Wagner LM, Capezuti E, Hamers JPH (2016) A Delphi consensus study to determine an internationally accepted definition on physical restraints. J Am Geriatr Soc. doi:10.1111/jgs.14435

Capezuti E (2004) Minimizing the use of restrictive devices in dementia patients at risk for falling. Nurs Clin N Am 39:625–647

Capezuti E, Wagner LM, Brush BL et al (2007) Consequences of an intervention to reduce restrictive side rail use in nursing homes. J Am Geriatr Soc 55:334–341

Castle NG (2006) Mental health outcomes and physical restraint use in nursing homes. Adm Policy Ment Health 33:696–704

De Veer AJE, Francke AL, Buijse R, Friele R (2009) The use of physical restraints in home care in the Netherlands. J Am Geriatr Soc 57:1881–1886

Engberg J, Castle NG, McCaffrey D (2008) Physical restraint initiation in nursing homes and subsequent resident health. Gerontologist 48:442–452

Evans LK, Strumpf NE, Allen-Taylor SL, Capezuti E, Maislin G, Jacobsen B (1997) A clinical trial to reduce restraints in nursing homes. J Am Geriatr Soc 45:675–681

Gulpers MJM, Bleijlevens MHC, Ambergen T, Capezuti E, Van Rossum E, Hamers JPH (2011) Belt restraint reduction in nursing homes: effects of a multi-component intervention program (EXBELT). J Am Geriatr Soc 59:2029–2036

Gulpers MJM, Bleijlevens MHC, Capezuti E, Van Rossum E, Ambergen T, Hamers JPH (2012) Preventing belt restraint use in newly admitted residents in nursing homes: a quasi-experimental study. Int J Nurs Stud 49:1473–1479

Gulpers MJM, Bleijlevens MHC, Ambergen T, Capezuti E, Van Rossum E, Hamers JPH (2013) Reduction of belt restraint use: long-term effects of the EXBELT intervention. J Am Geriatr Soc 61:107–112

Hamers JPH, Huizing AR (2005) Why do we use physical restraints in the elderly? Z Gerontol Geriatr 38:19–25

Hamers JPH, Gulpers MJM, Strik W (2004) Use of physical restraints with cognitively impaired nursing home residents. J Adv Nurs 45:246–251

Hamers JPH, Gulpers MJM, Bleijlevens M, Huizing AR, Scherder EJ, Houweling H, Van Rossum E (2009) Het reduceren van vrijheidsbeperking in verpleeghuizen (The reduction of physical restraints in nursing homes). T Ouderengeneesk 34:156–159

Hamers JPH, Bleijlevens MH, Gulpers MJ, Verbeek H (2016) Behind closed doors: involuntary treatment in care of persons with cognitive impairment at home in the Netherlands. J Am Geriatr Soc 64:354–358

Heinze C, Dassen T, Grittner U (2012) Use of physical restraints in nursing homes and hospitals and related factors: a cross sectional study. J Clin Nurs 21:1033–1040

Hofmann H, Hahn S (2013) Characteristics of nursing home residents and physical restraint: a systematic literature review. J Clin Nurs 23:3012–3024

Huizing AR, Hamers JPH, Candel M, De Jonge J, Berger MPF (2007) Organisational determinants of the use of physical restraints: a multilevel approach. Soc Sci Med 65:924–933

Huizing AR, Hamers JP, Gulpers MJ et al (2009a) A cluster-randomized trial of an educational intervention to reduce the use of physical restraints with psychogeriatric nursing home residents. J Am Geriatr Soc 57:1139–1148

Huizing AR, Hamers JP, Gulpers MJ et al (2009b) Preventing the use of physical restraints on residents newly admitted to psycho-geriatric nursing home wards: a cluster-randomized trial. Int J Nurs Stud 46:459–469

Kirkevold O, Sandvik L, Engedal K (2004) Use of constraints and their correlates in Norwegian nursing homes. Int J Geriatr Psychiatry 19:980–988

Koczy P, Becker C, Rapp K, Klie T, Beische D, Büchele G, Kleiner A, Guerra V, Rissmann U, Kurrle S, Bredthauer D (2011) Effectiveness of a multifactorial intervention to reduce physical restraints in nursing home residents. J Am Geriatr Soc 59:333–339

Köpke S, Mühlhauser I, Gerlach A, Haut A, Haastert B, Möhler R, Meyer G (2012) Effect of a guideline-based multicomponent intervention on use of physical restraints in nursing homes: a randomized controlled trial. JAMA 307:2177–2184

Kurata S, Ojima T (2014) Knowledge, perceptions, and experiences of family caregivers and home care providers of physical restraint use with home-dwelling elders: a cross-sectional study in Japan. BMC Geriatr 14:39. doi: 10.1186/1471-2318-14-39

Kuske B, Luck T, Hanns S et al (2009) Training in dementia care: a cluster-randomized controlled trial of a training program for nursing home staff in Germany. Int Psychogeriatr 21:295–308

Kwok T, Bai X, Chui MY, Lai CK, Ho DW, Ho FK, Woo J (2012) Effect of physical restraint reduction on older patients' hospital length of stay. J Am Med Dir Assoc 13:645–650

Lai CKY, Chan MH, Szeto SSL et al (2006) A retrospective study on the outcomes of a collaborative restraint reduction project by a residential home for older people and a hospital-based community geriatric assessment service. Hong Kong Nurs J 42:23–30

Mac Dermaid L, Byrne C (2006) Restraint reduction education. Can Nurs Home 17:10–14

Meyer G, Köpke S, Haastert B, Mühlhauser I (2008) Restraint use among nursing home residents: a cross-sectional study and prospective cohort study. J Clin Nurs 18:981–990

Milke DL, Kendall TS, Neumann I et al (2008) A longitudinal evaluation of restraint reduction within a multi-site, multi-model Canadian continuing care organization. Can J Aging 27:35–43

Möhler R, Richter T, Köpke S, Meyer G (2012) Interventions for preventing and reducing the use of physical restraints in long-term geriatric care – a Cochrane review. J Clin Nurs 21:3070–3081

Pellfolk TJ, Gustafson Y, Bucht G, Karlsson S (2010) Effects of a restraint minimization program on staff knowledge, attitudes, and practice: a cluster randomized trial. J Am Ger Soc 58:62–69

Pellfolk T, Sandman PO, Gustafson Y, Karlsson S, Lövheim H (2012) Physical restraint use in institutional care of old people in Sweden in 2000 and 2007. Int Psychogeriatr 24:1144–1152

Scheepmans K, Dierckx de Casterle B, Paquay L, Van Gansbeke H, Boonen S, Milisen K (2014) Restraint use in home care: a qualitative study from a nursing perspective. BMC Geriatr 14:17

Schüssler S, Dassen T, Lohrmann C (2014) Prevalence of care dependency and nursing care problems in nursing home residents with dementia: a literature review. Int J Caring Sci 7:338–352

Testad I, Aasland AM, Aarsland D (2005) The effect of staff training on the use of restraint in dementia: a single-blind randomised controlled trial. Int J Geriatr Psychiatry 20:587–590

Testad I, Ballard C, Bronnick K, Aarsland D (2010) The effect of staff training on agitation and use of restraint in nursing home residents with dementia: a single-blind, randomized controlled trial. J Clin Psychiatry 71:80–86

Verbeek H, Zwakhalen SMG, Schols JMGA, Hamers JPH (2013) Keys to successful embedding scientific research in nursing homes: a win-win perspective. J Am Med Dir Assoc 14:855–857

Wagner LM, McDonald SM, Castle NG (2012) Nursing home deficiency citations for physical restraints and restrictive side rails. West J Nurs Res 35:546–565

Care Dependency

Ate Dijkstra

Abstract

During the later stages of dementia, most people will become increasingly frail, which is one of the most common reasons for admission in a nursing home. Life in nursing homes can be characterized by a high degree of patients' dependency. Especially, many physical, cognitive, and social disabilities of demented in-patients result in dependency on nursing care. Care dependency and similar terms are frequently used in literature to understand and to give form and content to the care for elderly people with dementia. This chapter describes three aspects regarding the concept of care dependency: its conceptualization, operationalization, and utilization. The first paragraph gives the reason about "why" this chapter is written. In the next three paragraphs, an answer will be given on "what" is care dependency. The second paragraph gives a review about the literature on care dependency in an attempt to conceptualize what care dependency means and how it can be defined. The third paragraph focuses on how the definition can be operationalized to measure care dependency in patients admitted in a nursing home. The fourth paragraph explores "how" the measurement instrument can be utilized in daily practice of a nursing home. This chapter ends with a conclusion paragraph.

Keywords

Care dependency • Conceptualization • Operationalization • Utilization • Dementia • Nursing home

---

This chapter is based on an adaption of a previously published article "Operationalization of the Concept 'Nursing Care Dependency' for Use in Long-Term Care Facilities" (Dijkstra et al. 1998a).

A. Dijkstra, PhD MEd RN
NHL University of Applied Sciences, Leeuwarden, The Netherlands
e-mail: ate.dijkstra@icloud.com

© Springer International Publishing AG 2017
S. Schüssler, C. Lohrmann (eds.), *Dementia in Nursing Homes*,
DOI 10.1007/978-3-319-49832-4_17

17.1   Introduction

Dementia is one of the most common conditions treated in nursing homes (WHO 2012). Dementia can be described as a set of symptoms including memory loss and difficulties with thinking, problem-solving, or language (Alzheimer's Society 2013a). As one of the consequences of dementia, a decline in self-care abilities is a major component of the dementia syndrome and therefore closely related to the development and progression of care dependency (Schlüsser et al. 2014). These symptoms affect more and more daily life activities. McLaughlin et al. (2010) state that these functional impairments primarily result from cognitive impairment, with notable losses in the ability to perform self-care activities.

Patients with dementia will also gradually become dependent on others for all of their care, e.g., informal and/or professional carers (Alzheimer's Society 2013b). In nursing homes, several professional carers work together in an interdisciplinary context, each one with a focus on specific aspects of dementia. Clinicians, including physician, psychologist, physiotherapist, and speech therapist, tend to focus on physical illnesses, cognition, behavior, and/or function. Nurses mainly focus on the impact of dementia on the self-care abilities regarding activities of daily living.

Life in nursing homes can be characterized by the high degree of patients' dependency. Care dependency is a much used term in dementia care and closely related to the development of dementia. Care dependency means that the self-care abilities of a person in terms of their basic physical and psychosocial human needs (e.g., eating and drinking, hygiene, social contacts) have decreased to such an extent that the person is, to some degree, dependent on professional support (Dijkstra et al. 1998a, b).

It is imaginable that specifically patients who are admitted in a nursing home and their direct family members are more concerned with the daily consequences of dementia than with the disease itself, as described above in a set of symptoms. Because most of these daily consequences have to do with fulfilling basic human needs, the primary focus of this chapter will be on the concept of care dependency as it relates to the ability to perform self-care activities.

17.2   Care Dependency: Conceptualization

17.2.1 Introduction

The aim of this paragraph is to analyze and clarify the concept of care dependency. An essential step is to review relevant literature. From the concept under review, two elements can be derived for further literature review: *care* and *dependency*. *Care* is a key term related to the nurse as well as attributable to the patient; *dependency* is a patient-related key term (Stevens Barnum 1990). Two sources were consulted: dictionaries and related (nursing) literature. This paragraph ends with a recommendation to understand both concepts, *care* and *dependency*, as a social relationship.

17.2.2 Data Sources

Dictionaries Walker and Avant (1995) identify dictionaries as potential source for identifying uses of concepts. Three dictionaries were used to examine the uses of the two key terms mentioned above: *care* and *dependency*. They are *Cambridge International Dictionary of English* (Procter 1995), *Collins Cobuild English Language Dictionary* (Sinclair 1988), and *Compact Oxford English Dictionary* (2006).

According to Cambridge Dictionary (Procter 1995), the word *care* in the sense of "protection" means "the process of or responsibility for protecting and giving special attention to someone or something," and *care* in the sense of "attention" means "serious attention, especially to the details of a situation or something." Furthermore, this dictionary states that "dependence is a state of needing something or someone, especially in order to continue existing or operating." Collins Dictionary (Sinclair1988) describes *care* as "the act of constantly providing what a person (...) needs to keep them in good condition or to make them well, and to make sure that they do not come to any harm" and *dependency* as "a constant and regular need that someone has for something (in order to be able to survive or operate properly) or the need that someone has for another person, (...)." The Compact Oxford English Dictionary (2006) describes dependency as a state of being dependent, which is defined in its broadest sense as being "seeking support from."

As can be seen, the term *dependency* is "a state of" and the core of this state is a "need," which makes the person dependent on another person. The word *(nursing) care* contains the answer to a person's state of dependency by "protecting," "giving attention," and "providing what a person needs." *Care* is not passive, but it actively changes a person's current state.

Nursing Literature Concerning the two key terms, the following is found in the nursing literature by Abdellah, Henderson, and Orem. Abdellah and Levine (1986) describe healthy persons as having the ability to provide for the satisfaction of their own physical, emotional, and sociological needs. An impairment that limits the ability to satisfy these needs can cause a need for nursing care. Nursing care is directed toward making the patient better able to help himself. This implies that nursing care should aim at having the patient help himself to a state of independency.

Henderson (1966) notices the following about *care* and *dependence*. It was Henderson's belief that health is basic to all human functioning and equates with independence on a continuum that has illness equated with dependence. In this view, the desired outcome of nursing care is the patient's independence. Dependence on nursing care refers to nursing activities which patients will perform unaided if they have the necessary strength, knowledge, or will. Therefore, during a certain period of dependence, the nurses will do their utmost to meet the patients' needs, but they will only do this with a view to making their patients independent of nursing assistance as rapidly as possible. Before carrying out nursing interventions, nurses ask themselves what the patient can do on his own, independent of the nurse. Successful outcomes of nursing care are based on the speed with which the patient independently performs the activities that make, for the patient, a normal day. The nurse serves as a substitute for whatever the patient lacks in order to make him or her "complete," "whole," or "independent" (George 1990).

Orem's (1985) theory of self-care provides another contribution to clarifying the key terms *care* and *dependency*. According to Boggatz et al. (2007), the notion of care dependency is implied in the theoretical work of Orem (2001). Orem distinguishes between self-care as the "activities that individuals initiate and perform on their own behalf in maintaining life, health and wellbeing" (Orem 2001, p. 43) and dependent care as the "activities that responsible… persons initiate and perform on behalf of socially dependent persons" (Orem 2001, p. 515) who have limited, health-associated abilities to meet their self-care demands. Orem speaks of dependency when nursing assistance is needed. Dependency exists when the patient's self-care ability decreases and care demands make the patient wholly or partly dependent on nursing care.

The essence of Orem's ideas about care is formed by the constructs of self-care, self-care deficits, and nursing system. These are the main points where nursing converges on the health state of an individual. Orem (1985) defines self-care as actions which persons perform on their own behalf in maintaining life, health, and wellbeing. Self-care deficits exist when an individual's abilities to perform self-care are less than those required to meet specific health-care demands. The basic design of a nursing system is that of a helping system (Orem 1985). The term nursing system stands for all the actions and interactions of nurses and patients in nursing practice providing the necessary help for patients. Persons with a legitimate need for nursing are characterized by a demand for discernible kinds and amounts of self-care. There are three possible relationships between care abilities and care demands: greater than, equal to, or less than/not adequate (Hartweg 1991). Nursing is a legitimate service when self-care abilities are less than required, and also when these abilities exceed or are equal to those required for meeting the current self-care demands, but a future deficit can be foreseen.

Additional Literature When it concerns older people, or when diseases like dementia appear, "dependency always includes a negative evaluation of a situation or a set of characteristics of an individual, defined as such by the individual and/or people in the person's environment" (van den Heuvel 1976, p. 162). Van den Heuvel (1976) found the following meanings and descriptions of dependency. Dependency may refer to (1) a practical, almost physical, helplessness which necessitates attention or care by others; (2) helplessness or powerlessness in a social/personal relationship; and (3) a psychological (physical) need to be looked after, controlled, or nurtured. Boggatz et al. (2007) concluded that care dependency should then be characterized by the fact that someone feels a need for care but does not receive it, and self-reports would express unmet or under-met needs. There is some empirical support for this study. According to Boggatz et al. (2007), some authors (Nordgren and Fridlund 2001, Ellefsen 2002, Strandberg et al. 2003) have come to the conclusion that the meaning of dependency from the care recipient's perspective is associated with constraints, loss of freedom, and powerlessness. Pool (1995) distinguishes dependency from care dependency. Dependency is placed within the frame of common human relationships and care dependency is placed within the frame of professional and formal care assistance.

17.2.3 Sociological Perspective

Following Kittay (1999, cited in Fine and Glendinning 2005, p. 612), dependency is a fundamental and commonplace aspect of human life course, an aspect of the human condition encountered in early childhood, illness, disability, and frail old age. Contrary to the idea that individual dependency arises primarily from a person's health condition, the main element is that dependency implies a social relationship (Johnson 1993). "Deficit stands for the relationship between action that individuals should take and the action capabilities of individuals for self-care. Here deficit should be interpreted as a relationship, not as a human disorder" (Orem 1985, p. 39). And as George (1991, p. 178) states, "one cannot simply be dependent; one must be dependent upon someone for something else."

17.3 Care Dependency: Operationalization

17.3.1 Introduction

George (1991) notices a tendency to conceptualize dependency as a single quantity which can be measured across all populations, regardless of situation, or as a personal attribute rooted in illness, impairment, or old age. The aim of this paragraph is to clarify of the concept of care dependency. The first focus will be on the development of a general frame of reference for the concept of care dependency. Further, the selection of a measurement framework will be considered.

17.3.2 Frame of Reference

A frame of reference needs to be developed to enable understanding of what it means to say that a person is dependent or care dependent and to differentiate between these terms. According to Van den Heuvel (1976), dependency arises for two reasons. Either the individual defines his or her situation as dependent, or people in the person's environment define the person as dependent. Therefore, the first element for a frame of reference is the definition of the situation by the individual, and the second is the reaction to that definition by people in the person's environment. Van den Heuvel (1976) adds the following two elements. Objectivity versus subjectivity as a result of a discrepancy in perception of the definition of the situation between the individual on the one hand and the environment on the other is the third element. The fourth element is that either the individual or the environment or both evaluate the characteristics or situation of the individual as negative.

17.3.3 Operationalizing Nursing Concepts

Carper (1978) reminds nursing researchers of their responsibility to describe the concepts concerning nursing practice carefully and thoughtfully. Nursing concepts are thoughts, notions, or ideas about nursing or nursing practice and define the content of interest in measuring nursing phenomena (Waltz et al. 1991). McCormack (1992) views concept analysis as a process used to determine similarities and differences between concepts and to create a tentative operational definition. According to Waltz et al. (1991), concept operationalization is delineating what a concept means and how it can be measured. Kim (1983) distinguishes conceptualization and concept analysis. The former is an active generational process of theoretical thinking, whereas concept analysis is more reflective in nature and involves critical evaluation of conceptualization that has already occurred.

The process of operationalizing a concept has been influenced by the approach of Waltz et al. (1991). They suggest a multistep procedure, representing progression from the abstract to the concrete. The procedure in this paper involves the following interrelated steps:

1. Developing the theoretical definition
2. Specifying variable dimensions derived from the theoretical definition
3. Identifying observable indicators
4. Developing a means for measuring these indicators

17.3.4 Developing the Theoretical Definition

The preliminary definition will mainly be based on the work by Abdellah, Henderson, and Orem. Such "needs theorists" focus on problems and needs of patients as seen by health-care providers and on the role of nurses in assessing these needs and meeting need requisites (Meleis 1991).

Literature on Abdellah's, Henderson's, and Orem's nursing theories reveals the following definitions and descriptions of synonyms which fit within the boundaries of the concept of nursing care dependency. For Abdellah, *nursing care* is doing something to or for the person or providing information to the person with the goal of meeting needs, increasing or restoring self-help ability, or alleviating an impairment (Marriner-Tomey 1988). Henderson (cited in: Halloran 1995, p. 89–90) views *nursing need* as whatever the person requires in knowledge, will, or strength to perform his or her daily activities and to carry out treatments prescribed for him or her. And Henderson describes need for care as a self-help deficit (Halloran 1995, p. 30). For Orem (1985) a *care demand* exists when care abilities are less than those required for meeting a known self-care demand. In Orem's view (1985), *nursing assistance* is a form of help given by nurses to persons with a legitimate need for it, by promoting self-care and motivating attempts toward independence. Basing her description in Orem (1985), Meleis (1991) defines the term *self-care deficit* as the balance between self-care demands and self-care capabilities and an indication of a state of social independence.

In view of these findings, care dependency is preliminary defined as: *a nurse-patient relationship resulting from a person's decrease in self-care and a simultaneous increase in dependency on nursing care whenever needs must be satisfied.*

The starting point for defining care dependency is the frame of reference of dependency described by Van den Heuvel (1976). This frame consists of four elements:

1. Definition of the situation
2. Reaction to that definition
3. Discrepancy in perceptions
4. Negative evaluation

These four elements fit a frame of reference regarding the concept of care dependency. Instead of the general term for the first element – "definition of the situation" – the more specific terms "patient system" and "professional system" will be used. The patient system communicates its disabilities, needs, or deficits in regard to self-care to the professional system in terms of care demands. And because of cognitive and communicative limitations in the way in which psychogeriatric patients express their care demands, a distinction will be made between explicit and implicit care demands. Regarding the second element, Goffman (1961) and Lasch (1979) have cautioned against patients' dependency on the professional system and against the helping professions reducing the patient to incompetence and relieving him of responsibility. According to Jirovec and Kasno (1993), unnecessary dependency is also fostered because institutionalized persons are not encouraged to maintain any remaining independent, self-care behavior. Miller (1985a, b) notices that, while nursing is normally a direct result of patient dependency, prolonged exposure to nursing activities can result in increased patient dependency. Especially in the long-term care facilities, professional workers such as nurses have a key role in assessing the patient's care demands. By "affirming" or "denying" these care demands, the professional worker decides what will be done and what not: in other words, the carer determines the beginning of a caring process. Regarding the third and fourth element, professional workers like nurses have a critical role in maintaining the patient's dependency status or turning his/her dependency into independence. Therefore, agreement about the care demand and a joint goal for action are needed. As Paterson and Zderad (1988, p.24) state: "Both patient and nurse have a goal or an expectation in mind. Therefore, the intersubjective transaction has meaning for them; the event is experienced in the light of their goals." The patient's expectation has been translated into the perspective of working on his independence. Theoretically, three outcomes can be expected: dependency increases, remains unchanged, or decreases.

So the following frame of reference can be developed. Table 17.1 reveals the train of thought which led to defining the theoretical concept of nursing care dependency. This framework concerns persons who are not able to manage their mental health problems and, consequently, need care assistance in a long-term care facility. For nurses, this is the starting point of a caring relationship with the patient. From the viewpoint of the patient, there is a care demand resulting from an absence or

Table 17.1 Frame of reference of care dependency

Patient system		Professional system	
Assessment		Agreement	Perspective
The patient communicates his care demand explicitly (real or unreal)	The nurse affirms the care demand	Joint goal for action	Decreased patient's dependency
	The nurse denies the care demand	Separate goal for action	Unchanged or increased patient's dependency
The patient communicates his care demand implicitly (real or unreal)	The nurse denies the care demand	Separate goal for action	Unchanged or increased patient's dependency
	The nurse affirms the care demand	Joint goal for action	Decreased patient's dependency

inadequacy of required self-care, which makes him/her wholly or partly dependent on nursing care. For a nurse, the patient's care demand is the starting point of a process in which he/she takes care of that particular patient. This means taking responsibility for providing the patient with what he/she needs. The purpose of nursing care is changing the patient's state of dependence into a state of independence. It is a movement of the patient away from nursing care toward self-care without direct assistance. In summary, the following theoretical definition can be posed: *care dependency is a process in which the professional offers support to a patient whose self-care abilities have decreased and whose care demands make him/her to a certain degree dependent, with the aim of restoring this patient's independence in performing self-care.*

17.3.5 Specifying Variable Dimensions

The second step in the present study will be to determine which framework is useful in specifying the variable properties of the concept of care dependency as established in the theoretical definition. The following aspects of care dependency were measured in the literature reviewed. Benoniel et al. (1980) developed a social dependency scale, which measures three capacities of patients with chronic illnesses: everyday self-care competence, mobility competence, and social competence. Hardy et al. (1982) examined the effect of care programs on the dependency status of elderly residents in an extended care setting. Among other things, a tool to measure the patient's nursing dependency status was used. This tool measures requirements for nursing staff time in terms of workload generated by patients' needs. Miller (1985a, b) studied the dependency of elderly patients in wards using different methods of nursing care. The incidence of dependency in elderly people and patient dependency in relation to nursing care was discussed. Patient dependency was measured by using a scale which rated the patients' level of physical dependency, apathy, social disturbance, communication difficulties, and incontinence. For policy purposes as well as for the provision of individual care, Maaskant (1993) investigated the care dependency of elderly, mentally handicapped people. Jirovec and Kasno (1993) studied predictors of self-care abilities among the institutionalized elderly. Self-care abilities were measured using the Appraisal of self-Care Agency (ASA-A) scale (Evers 1989). Dijkstra et al. (1995) compared the need for care in three types of Dutch institutions: nursing homes, old people's homes, and home care. For that purpose, the authors measured the degree of dependence for self-care activities, incontinence, and mobility. In all these studies, the care dependency concept was used to search for a method by which the dependency of a population can be measured. Similarly, George (1991, p. 178) concluded that "researchers and planners have attempted to define the quality of dependency in ways which will help them to assess the need for, and calculate the workload entailed in providing, continuing or long-stay accommodation for the elderly population."

In contrast to a medical orientation, the ideas of the "needs theorists" may be characterized as based on Maslow's hierarchy of needs and influenced by Erikson's stages of development (Fitzpatrick and Whall 1989; Riehl 1989; George 1990; Meleis 1991). Maslow (1970) identified basic human needs as physiological needs, safety needs, belongingness and love needs, esteem needs, and the need for self-actualization. The influence of Maslow is evident in the work of Abdellah, Henderson, and Orem. Although their formulations are different, each of the three "needs theorists" identifies need requisites which correspond to Maslow's basic human needs.

In Abdellah's model (1960), the concept of nursing is expressed in a typology of 21 nursing problems which encompass the physical, sociological, and emotional needs of the patient. The nursing activity typology of 21 nursing problems represents the categories or classifications of nursing action that can influence responses in the patient condition (Fitzpatrick and Whall 1989).

Henderson (1966, 1985) specified 14 components of basic nursing care. They remain comprehensive, complete, and consistent with various hierarchies and levels of human need (Yura and Walsh 1983). The components start with physiological functioning and move to the psychosocial aspects, which may convey that bodily operation takes priority over emotional or cognitive status (George 1990). These basic needs address not health problems of the patient, but areas in which actual or potential problems might occur (Gordon 1994). According to Fitzpatrick and Whall (1989), assessment of Henderson's 14 components of care helps the nurse move the patient from a state of dependence to a state of independence.

Orem (1985, 1995) identified three types of self-care requisites: universal, developmental, and health deviation. Each type of requisites represents a category of deliberate actions to be taken by or for the patient because of his or her needs as a human being. Universal self-care requisites are common to all human beings. Developmental self-care requisites are associated with human developmental processes, or they are new requisites derived from a condition or associated with an event. Health-deviation self-care requisites are associated with genetic and constitutional defects. Orem's eight universal self-care requisites, common to all human beings, more or less coincide with Henderson's 14 human basic needs (Meleis 1991).

Characteristics of basic human needs cover a broad range of physical and psychosocial needs. In the frameworks presented, physical needs dominate. "Needs theorists" associate these needs with air, food, elimination, sleep, exercise, and temperature. As long as these physical needs are unsatisfied, all other needs get low priority in need fulfillment. "Needs theorists" identify psychosocial needs such as self-concept, role function, interdependence, education, and family.

For the following reasons, Henderson's framework provides a good starting point to specifying the variable aspects of the concept of care dependency.

1. As stated, it was Henderson's belief that health is basic to all human functioning and equates with independence on a continuum that has illness equated with dependence. In this view, the desired outcome of nursing care is the patient's independence. The 14 human needs help the nurse move the patient from a state of dependence (...) to a state of independence (Fitzpatrick and Whall 1989).
2. Henderson speaks about *fundamental* human needs which appear in every patient-nurse relationship, independent of the patient's age and/or the type of care setting.
3. Henderson's ideas are frequently applied in practice and in the curriculum for educating nursing students working in long-term care facilities.

So Henderson's components of nursing care are used to specify the 14 variable aspects of the concept of care dependency. To allow them to be useful in the context of the research project, Henderson's 14 human needs have been translated into 15 care dependency items (see Table 17.2).

Table 17.2 Translation of Henderson's 14 human needs into 15 care dependency items of nursing care

Henderson's 14 human needs	Fifteen care dependency items of nursing care
1. Breathing normally	1. Eating and drinking
2. Eat and drink adequately	2. Incontinence
3. Eliminate body wastes	3. Mobility
4. Move and maintain desirable postures	4. Body posture
5. Sleep and rest	5. Rest and sleep
6. Suitable clothes – dress and undress	6. Getting dressed and undressed
7. Maintain body temperature within normal range by adjusting clothing and modifying the environment	7. Body temperature
8. Keep body clean and well groomed and protect the integument	8. Hygiene
9. Avoid dangers in the environment and avoid injuring other	9. Avoidance of danger
10. Communicate with others in expressing emotions, needs, fears, or opinions	10. Communication

Table 17.2 (continued)

Henderson's 14 human needs	Fifteen care dependency items of nursing care
11. Worship according to one's faith	11. Contact with others
12. Work in such a way that there is a sense of accomplishment	12. Sense of standards and values
13. Play or participate in various forms of recreation	13. Daily activities
14. Learn, discover, or satisfy the curiosity that leads to normal development and health and use the available health facilities	14. Recreation
	15. Learning ability

From Henderson (1966) The Nature of Nursing. New York, Macmillan

17.3.6 Identifying Observable Indicators

According to Challis et al. (1996), it is widely agreed that the best way to address the patient's care needs is by thorough and systematic assessment. The importance of regular assessments is evidenced by the frequency of acute and subacute changes in health status which may occur in patients in long-term care settings (Bernadini et al. 1993). Iyer et al. (1986) identified four types of assessment data: subjective, objective, historical, and current data. Here, where patients with cognitive and communicative dysfunctions are unable to share reliable information about their care dependency with their nurse, the focus is on objective data. Cox et al. (1993) define objective data as those facts that are observable and measurable by the nurse.

When selecting observable and measurable indicators, Waltz et al. (1991) suggest that it is important to determine whether the concept represents an either-or phenomenon or one that varies. Care dependency can be defined as variable in intensity. The described theoretical definition represents one end of a continuum, ranging from total patient dependency to total independence, in activities related to the specified 15 variable properties of the concept of care dependency.

In order to measure the patient's degree of care dependency, the number of indicators must be determined. Nursing literature refers to a number of indicators, varying from three to five. For example, Cox et al. (1993) mention five dimensions for rating areas of self-care: completely independent; requires use of equipment or device; requires help from another person, for assistance, supervision, or teaching; requires help from another person and equipment device; and dependent (does not participate in activity) (Code adapted by NANDA from E. Jones et al., Patient Classification for Long-Term Care: User's Manual. HEW Publication No. HRA-74-3107, November 1974). For each of the 15 dimensions of care dependency, it was decided to conceptualize five written indicators, ranging from totally dependent to totally independent. With these indicators the patient's care dependency can be evaluated.

17.3.7 Developing Means for Measuring the Indicators

Structured assessment instruments can assist in screening for problems that often remain undetected in older patients, and they can be adopted as part of everyday practice (Applegate et al. 1990). Assessment instruments may be helpful to complete the measurements of patients' indicators. Two instruments have been designed as means for measuring the 15 dimensions of nursing care dependency. Each version consists of the following components: (1) a label, (2) a description of the given label, and (3) five indicators to determine the degree to which patients depend on nursing care. The difference between the two versions is the way in which care dependency is assessed.

Responses on the clinical scale are rated on the basis of five written criteria (e.g., see Table 17.3), whereas all ratings of the research version are on a five-point Likert-scale, ranging from 1 (completely care dependent) to 5 (almost independent) (e.g., see Table 17.4).

The present paragraph can be ended by stating an operational definition of care dependency for use in nursing practice: *the degree of dependency on nursing care with regard to the 15 dimensions of human need, experienced by a long-term care patient.* And the mean to measure care dependency can be done by the care dependency scale.

Table 17.3 Example of a CDS item of the English-USA proxy version

Eating and drinking	
The extent to which the patient is able to satisfy his/her need for food and drink	
1	Patient is unable to take food and drink unaided
2	Patient is unable to prepare food and drink unaided; patient is able to put and drink into his/her mouth unaided
3	Patient is able to prepare food and drink and put food and drink into his/her mouth unaided with supervision; has difficulty determining quantity
4	Patient is able to eat and to drink unaided with some supervision
5	Patient is able to prepare meals and to satisfy his/her need for food unaided

Table 17.4 Example of a CDS item of the English-USA research version

Eating and drinking	
The extent to which the patient is able to satisfy his/her need for food and drink	
1	Completely care dependent (missing all initiative to act; therefore care and assistance is always necessary)
2	To a great extent care dependent (many restrictions to act independently, therefore to a great extent dependent on care and assistance)
3	Partially care dependent (there are restrictions to act independently, therefore partially dependent on care and assistance)
4	To a limited extent care dependent (few restrictions to act independently, therefore only to a limited extent dependent on care and assistance)
5	Almost independent (almost everything can be done without assistance)

17.4 Care Dependency Scale: Utilization

17.4.1 Introduction

The question to be answered in this paragraph is the additional value of the care dependency scale (CDS) for use in nursing home practice. First, general instructions will be given for use of the CDS in clinical practice. Subsequently, the use of the CDS will be discussed in clinical reasoning.

17.4.2 Instruction for Use in Clinical Practice

Instruction For completion of the CDS, the following guidelines must be observed: (1) in case of use by professional health carers, the CDS should be filled in by the nurse or another health carer who is most familiar with the daily care of the patient; (2) the scale consists of 15 items, each of which has five item-criteria relating to the aspect of dependency being rated; and (3) for each item an assessment should be made of the patient's level of dependency, and the item-criterion that best describes the patient's should be circled. Only one of the five item-criteria should be selected (Dijkstra et al. 2000b).

Scoring of Items In quality of life questionnaires, the experience of impairments, dysfunction, or social handicaps can be formulated either in the actual mode (e.g., is the patient incontinent?) or from the experienced burden perspective (e.g., to what extent is the patient able to control the discharge of urine and feces voluntarily?). In the CDS the level of care dependency is formulated from the experienced burden perspective. The person who fills in the CDS is asked to what extent the patient is able to perform activities.

The CDS sum score can be computed by adding the outcome of each of the 15 items of care dependency. Low sum scores on the CDS indicate that the patient is dependent on care from others. On the other hand, a high sum score means that the patient is almost independent of care. Repeated assessments with the CDS provide data for monitoring change in patient status and, potentially, assessing the success of interventions in decreasing patient dependency. By using the CDS scoring chart (see Fig. 17.1), the CDS score on each separate item can be seen (Dijkstra et al. 2006).

Time Frame In general, the time frame for assessment by proxy covers "the last week." Regarding assessment by proxy, the time frame depends on the period that the respondent is able to determine the patient's care dependency. The decision to opt for a longer period or repeated assessment can be based on the wish to assess more fully the abilities of the patient (Dijkstra et al. 2006).

Time Needed The CDS is easy to use and quick to complete, normally taking less than 5 min. Patients take, on average, 15 min to complete the CDS (Dijkstra et al. 2006).

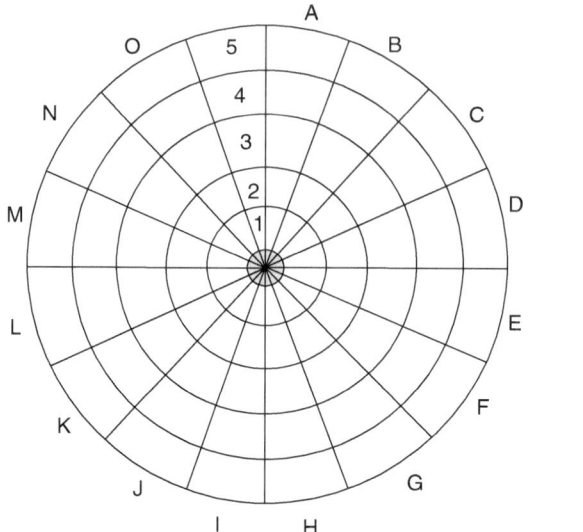

A = Eating and drinking
B = Continence
C = Body posture
D = Mobility
E = Day/night pattern
F = Getting (un) dressed
G = Body temperature
H = Hygiene
I = Avoidance of danger
J = Communications
K = Contact with others
L = Sense of rules and values
M = Daily activities
N = Recreational activities
O = Learning ability

1 = Completely care dependent
2 = To a great extent care dependent
3 = Partially care dependent
4 = To a limited extent care dependent
5 = Almost independent

Fig. 17.1 CDS scoring chart

17.4.3 Clinical Reasoning

Clinical reasoning, which has become synonymous with the nursing process or practice, refers to the processes by which nurses (and other clinicians) make their judgments to determine how to prevent, reduce, or resolve the identified patient needs and care demands (Tanner 2006). To support the process of clinical reasoning, assessment is valuable and necessary in order to gain essential information for individual care planning (Bartholomeyczik 2009). Following the steps of clinical reasoning, beginning with collecting cues, nurses identify identifiable changes experienced by the patient, perceived through history or assessing patients' self-care needs (with use of the CDS) and the degree of professional assistance required meeting these self-care needs. This knowledge may enable nurses, in processing this information, to develop a draft care plan, which they may discuss in the interdisciplinary consultation with the involved clinicians. Levett-Jones et al. (2010) refer to "clinical reasoning" as the process by which nurses (and other clinicians) collect cues, process the information, come to an understanding of a patient problem or situation, plan and implement interventions, evaluate outcomes, and then reflect on and learn from the process. Clinical reasoning helps nurses to choose the right care in a methodical manner by "knowing what to do" and "knowing how to do."

In practice, the CDS is intended to be used in clinical reasoning process as a self-care assessment and/or a case finding tool to help nurses in "knowing what to do."

The scale gives no direct answers, but indicates directions so that nurses and other health carers can focus on care needs amenable to nursing or caring diagnoses. The CDS is a scale derived from observed behavior, so the accuracy of the assessment depends on the degree to which the health carer is familiar with the daily functioning, care demands, and needs of the patient. Therefore, practicing nurses or health carers are in the best position to assess patients, especially in situations where the latter are unable to communicate or have limited communication capabilities.

The CDS is an aid to assessing patient's needs and the degree of professional assistance required to meet these needs. This knowledge may enable health carers to develop a draft care plan, which they may discuss in a multidisciplinary consultation. The aim of this consultation would be to determine joint diagnoses, objectives, and interventions that specify the input of different professionals to patient care. Repeated assessments with the CDS provide data for monitoring change in patient status and, potentially, assessing the success of interventions in decreasing patient's dependency.

Besides need assessment, the CDS can also be used in case finding patients with or without care dependency. The CDS has been validated in establishing care dependency and a cutoff score for care dependency must be chosen to indicate the presence or absence of "needs." Dijkstra et al. (2005) found that nursing home patients with various care needs with a CDS sum score ≤ 68 (rule-out cutoff point) were classified as care dependent and all others as independent. The prevalence in their sample study was very high (84%). The area under the receiver operating characteristics curve for the care dependency scale was 0.81, which indicates moderate diagnostic accuracy. The determination of the appropriate cutoff point was based on sensitivity (0.85) and positive predictive value (0.90).

17.4.4 Care Dependency and Nursing Care Problems

In the course of dementia, nursing home patients can develop, in addition to care dependency, various nursing care problems like pressure ulcer, incontinence, fall, malnutrition, and restraints (Schlüsser et al. (2014). Berger et al. (2012) define nursing care problems as impairments or risks related to health or interventions that the person cannot manage or resolve themselves and that restricts their independence. As Schlüsser et al. (2014) state, care dependency and nursing care problems can influence each other negatively. Detailed and valid information about the degree of care dependency and the risk on having a nursing care problem is essential input to tailor care plans in preventing, improving, or stabilizing both care dependency and nursing care problems. Regarding pressure ulcer, the CDS can be used as risk assessment instrument in nursing homes. A cutoff point of ≤ 58 was chosen for a first risk assessment of pressure ulcer in nursing homes (Dijkstra et al. 2015). These values were almost the same as found in a study by Mertens et al. (2008). Balzer et al. (2007) emphasize that in practice, the use of (risk) assessment instruments must always be combined with the individualized assessment based on nurses' clinical experience and judgment, especially because the usefulness of the CDS for pressure ulcer detection is limited.

17.4.5 Practical Application of the CDS

Following the steps of clinical reasoning, nurses start to collect information about the patient's health condition and the extent to which the patient can provide for its own self-care activities. The aim will be to come to an understanding of the patients self-care needs with the aid of the results of the CDS assessment. This knowledge may enable nurses to develop a draft care plan and to discuss this plan in an interdisciplinary consultation. The aim of the interdisciplinary consultation is to determine nursing diagnoses and to select goals as a desired outcome and a guidepost of interventions, which concretize the care tasks of nurses. The selected nursing interventions should be recorded in the individual care plan. Regularly evaluating the effects of the interventions is important to answer the question: do the interventions contribute to the measures as recorded in the care plan? The CDS can also play a role in evaluating the effects of the interventions in comparing historical with present outcomes. Repeated assessments with the CDS provide data for monitoring change in patient status and, potentially, assessing the success of interventions in decreasing patient dependency. In many cases, there will be stabilization or deterioration in care dependency (e.g., see Fig. 17.2). In addition, the CDS sum score is useful to generate management information on a population level.

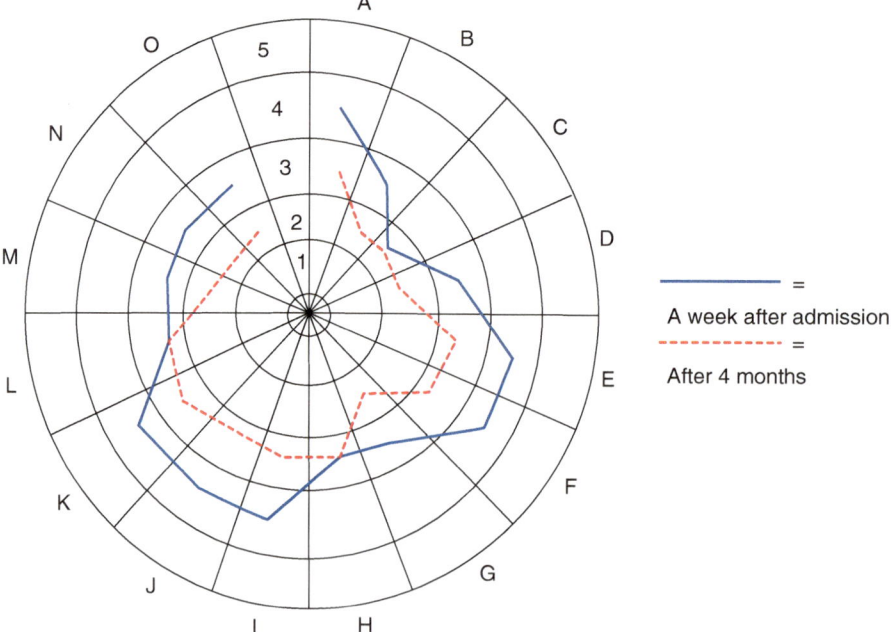

Fig. 17.2 Repeated assessment for monitoring changes in self-care abilities

Conclusion

Summarizing, the care dependency scale (CDS) provides a reliable and valid tool for assessing the care dependency status of nursing home patients. It measures 15 human needs: eating and drinking, continence, body posture, mobility, day/night pattern, getting dressed and undressed, body temperature, hygiene, avoidance of danger, communication, contact with others, sense of rules and values, daily activities, recreational activities, and learning ability. The instrument consists of these 15 care dependency items, each one of which has an item description and five care dependency criteria. Nurses rate all items by selecting one criterion out of the five. Low scores on the items indicate that patients are completely dependent on care. On the other hand, high scores mean that patients are almost independent of care. Development and psychometric testing of the CDS have been described in several studies (Dijkstra et al. 1996, 1998a, b, 1999, 2000b). Besides these studies, the international psychometric properties of the CDS were determined using data sets from Canada, Italy, Norway and the Netherlands (Dijkstra et al. 2000a), Finland, Spain and the United Kingdom (Dijkstra et al. 2003), Germany (Lohrmann et al. 2003), Japan (Suzuki et al. 2010), Poland (Dijkstra et al. 2010), and Turkey (Hakverdioğlu-Yönt et al. 2010, Dijkstra et al. 2012). The outcomes confirm that the CDS proved to be a reliable and valid scale in terms of internal consistency, inter-item correlation, and principal component analysis.

References

Abdellah FG, Beland IL, Martin A et al (1960) Patient-centered approaches to nursing. Macmillan, New York

Abdellah FG, Levine E (1986) Better Patient Care Through Nursing Research,. 3rd edn. Macmillan, New York

Alzheimer's Society (2013a) What is dementia? Factsheet 400LP. https://www.alzheimers.org.uk/site/scripts/download_info.php?downloadID=1092. Assessed 30 Mar 2016

Alzheimer's Society (2013b) The later stages of dementia. Factsheet: https://www.alzheimers.org.uk/site/scripts/documents_info.php?documentID=101. Assessed 30 Mar 2016

Applegate WB, Blass JP, Williams TF (1990) Instruments for the functional assessment of older patients. N Engl J Med 322:1207–1214

Balzer K, Pohl C, Dassen T et al (2007) The norton, waterlow, braden and care dependency scale: comparing their validity when identifying patients' pressure sore risk. J Wound Ostomy Continence Nurs 34:389–398

Bartholomeyczik S (2009) Standardisierte Assessmentinstrumente: Verwendungsmöglichkeiten und Grenzen [Standardized assessment instruments: use opportunities and borders]. In: Bartholomeyczik S, Halek M (EDS). Assessmentinstrumente in der Pflege. Schlütersche Verlaggesellschaft mbH & COKG, Hannover

Berger S, Helmbold A, Mosebach H et al. (2012) Wissenschaftliche Hintergründe ENP – Version 2.7. RECOM, Baar-Ebenhausen, Germany

Bernadini B, Meinecke C, Zaccarini C et al (1993) Adverse clinical events in dependent long-term nursing home residents. J Am Geriatr Soc 41:105–111

Boggatz T, Dijkstra A, Lohrmann C et al (2007) The meaning of care dependency as shared by care givers and care recipients: a concept analysis. J Adv Nurs 60(5):561–569. doi:10.1111/j.1365-2648.2007.04456.x

Benoniel JQ, McCorkle R, Young K (1980) Development of a Social Dependency Scale. Res Nurs Health 3:3-10

Carper B (1978) Fundamental patterns of knowing. Adv Nurs Sci 1:13–23

Challis D, Carpenter I, Traske K (1996) Assessment in continuing care homes: towards a national standard instrument. PSSRU, Canterbury

Compact Oxford English Dictionary (2006) Dependent/Dependency. http://www.askoxford.com/dictionaries/?view=uk. Assessed on 27 Apr 2016

Cox HC, Hinz MD, Lubno MA et al (1993) Clinical applications of nursing diagnoses: adult, child, women's, psychiatric, gerontic and home health considerations, 2nd edn. FA Davis, Philadelphia

Dijkstra GJ, Groothoff JW, Dassen TWN (1995) Vergelijking van lichamelijke zorgbehoefte van ouderen in drie typen instellingen. Tijdschr Soc Gezondheidsz 73:135–140

Dijkstra A, Buist G, Dassen T (1996) Nursing-care dependency: development of an assessment scale for demented and mentally handicapped patients. Scand J Caring Sci 10:137–143

Dijkstra A, Buist G, Dassen T (1998a) Operationalization of the concept of 'nursing-care dependency' for use in long-term care facilities. Aust N Z J Ment Health Nurs 7:142–151

Dijkstra A, Buist G, Dassen T (1998b) A criterion-related validity study of the Nursing-Care Dependency (NCD) scale. Int J Nurs Stud 35:163–170

Dijkstra A, Buist G, Moorer P et al (1999) Construct validity of the nursing care dependency scale. J Clin Nurs 8:380–388

Dijkstra A, Brown L, Havens BS et al (2000a) An international psychometric testing of the Nursing-Care Dependency (NCD) Scale. J Adv Nurs 31:944–952

Dijkstra A, Buist G, Moorer P et al (2000b) A reliability and utility study of the care dependency scale. Scand J Caring Sci 14:155–161

Dijkstra A, Coleman M, Tomas C et al (2003) Cross-cultural psychometric testing of the care dependency scale with data. J Adv Nurs 43:181–187

Dijkstra A, Tiesinga LJ, Plantinga L et al (2005) Diagnostic accuracy of the care dependency scale. J Adv Nurs 50(4):410–416

Dijkstra A, Smith J, White M (2006) Measuring care dependency with the Care Dependency Scale (CDS): a manual. Noordelijk Centrum voor Gezondheidsvraagstukken, Groningen

Dijkstra A, Muszalik M, Kędziora-Kornatowska K et al (2010) Care dependency scale: psychometric testing of the polish version. Scand J Caring Sci 24:62–66

Dijkstra A, Hakverdioğlu-Yönt G, Akın-Korhan E et al (2012) The care dependency scale for measuring basic human needs: an international comparison. J Adv Nurs 68:2341–2348

Dijkstra A, Kazimier H, Halfens RJG (2015) Using the care dependency scale for identifying patients at risk for pressure ulcer. J Adv Nurs 71(11):2529–2539. doi:10.1111/jan.12713

Ellefsen B (2002) Dependency as disadvantage – patients' experiences. Scand J Caring Sci 16:157–164

Evers GCM (1989) Appraisal of Self-Care Agency (A.S.A) Scale. Van Gorcum, Assen/Maastricht

Fine M, Glendinning C (2005) Dependence, independence or inter-dependence? Revisiting the concepts of 'care' and 'dependency'. Ageing Soc 25(4):601–621 . http://dx.doi.org/10.1017/S0144686X05003600

Fitzpatrick JJ, Whall AL (1989) Conceptual models of nursing: analysis and application. Appleton & Lange, Norwalk

George JB (1990) Nursing theories: the base for professional nursing practice. Prentice-Hall, Englewood Cliffs

George S (1991) Measures of dependency: their use in assessing the need for patiential care for the elderly. J Public Health Med 13:178–181

Goffman E (1961) Asylums. Doubledy, New York

Gordon M (1994) Nursing diagnosis: process and application. McGraw-Hill, New York

Hakverdioğlu-Yönt G, Akın-Korhan E, Khorshid L et al (2010) Bakım bağımlılığı ölçeğinin yaşlı bireylerde geçerlik ve güvenirliğinin incelenmesi. Turk J Geriatr 13:71

Halloran EJ (1995) A Virginia Henderson reader: excellence in nursing. Springer Publishing Company, New York

Hardy VM, Capuano EF, Worsam BD (1982) The effect of care programmes on the dependency status of elderly residents in an extended care setting. J Adv Nurs 7:295–300

Hartweg DL (1991) Dorothea Orem: self-care deficit theory. Sage Publications, Newbury Park

Henderson V (1966) The nature of nursing: a definition and its implications for practice, research and education. MacMillan Press, New York

Henderson V (1985) The essence of nursing in high technology. Nurs Adm Q 9:1–9

Iyer PW, Taptich BJ, Bernocchi-Losey D (1986) Nursing process and nursing diagnosis. WB Saunders, Philadelphia

Jirovec MM, Kasno J (1993) Predictors of self-care abilities among the institutionalized elderly. West J Nurs Res 15:314–326

Johnson M (1993) Dependency and interdependency. In: Bond J, Coleman P, Peace S (eds) Ageing in society. Sage, London, pp 255–279

Kim HS (1983) The nature of theoretical thinking in nursing. Appleton-Century-Crofts, Norwalk

Kittay EF (1999) Love's labor: essays on women, equality, and dependency. Routledge, New York

Lasch C (1979) The culture of narcissism. Warner Books, New York

Levett-Jones T, Hoffman K, Dempsey Y et al (2010) The 'five rights' of clinical reasoning: an educational model to enhance nursing students' ability to identify and manage clinically 'at risk' patients. Nurse Educ Today 30(6):515–520

Lohrmann C, Dijkstra A, Dassen T (2003) Care dependency: testing the German version of the care dependency scale in nursing homes and on geriatric wards. Scand J Caring Sci 17: 51–56

Maaskant MA (1993) Mental handicap and ageing. Kavanah, Dwingeloo

Marriner-Tomey A (1988) Nursing theorists and their work, 2nd edn. Mosby, St. Louis

Maslow A (1970) Motivation and personality. Harper & Row, New York

McCormack B (1992) Intuition: concept analysis and application to curriculum development. 1. Concept analysis. J Clin Nurs 1:339–344

McLaughlin T, Feldman H, Fillit H et al (2010) Dependence as a unifying construct in defining Alzheimer's disease severity. Alzheimers Dement 6:482–493

Meleis AI (1991) Theoretical nursing: development and progress. Lippincott, Philadelphia

Mertens EI, Halfens RJG, Dietz E et al (2008) Pressure ulcer risk screening in hospital and nursing homes with a general nursing assessment tool: evaluation of the care dependency scale. J Eval Clin Pract 14:1018–1025

Miller A (1985a) A study of the dependency of elderly patients in wards using different methods of nursing care. Age Ageing 14:132–138

Miller A (1985b) Nurse/patient dependency-is it iatrogenic? J Adv Nurs 10:63–69

Nordgren S, Fridlund B (2001) Patient's perceptions of selfdetermination in the context of care. J Adv Nurs 35(1):117–125

Orem DE (1985) Nursing: concepts of practice, 3rd edn. McGraw-Hill, New York

Orem DE (1995) Nursing: concepts of practice, 5th edn. Mosby, St. Louis

Orem DE (2001) Nursing Concepts of Practice. 6th edn. Mosby, St Louis

Paterson JG, Zderad LT (1988) Humanistic nursing. National League for Nursing, New York

Pool ASG (1995) Autonomie, Afhankelijkheid en Langdurige Zorgverlening. Lemma, Utrecht

Procter P (Ed) (1995) Cambridge International Dictionary of English. 18th edn. Cambridge University Press, Cambridge

Riehl-Sisca J (1989) Conceptual models for nursing practice. Appleton & Lange, Norwalk

Schlüsser S, Dassen T, Lohrmann C (2014) Prevalence of care dependency and nursing care problems in nursing home residents with dementia: a literature review. Int J Caring Sci 7:338–352

Sinclair J (Ed) (1988) Collins Cobuild English Language Dictionary. Williams Collins Sons & Co Ltd, Glasgow

Stevens Barnum BJ (1990) Nursing theory: analysis, application, evaluation. Scott, Foresman, and Company, Glenview

Strandberg G, Norberg A, Jansson L (2003) Meaning of dependency on care as narrated by 10 patients. Res Theory Nurs Pract 17(1):65–84

Suzuki M, Mizuno Y, Fukahori A et al (2010) Development of a Japanese version of the care dependency scale. Jpn J Geriatr Psy 21:241–251

Tanner CA (2006) Thinking like a nurse: a research-based model of clinical judgment in nursing. J Nurs Educ 45(6):204–211

Walker LO, Avant KC (1995) Strategies for theory construction in nursing, 3rd edn. Appleton & Lange, Norwalk

Waltz CF, Strickland OL, Lenz ER (1991) Measurement in nursing research, 2nd edn. F.A. Davis, Philadelphia

WHO (2012) Dementia: a public health priority. World Health Organization, Geneva

Yura H, Walsh MF (1983) The nursing process. Appleton-Century-Crofts, Norwalk

van den Heuvel WJA (1976) The meaning of dependency. In: Munnichs JMA, Heuvel van den WJA (eds) Dependency or interdependency in old age. Martinus Nijhoff, The Hague, pp 162–173